Stereotactic and Functional Neurosurgery

Official Journal of the World Society for Stereotactic and Functional Neurosurgery

Official Journal of the American Society for Stereotactic and Functional Neurosurgery

Founded 1938 as 'Confinia Neurologica' by E.A. Spiegel
Continued 1975–1988 as 'Applied Neurophysiology'

KARGER

Printed in Switzerland
on acid-free paper by
Thür AG Offsetdruck, Pratteln

Appears 6-weekly;
2 volumes per year (8 issues)

Stereotactic and Functional Neurosurgery

Submission: Only original papers written in English are considered and should be sent to:

Prof. Dr. Ph.L. Gildenberg
6624 Fannin, Suite 1620
Houston, TX 77030 (USA)

Manuscripts should be submitted in triplicate (with three sets of illustrations of which one is an original), typewritten double-spaced on one side of the paper, with a wide margin.

Conditions: All manuscripts are subjected to editorial review. Manuscripts are received with the explicit understanding that they are not under simultaneous consideration by any other publication. Submission of an article for publication implies the transfer of the copyright from the author to the publisher upon acceptance. Accepted papers become the permanent property of 'Stereotactic and Functional Neurosurgery' and may not be reproduced by any means, in whole or in part, without the written consent of the publisher. It is the author's responsibility to obtain permission to reproduce illustrations, tables, etc. from other publications.

Arrangement

Title page: The first page of each paper should indicate the title (main title underlined), the authors' names, and the institute where the work was conducted. A short title for use as running head as well as the full address of the author to whom correspondence should be sent are also required.

Full address: The exact postal address complete with postal code must be given at the bottom of the title page. Please also supply Phone, Fax, and E-mail numbers.

Key words: For indexing purposes, a list of 3–10 key words in English is essential.

Abstract: Each paper needs an abstract of up to 10 lines.

Small type: Paragraphs which can or must be set in smaller type (case histories, test methods, etc.) should be indicated with a 'p' (petit) in the margin on the left-hand side.

Footnotes: Avoid footnotes. When essential, they are numbered consecutively and typed at the foot of the appropriate page.

Tables and illustrations: Tables and illustrations (both numbered in Arabic numerals) should be prepared on separate sheets. Tables require a heading and figures a legend, also prepared on a separate sheet. For the reproduction of illustrations, only good drawings and original photographs can be accepted; negatives or photocopies cannot be used. Due to technical reasons, figures with a screen background should not be submitted. When possible, group several illustrations on one block for reproduction (max. size 113 × 174 mm) or provide crop marks. On the back of each illustration, indicate its number, the author's name, and 'top' with a soft pencil.

Color illustrations: Up to 6 color illustrations per page can now be integrated with the text at the reduced price of CHF 600.– / USD 545.00 per page. Color illustrations are reproduced at the author's expense.

References: In the text identify references by Arabic numerals [in square brackets]. Material submitted for publication but not yet accepted should be noted as 'unpublished data' and not be included in the reference list. The list of references should include only those publications which are cited in the text. Do not alphabetize; number references in the order in which they are first mentioned in the text. The surnames of the authors followed by initials should be given. There should be no punctuation other than a comma to separate the authors. Cite all authors, 'et al' is not sufficient. Abbreviate journal names according to the Index Medicus system. (Also see International Committee of Medical Journal Editors: Uniform requirements for manuscripts submitted to biomedical journals. Br Med J 1988;296:401–405.)

Examples

(a) Papers published in periodicals: Kauffman HF, van der Heide S, Beaumont F, Blok H, de Vries K: Class-specific antibody determination against *Aspergillus fumigatus* by means of the enzyme-linked immunosorbent assay. III. Comparative study: IgG, IgA, IgM ELISA titers, precipitating antibodies and IgE binding after fractionation of the antigen. Int Arch Allergy Appl Immunol 1986;80:300–306.

(b) Monographs: Matthews DE, Farewell VT: Using and Understanding Medical Statistics. Basel, Karger, 1985.

(c) Edited books: Hardy WD Jr, Essex M: FeLV-induced feline acquired immune deficiency syndrome: A model for human AIDS; in Klein E (ed): Acquired Immunodeficiency Syndrome. Prog Allergy. Basel, Karger, 1986, vol 37, pp 353–376.

Further details: Authors may consult our leaflet 'Rules for the Preparation of Manuscripts', available on request from the Publisher, S. Karger AG, P.O. Box, CH–4009 Basel (Switzerland).

Page charges: There is no page charge for papers of 8 or fewer printed pages (including tables, illustrations and references). Each additional complete or partial page is charged to the author at CHF 245.– / USD 196.00. The allotted size of a paper is equal to approx. 16 manuscript pages (including tables, illustrations and references).

Galley proofs: Unless indicated otherwise, galley proofs are sent to the first-named author and should be returned with the least possible delay. Alterations made in galley proofs, other than the correction of printer's errors, . are charged to the author. No page proofs are supplied.

Reprints: Order forms and a price list are sent with the galley proofs. Orders submitted after the issue is printed are subject to considerably higher prices. Allow five weeks from date of publication for delivery of reprints.

KARGER
E-Mail karger@karger.ch
Fax +41 61 306 12 34
http://www.karger.ch

General Information
http://www.karger.ch/journals/sfn/sfndes.htm

Stereotactic and Functional Neurosurgery

Publication data: 'Stereotactic and Functional Neurosurgery' is published 8 times annually. Volumes 66–67 with 4 issues each appear in 1996.

Subscription rates: Subscriptions run for a full calendar year. Prices are given per volume.

Personal subscription:

Subscription	+ *postage and handling*
CHF 148.80	+ CHF 14.70 Europe
CHF 148.80	+ CHF 22.40 Overseas
USD 114.60	+ USD 14.70

(Must be in the name of, billed to, and paid by an individual. Order must be marked 'personal subscription'.)

Institutional subscription:

Subscription	+ *postage and handling*
CHF 248.–	+ CHF 18.40 Europe
CHF 248.–	+ CHF 28.– Overseas
USD 191.00	+ USD 18.40

Airmail postage: CHF 24.–, USD 20.00. (Extra per volume.)

Discount subscription prices: Societies for Stereotactic and Functional Neurosurgery are requested to apply for appropriate discounts.

Microforms: Please direct all enquiries and orders to:
University Microfilms Inc.
300 North Zeeb Road, P.O. Box 1346
Ann Arbor, MI 48106-1346 (USA)

Subscription orders: Orders can be placed at agencies, bookstores, directly with the Publisher S. Karger AG, P.O. Box, CH – 4009 Basel (Switzerland) or with any of the following distributors:
Deutschland: S. Karger GmbH, Postfach
D – 79095 Freiburg
France: Librairie Luginbühl
36, bd de Latour-Maubourg
F–75007 Paris
Great Britain, Ireland: S. Karger Publishers
11 Ravenscroft Road
Beckenham, Kent BR3 4TP
USA: S. Karger Publishers, Inc.
26 West Avon Road, P.O. Box 529
Farmington, CT 06085
India, Bangladesh, Sri Lanka:
S. Karger India Subscription Agency
B – 5/132 Safdarjung Enclave
New Delhi-110029
Japan: Katakura Libri, Inc.
Take 1 Bldg, 2nd Floor
4-5-7 Yushima, Bunkyo-ku
Tokyo 113

Change of address: Both old and new address should be sent to the subscription source.

Single issues and back volumes: Information can be obtained through the Publisher.

Advertising: Correspondence and rate requests should be addressed to the Publisher.

Bibliographic indices: This journal is regularly listed in bibliographic services, including *Current Contents®*.

Book Reviews: Books are accepted for review by special agreement.

KARGER
E-Mail karger@karger.ch
Fax + 41 61 306 12 34
http://www.karger.ch

State-of-the-art knowledge in radiosurgery

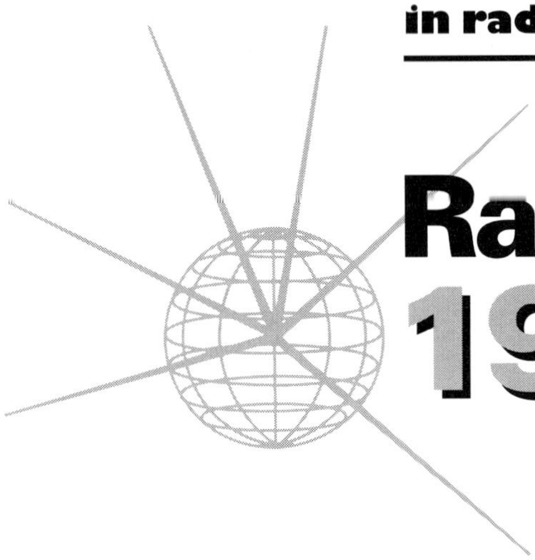

Radiosurgery 1995

Editor: D. Kondziolka

This book is the first official publication of the International Stereotactic Radiosurgery Society (ISRS). It marks the start of a unique, peer reviewed high quality book series, with a new volume published after each main congress of the society which takes place every two years. It will serve as the current standard for work in radiosurgery during this period of time.
The initial volume in this series features efforts from institutes across the world applying different technology and using the latest knowledge in radiosurgery for various intracranial disorders. Important results on how to avoid and manage complications as well as essential findings on refinements and developments in stereotactic techniques are presented by experts in their fields. Targeted to neurosurgeons, radiation oncologists and medical physicists, the book will provide up-to-date and precise information in radiobiology, radiation physics, computer dose planning and expansion of indications.

Selected Contents

The History of Radiosurgery: The Early Years (1950–1970) • Radiosurgery: Where Does the Future Lead?

Benign Tumors
Radiosurgery versus Radiotherapy for Benign Intracranial Tumors • LINAC Radiosurgery for Acoustic Neuromas • Stereotactic Radiosurgery for Pituitary Tumors • Craniopharyngioma: Preliminary Results of Stereotactic Radiation Therapy

Malignant Tumors
Stereotactic Radiosurgery for the Treatment of Brain Metastases. An Update • Results of Radiosurgery for Recurrent Gliomas • The Evolving Use of Gamma Knife Radiosurgery for Malignant Brain Tumors in Japan • Hypofractionated Stereotactic Radiotherapy for Recurrent Gliomas in Children and Adults: A Biological Compromise between Radiosurgery and Conventionally Fractionated Radiotherapy

Cost-Effective Analysis
Cost Analysis of Radiosurgery versus Resection for Single Brain Metastases • The Cost-Effectiveness for Alternative Treatments for Single Brain Metastases

Vascular Malformations
Long-Term Angiographic Outcome of Arteriovenous Malformations Responding Incompletely to Gamma Knife Surgery • Stereotactic Radiosurgery for Arteriovenous Malformations of the Posterior Fossa

Functional Disorders
Functional Neurosurgery with the Leksell Gamma Knife

Complication Management
Radiosurgery-Related Imaging Changes in Surrounding Brain: Multivariate Analysis and Model Evaluation • Unusual Complications following Gamma Knife Radiosurgery • Informed Consent for Radiosurgery

Radiobiology
Radiosurgery and Fractionation • A Dynamic Collimator System for Conformal Stereotactic Radiosurgery and Radiotherapy • Exploring the Boundary between 3-D Conformal Radiotherapy and Stereotactic Radiosurgery

Technology and Techniques
Preliminary Clinical Experience with the Cyberknife: Image-Guided Stereotactic Radiosurgery • Cranial Nerve Imaging for Radiosurgery at the Base of the Skull

Radiosurgery, Vol. 1
Series Editors: Alexander, E., III (Boston, Mass.);
Kondziolka, D. (Pittsburgh, Pa.);
Lindquist, C. (Stockholm);
Loeffler, J.S. (Boston, Mass.)
ISSN 1024–2651
Fields of Interest: Neurosurgery; Surgery; Radiology; Neurology, Radiobiology, Neuropathology, Roentgenology

Radiosurgery 1995
2nd International Stereotactic Radiosurgery Society Meeting, Boston, June 1995
Editor: Kondziolka, D. (Pittsburgh, Pa.)
XII + 350 p., 119 fig., 65 tab., hard cover, 1996
CHF 339.– / DEM 406.– / USD 295.00
Prices subject to change
DEM price for Germany, USD price for USA only
ISBN 3–8055–6236–5

KI 96441

KARGER

Stereotactic and Functional Neurosurgery

Proceedings of the 7th International Meeting of the

Leksell Gamma Knife® Society

Island of Lana'i, Hawaii, November 12–15, 1995

Editors
Jeremy C. Ganz, Graz
Ronald F. Young, Seattle, Wash.
Philip L. Gildenberg, Houston, Tex.
Patricia O. Franklin, Houston, Tex.

144 figures, 10 in color, and 72 tables, 1997

KARGER

Leksell Gamma Knife® is a registered trademark of Elekta Instruments, Inc., Atlanta, Ga.

KARGER

S. Karger · Medical and Scientific Publishers
Basel · Freiburg · Paris · London · New York · New Delhi · Bangkok · Singapore · Tokyo · Sydney

Drug Dosage. The authors and the publisher have exerted every effort to ensure that drug selection and dosage set forth in this text are in accord with current recommendations and practice at the time of publication. However, in view of ongoing research, changes in government regulations, and the constant flow of information relating to drug therapy and drug reactions, the reader is urged to check the package insert for each drug for any change in indications and dosage and for added warnings and precautions. This is particularly important when the recommended agent is a new and/or infrequently employed drug.

Printed in Switzerland on acid-free paper by Thür AG Offsetdruck, Pratteln
ISBN 3-8055-6446-5

Contents Vol. 66, Supplement 1, 1996

Stereotactic and Functional Neurosurgery

KARGER

E-Mail karger@karger.ch
Fax + 41 61 306 12 34
http://www.karger.ch

The list of contents is available at:
http://www.karger.ch/journals/sfn/sfncont.htm

Proc 7th Int Meeting Leksell Gamma Knife® Society,
Island of Lana'i, Hawaii, November 1995
Stereotact Funct Neurosurg 1996;66(suppl 1):1–3

Stereotactic and Functional Neurosurgery

Editorial Introduction

J.C. Ganz

Department of Neurosurgery, Karl Franzens University School of Medicine,
Graz, Austria

This is the third volume of proceedings from the meetings of what has become the Leksell Gamma Knife Society. The first proceedings came from the meeting in Buenos Aires in 1992 and was published in 1993. The second came from the meeting in Kyoto in 1994 and was published in 1995. There were no proceedings from the meeting in 1993. The contents of the proceedings reflects changes in direction and emphasis within this developing milieu and these changes are the subject of this editorial. Simple charts give an initial illustration of the changes which are taking place.

The most impressive difference has been in the number of articles submitted. This is the first time where there were so many that some, regretfully, had to be refused. The changes can be easily perceived from a number of simple illustrations. Figure 1 shows the increasing number of papers and reflects the spread of the Gamma Knife around the world. Gamma Knife centers need, of course, to be in operation for at least 3 years before they can accumulate experience which may form the basis for a paper. It is noteworthy how the Far East centers have increased their contribution over the last 3 years.

Figure 2 and 3 reflect the increasing interest in treating tumors. Only a few years ago, arteriovenous malformations (AVMs) accounted for more than 50% of all treated cases. This no longer true, and the number of tumor papers far exceeds the number of AVM reports. On the other hand, the vascular papers reflect the long experience in this field, because they are mainly concerned with reporting increasingly sophisticated techniques. The tumor papers to a larger degree are still concerned with reporting clinical results. Functional papers form a significant part of the total as well, even if relatively few patients have been treated to date, and all authors are cautious in the conclusions that they draw.

KARGER

E-Mail karger@karger.ch
Fax + 41 61 306 12 34
http://www.karger.ch

1011–6125/96/0665–0001$10.00/0

Jeremy C. Ganz, MA, PhD, FRCS
Department of Neurosurgery, Karl Franzens University
School of Medicine
A–8036 Graz (Austria)

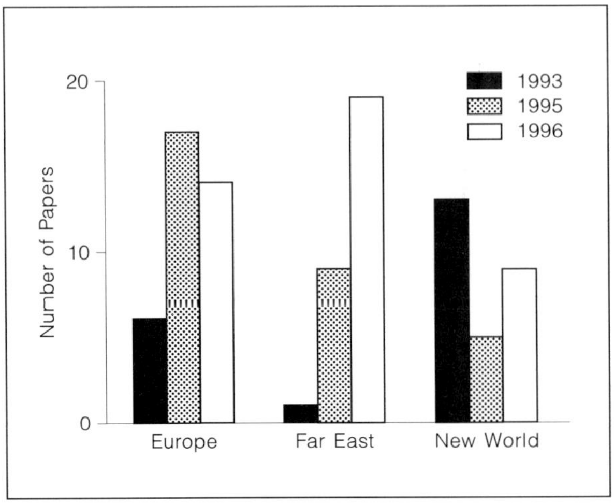

1

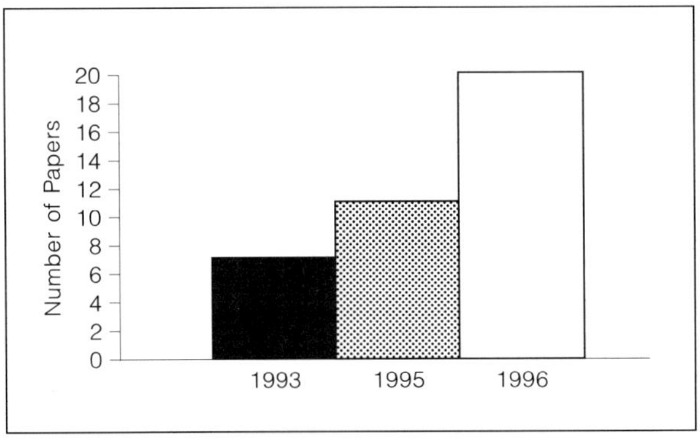

2

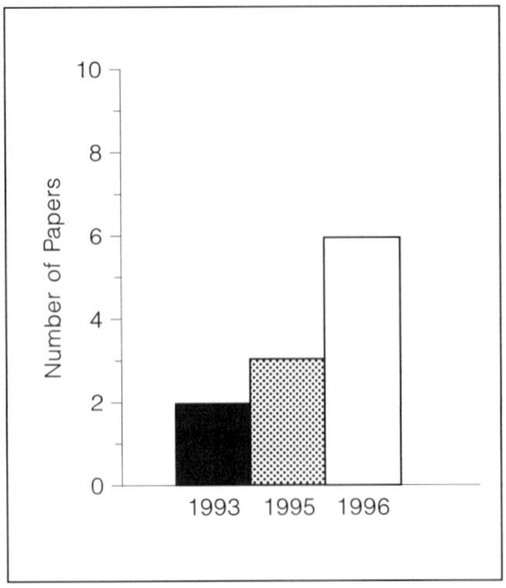

3

Fig. 1. Distribution of papers according to region in 1993, 1995 and 1996.

Fig. 2. Number of papers on tumors in 1993, 1995 and 1996.

Fig. 3. Number of papers on AVMs in 1993, 1995 and 1996.

There was one disappointing aspect. The first proceedings carried seven papers on physics. In the 1995 proceedings there were none and in the current edition there is only one. Physicists are a vital part of a Gamma Knife radiosurgery team and it is hoped that in subsequent meetings there will be more written contributions from them. These proceedings are their forum too, even if what they write is not readily understood by physicians.

There is increasing interest in the radiobiology of radiosurgery. This is examined in a variety of ways, studying such diverse processes as apoptosis on the one hand to the increased sensitivity of single photon emission computed tomography to early changes in AVMs on the other. There is also an account of an experimental analysis of the changes in neurotransmitters following a radiosurgical dose. Improvements in technique range from accounts of straightening up the inherent distortions of digital subtraction angiography to paying attention to the size of the matrix in functional cases.

This is a changing and evolving field, with each new set of proceedings being characterized by increasing knowledge and creative endeavor. This editor would like to thank all the participants for allowing him to perform an interesting task. It was a most interesting meeting.

Proc 7th Int Meeting Leksell Gamma Knife® Society,
Island of Lana'i, Hawaii, November 1995
Stereotact Funct Neurosurg 1996;66(suppl 1):4–16

Stereotactic and Functional Neurosurgery

Radiobiological Effects of Gamma Knife Radiosurgery on Brain Tumors Studied in Autopsy and Surgical Specimens

M. Hirato[a], *J. Hirato*[b], *A. Zama*[a], *H. Inoue*[a], *C. Ohye*[a], *T. Shibazaki*[c], *Y. Andou*[c]

Departments of [a] Neurosurgery,
[b] Pathology, Gunma University School of Medicine, and
[c] Hidaka Hospital, Maebashi, Japan

Key Words

Gamma Knife · Radiosurgery · Radiobiological effect · Histology · Pathology · Tumor · Immunohistochemical staining

Abstract

To elucidate the radiobiological effect of Gamma Knife radiosurgery on brain tumors, we performed a histological study on nine cases. In two, the material was obtained at autopsy and in seven following surgery. In the central region of the radiation field, destructive changes occurred both in tumor cells and in vessels. In the peripheral area, destructive and proliferative vascular changes were intermingled with residual tumor tissue. Immunohistochemical staining of surgical specimens showed that the vascular proliferative changes consisted of pericytic proliferation with or without endothelial proliferation. These characteristic changes might suppress tumor growth, at least in the short-term.

Introduction

Leksell [1] developed the Gamma Knife in 1951, and with it the concept of radiosurgery [2], a treatment modality which has now become available for various neurological diseases [3, 4]. However, the radiobiology of high-dose, small-volume, single-fraction irradiation for the human brain or brain tumors (BTs) remains poorly understood [3–7]: the characteristic changes following radio-

KARGER
E-Mail karger@karger.ch
Fax + 41 61 306 12 34
http://www.karger.ch

1011–6125/96/0665–0004$10.00/0

Dr. M. Hirato
Department of Neurosurgery
Gunma University School of Medicine
3-39-15, Showa-machi
Maebashi, Gunma 371 (Japan)

Table 1. Autopsy cases

Diagnosis	Case	Age years	Sex	Location	Side	Central dose, Gy	Marginal dose, Gy	Duration months	Pathological diagnosis
Metastasis No. 1	TA	53	F	frontal	L	45	18	12	adenocarcinoma (breast)
				occipital	R	50	25	12	
				parietal	R	50	25	12	
						40	20	7	
				temporal	R	40	16	7	
				occipital	R	40	12	7	
				occipital	L	40	20	7	
Metastasis No. 2	YM	30	M	parietal	L	45	22.5	12	alveolar soft-tissue sarcoma
				occipital	L	30	21	12	
				occipital	R	40	20	12	
				temporal	L	30	21	9	

L = Left; R = right.

surgery are not clear. Neither is it clear what mechanisms are essential to suppress tumor growth. There are few studies in humans clarifying the temporal course of radiosurgical lesions histologically [8, 9]. A few experimental studies on the effects of radiosurgery on normal brain tissue or BTs are now in progress using animal models [10–13].

To elucidate the radiobiological effects of Gamma Knife radiosurgery on BTs, we performed a histological study on autopsy and surgical specimens after treatment.

Materials and Methods

Autopsy specimens were studied in two cases with metastatic BT obtained 12 months after treatment (table 1). Surgical specimens were studied in seven cases with BT: four with glioma, one with metastatic BT and two with acoustic schwannoma. The specimens were obtained from 2 to 10 months after radiosurgery (table 2). The central dose was between 30 and 50 Gy for metastatic BTs, between 20 and 33 Gy for gliomas and between 24 and 34 Gy for schwannomas. The margin was between 12 and 25 Gy for metastatic BTs, between 9 and 16.5 Gy for gliomas and between 12 and 17 Gy for acoustic schwannomas. In one case of glioma, fractionated Gamma Knife radiosurgery with a low marginal dose (10 Gy) was carried out three times over 5 days. Moreover, Gamma Knife radiosurgery was carried out twice in the same lesion in one case of metastatic BT. Neuroimaging studies were performed

Table 2. Surgical cases

Diagnosis	Case	Age years	Sex	Central dose, Gy	Marginal dose, Gy	Duration months	Pathological diagnosis
Metastasis No. 1	NT	59	F	40	12	5	adenocarcinoma (clear cell)
Glioma No. 1	SN	31	F	20[a]	10[a]	2	fibrillary astrocytoma (grade 2)
Glioma No. 2	MK	7	F	30	12	6	fibrillary astrocytoma (grade 2)
Glioma No. 3	IC	13	F	33	16.5	8	fibrillary astrocytoma (grade 2)
Glioma No. 4	CV	3	F	30	9	10	ependymoma
Schwannoma No. 1	AY	51	F	34	17	5	schwannoma
Schwannoma No. 2	SM	58	M	24	12	4	schwannoma

[a] Fractionated Gamma Knife treatment – 3 fractions over 5 days.

periodically after treatment, using magnetic resonance imaging (MRI) and a computed tomography (CT) scan. Histological studies included immunohistochemical staining for vascular endothelial or pericytic cells. Electron microscopic studies were sometimes performed.

Results

Mestastatic BT

Case TA

This was a 53-year-old female, who suffered from breast cancer. The tumor was removed and the histological diagnosis was adenocarcinoma. Four years after treatment, multiple metastatic brain lesions were found in the left frontal, right parietal and right occipital lobes. She received Gamma Knife radiosurgery. Five months after treatment, metastatic brain lesions were found in the right parietal region (at the same site as the previously treated lesion). New metastases were found in the temporal, right occipital and left occipital lobes. These lesions were also treated with the Gamma Knife. The tumors located in the right occipital and temporal lobes disappeared. The tumor in the right parietal lobe was slightly enlarged at 5 months follow-up but was diminished in size 11 months after treatment.

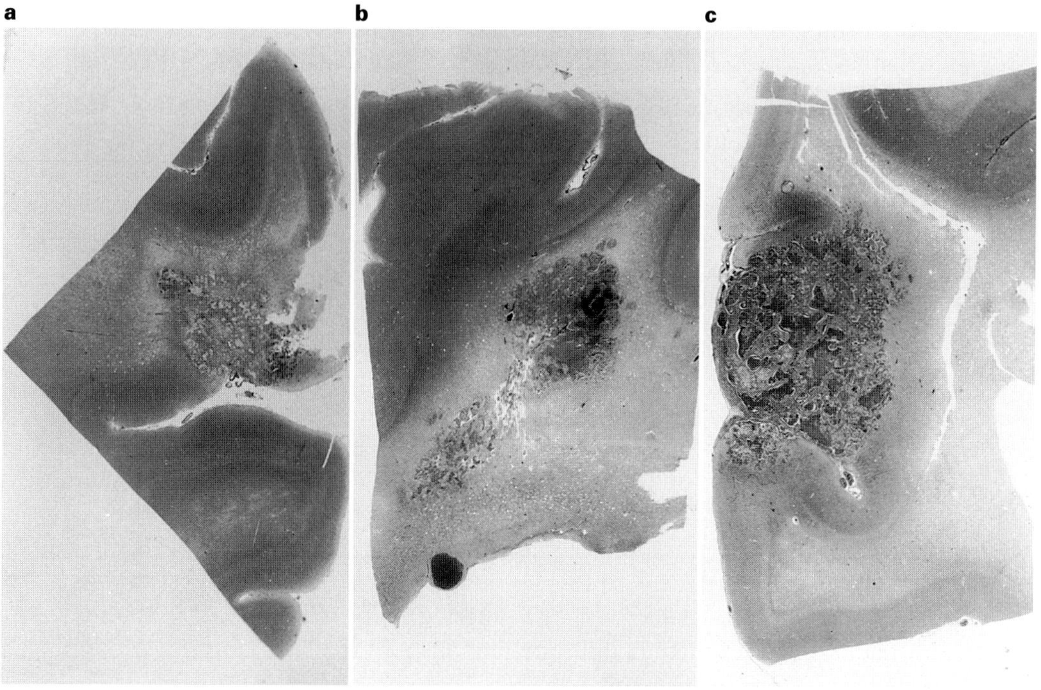

Fig. 1. Macroscopic histological study of a metastatic BT (adenocarcinoma, breast) after Gamma Knife radiosurgery (case TA). An increase of fibrous stroma was seen in each lesion treated by Gamma Knife. Masson trichrome staining. **a** Left occipital lesion. × 2.3. **b** Right temporal lesion. × 2.3. **c** Right parietal lesion. × 2.7.

MR images demonstrated that the tumors in the left frontal and occipital lobes remained unchanged in size and showed only a central signal change. The patient died of respiratory failure 1 year after the first treatment. In both the left occipital and right temporal lesions, histological study revealed a marked decrease in the tumor cell population. There was also an increase in fibrous stroma and fibrous thickening of the vascular walls in the tumor (fig. 1a, b). Adjacent to the tumor, fibrous thickening of vascular walls, infiltration of foamy macrophages, an increase in edema and small amounts of residual tumor cell nests were observed. In the right parietal lesion, tumor necrosis with a marked increase in fibrous stroma was observed on both the surface and the base of the tumor, being more obvious on the surface (fig. 1c). In the periphery of the tumor, fibrinoid necrosis of vascular walls was seen, but there were also residual tumor cells. In the left frontal and the right occipital lesions, necrosis was found in the tumor. However, many tumor cells remained in the peritumoral region, where small amounts of fibrinoid necrosis and fibrous thickening of vascular walls were observed.

Case YM

This 30-year-old male had a left hemiparesis. MRI showed a right parietal lobe tumor which was removed at craniotomy. The histological diagnosis was alveolar soft-tissue sarcoma. Further examination revealed a primary lesion in the right leg (tibia). Two years after treatment, other new metastatic lesions were found in the left parietal, occipital, temporal and right occipital lobes. Three of four lesions were treated using the Gamma Knife. Three months after the first treatment, the residual left temporal lesion was also treated with the Gamma Knife. In MR images, the temporal tumor and the bilateral occipital lesions had disappeared.

The right parietal tumor, which was the largest, had enlarged at 3 months after treatment but diminished in size by 12 months (fig. 2a–d). The patient died of respiratory failure 12 months after treatment. A histological study of the left parietal tumor was performed. It revealed a decrease in tumor cell population, fibrous thickening of the vascular walls and obliteration of the vessels in the center of the tumor. Masson trichrome staining showed an increase of fibrous stroma and fibrinoid necrosis of the vascular walls in the same region. In the tumor periphery, an increase of fibrous stroma was observed together with fibrous thickening and fibrinoid necrosis. Also detected were an increase in peritumoral edema, fibrinous exudation, infiltration of macrophages and astrocytosis (fig. 2e).

Case NT

In this 59-year-old female, the tumor was located in the left temporal lobe. The patient refused an operation and was treated with the Gamma Knife. Five months after radiosurgery, MRI showed an enlarged heterogeneously enhanced tumor and the mass effects had increased. The tumor was removed at craniotomy. The histological diagnosis was clear cell adenocarcinoma. Histological study of the surgical specimens revealed parenchymal coagulation necrosis and various vascular changes. These included vascular proliferation and fibrous thickening of vascular walls, marked lymphocyte infiltration, hemosiderin deposits and hemorrhages.

Glioma

Case SN

This patient was a 31-year-old female with a tumor located in the midbrain. After partial removal of a cystic tumor at craniotomy, she was treated by fractionated Gamma Knife radiosurgery three times over a 5-day period. The histological diagnosis was fibrillary astrocytoma grade 2. Two months after radiosurgery, MRI revealed that the cyst in the tumor had enlarged, although its solid part remained unchanged. Because the mass effects had increased, the tumor was

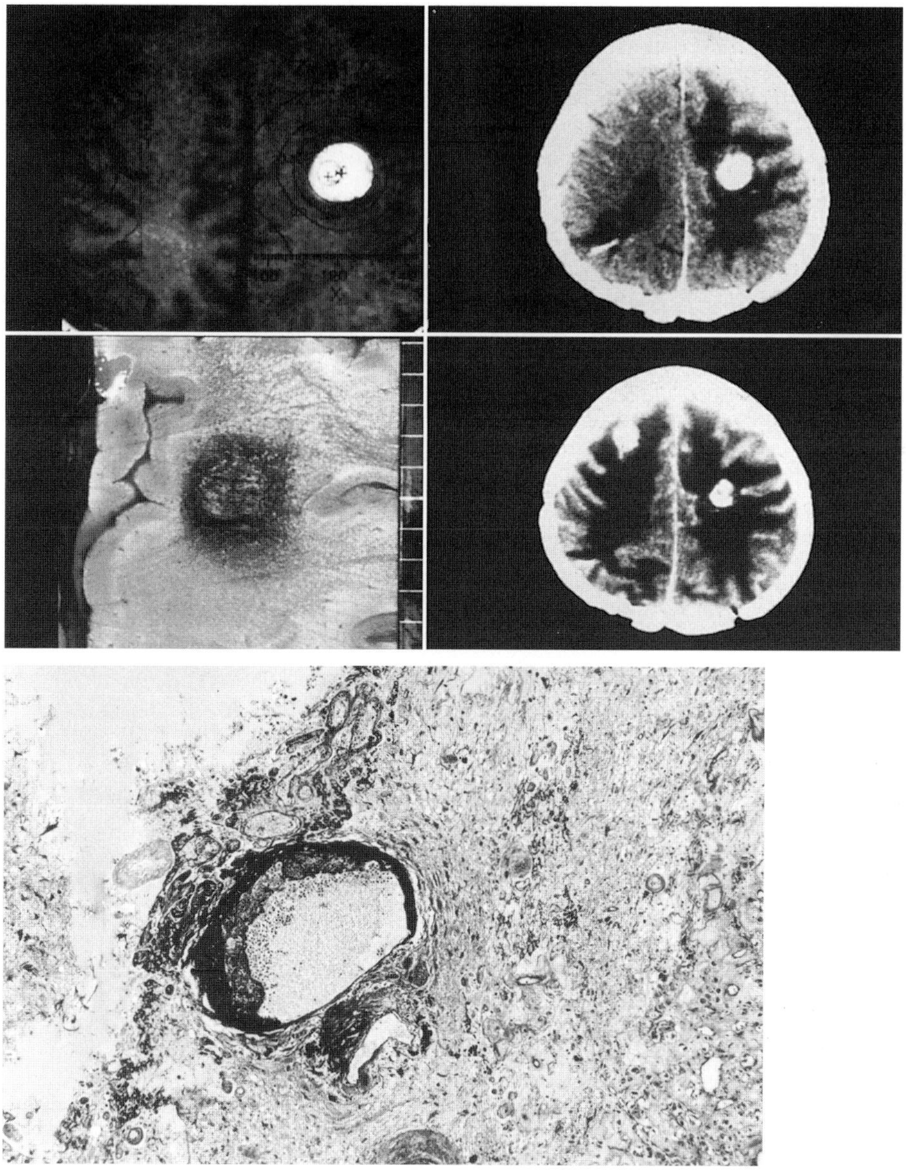

Fig. 2. Neuroimaging study and autopsy specimens of metastatic BT treated by Gamma Knife (case YM). **a** Dose planning at the treatment. **b** CT scan 3 months after treatment. **c** CT scan 1 year after treatment. **d** Autopsy specimen. **e** Histological specimen after Gamma Knife radiosurgery. An increase in fibrous stroma, fibrous thickening and fibrinoid necrosis of the vascular wall, and an increase in peritumoral edema and fibrinous exudation in the periphery of the tumor were found. Pathological diagnosis: alveolar soft-tissue sarcoma. Masson trichrome staining. × 39.

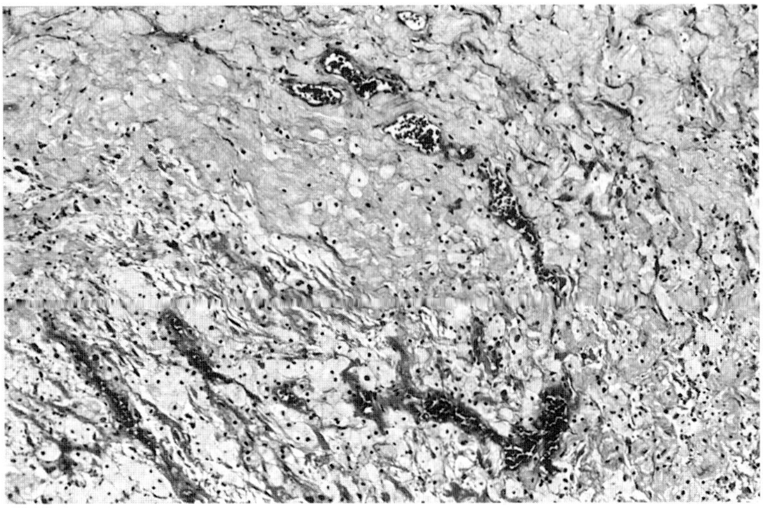

Fig. 3. Histological study of glioma after fractionated Gamma Knife radiosurgery (case SN). Prominent fibrosis and infiltration of foamy macrophages were found. Pathological diagnosis: fibrillary astrocytoma grade 2. Masson trichrome staining. × 150.

removed. Histological study revealed a decrease in the tumor cell population, infiltration of foamy macrophages, and fibrous thickening, degeneration of vascular walls and hemorrhages in the tumor. Masson trichrome staining showed prominent fibrosis in the tumor (fig. 3).

Case MK

The cystic tumor in a 7-year-old girl was located in the left medial occipital lobe close to the posterior horn of the lateral ventricle. Gamma Knife radiosurgery was planned following stereotactic biopsy. The histological diagnosis was astrocytoma grade 2. Six months after radiosurgery the tumor was removed because the cyst had enlarged. Histological study revealed necrosis of the tumor cells in the center of the tumor. Vascular proliferation was observed in the tumor periphery, together with fibrinoid necrosis of the vessels, hemorrhage and infiltration of lymphoid cells. PAM staining, specific for the basement membrane, demonstrated endothelial proliferation in the region of vascular proliferation (fig. 4).

Case IC

In this 13-year-old girl, a cystic tumor was located in the left parasellar region extending to the basal ganglia. The tumor had been partially removed 3 years

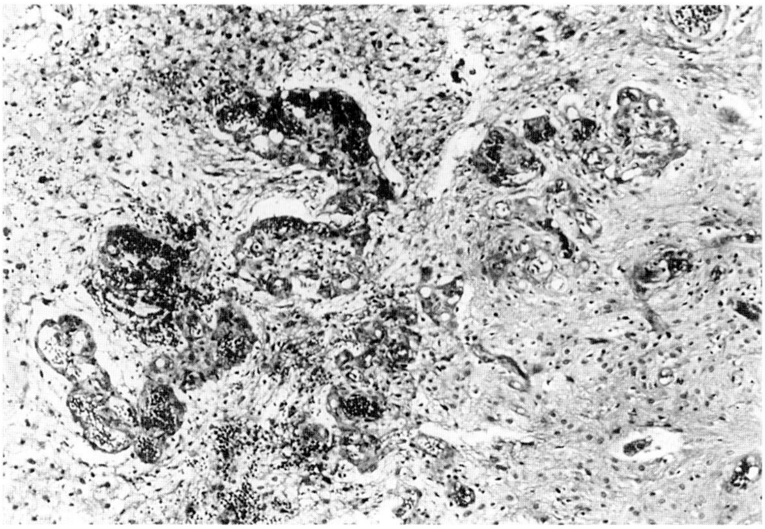

Fig. 4. Histological study of glioma after Gamma Knife radiosurgery (case MK). Marked proliferation of the vascular components surrounding the necrosis of the tumor cells was shown in the tumor periphery. Pathological diagnosis: fibrillary astrocytoma grade 2. HE. ×96.

before, mainly in the parasellar region. The histological diagnosis was astrocytoma grade 2. After the operation, Gamma Knife radiosurgery was planned, because the tumor continued to enlarge. Eight months after the treatment, because the cyst in the tumor had enlarged and mass effects appeared, the tumor was removed. Histological study revealed necrosis of the tumor cells in the center of the tumor. Residual tumor cells surrounded these areas, showing pseudopalisading. Tumor cell atypia was occasionally encountered. In the region surrounding the vessels, unusually prominent fibrosis was found, intermingled with residual tumor cells, showing a strand-like arrangement. Close to this region at a location where fibrosis was not prominent, vascular proliferation was seen. Immunohistochemical staining using smooth muscle α-actin indicated that this proliferation was mainly pericytic.

Case CV

The tumor was located in the occipital lobe of this 3-year-old girl. After stereotactic biopsy, she was treated by Gamma Knife. The histological diagnosis was ependymoma. Ten months after radiosurgery, MRI revealed that the cyst in the tumor had enlarged, although its solid part remained unchanged. Because the mass effects had increased, the tumor was removed. Histological study revealed

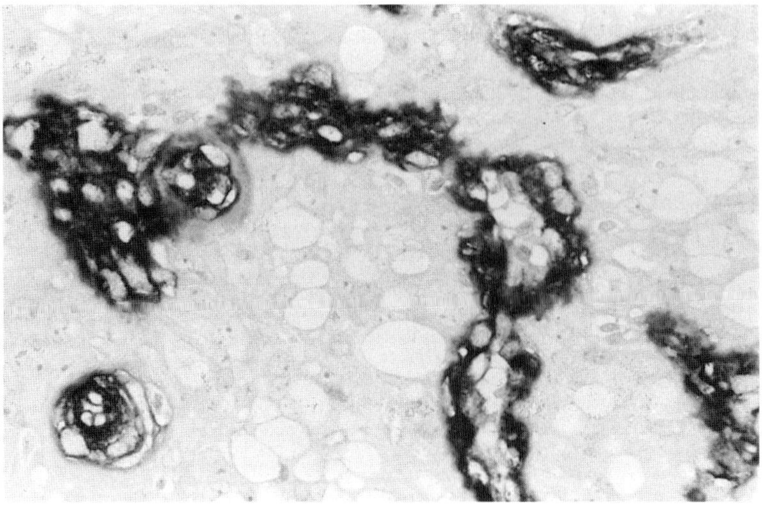

Fig. 5. Immunohistochemical study of glioma after Gamma Knife radiosurgery (case CV). Marked proliferation of endothelial cells was found in the periphery of the tumor. Pathological diagnosis: ependymoma. Factor-8-related-antigen staining. × 600.

fibrosis and focal cell loss in the center of the tumor. The most prominent findings were various vascular changes in the periphery. We found vascular wall thickening, endothelial cell swelling and infiltration of foamy macrophages in the perivascular spaces. Endothelial proliferation was shown using factor-8-related-antigen staining, which is specific for endothelial cells (fig. 5). However, with smooth muscle α-actin staining, which is specific for pericytes and smooth muscle cells, we found no immunopositive pericytes in the vascular walls. In one region, hematoxylin-eosin (HE) staining demonstrated thrombosis.

Neurinoma

Case AY

In this 51-year-old female, the cystic tumor was located in the left cerebellopontine angle. It was treated with the Gamma Knife. Five months after radiosurgery, MRI revealed that the cyst in the tumor had enlarged. Because the mass effects had increased, the tumor was removed surgically, and the diagnosis of schwannoma confirmed. Histological study revealed various kinds of tissue reactions. Parenchymal necrosis and fibrosis were observed in the center of the tumor. However, the most prominent findings were various vascular changes at the tumor periphery.

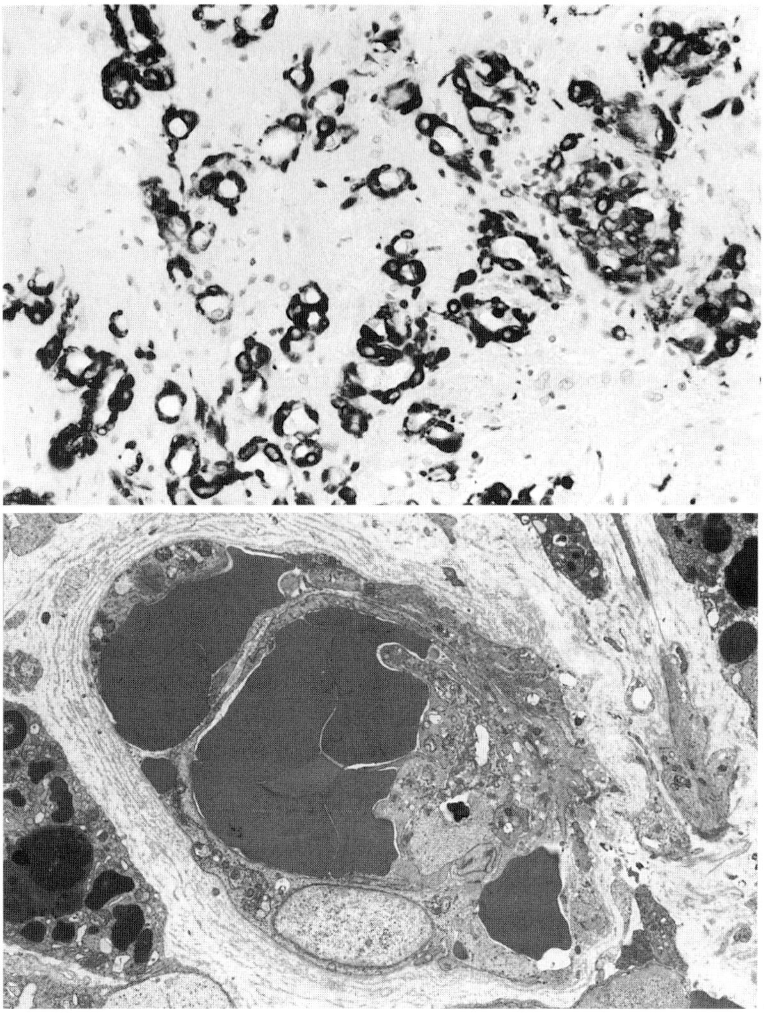

Fig. 6. Case AY after Gamma Knife radiosurgery. **a** Immunohistochemical study of schwannoma. Marked proliferation of pericytes was found on the vascular wall. Smooth muscle α-actin staining. × 195. **b** Electron microscope study of schwannoma. Fenestration and stratification of endothelial cells of the vascular wall were seen. × 3,350.

There were fibrin deposits in the vascular walls and thrombus formation. Infiltration of macrophages and small lymphoid cells around the vessels was detected with HE staining. Basement membrane degradation was associated with thrombosis in one region, as demonstrated with PAM staining, which is specific for the basement membrane of the vascular wall. However, in another region, there were also vascular proliferative changes. Periodic acid-Schiff staining showed thickening of the vascular wall. With factor-8-related-antigen staining, endothelial proliferation was shown in the same location. With smooth muscle α-actin staining, pericytic proliferation was also seen (fig. 6a). Therefore, vascular proliferation was the result of both endothelial and pericytic proliferation in this region. Corresponding with these findings, an electron microscopic study showed stratification of endothelial cells and, sometimes, fenestration of the vascular wall (fig. 6b).

Case SM

This 58-year-old male had a cystic tumor located in the right cerebellopontine angle. It was treated with the Gamma Knife. Four months after radiosurgery, because the mass effects had increased and MRI revealed that the cyst in the tumor had enlarged, the tumor was removed. Histological study revealed necrosis, which was sharply demarcated with surrounding residual tumor cells. Around the necrosis, HE staining could not show definite changes in the vascular components. However, an immunohistochemical study using factor-8-related antigen and smooth muscle α-actin revealed marked pericytic proliferation of the vascular wall.

Discussion

This study included several kinds of tumor pathology and was based on different types of specimens obtained from autopsy or surgery. Nonetheless, several characteristic histological changes were noted, which might be related to the mechanisms of tumor growth suppression. In two autopsy cases, we could study a precise relationship between radiation dosage and the histological changes in the tumor and surrounding brain tissues. In the high-dose (central) region, destructive changes occurred both in tumor cells and vessels. Coagulation necrosis, a decrease in the tumor cell population and an increase in fibrous stroma or fibrinoid necrosis of the vascular wall were observed. In the low-dose (peripheral) region, vascular changes were often recognized intermingled with residual tumor tissues. Here, fibrous thickening or fibrinoid necrosis of vascular walls could be detected, sometimes associated with vascular proliferative changes.

The findings outlined above correspond well with previous histological studies in humans [8, 9]. Moreover, such findings are in keeping with experimental studies following radiosurgery [10]. In the latter study, gadolinium-enhanced MRI and histological examinations were performed on brain tumors following radiosurgery. It was demonstrated that peripheral enhanced regions correlated histologically with areas of vascular proliferation, and central nonenhancing areas with radiation necrosis [10]. From these experimental findings, the radiobiological effects of radiosurgery on normal brain tissue were classified into three stages. In our series, as the specimens were obtained from 2 to 12 months, they correspond to the intermediate stage [4, 10]. In this stage, chronic inflammatory reactions occurred: resorption of the necrotic debris as shown by progressive cavitation, microglial response and increased perilesional vascularity. There were congested vessels, new capillary formation and endothelial thickening at the marginal zone. In addition to these findings, an increase in fibrous stroma was characteristic in our study. This might be related to the response to injury caused by radiosurgery and indicate radionecrosis [4]. These changes were particularly notable in the glioma that underwent fractionated Gamma Knife treatment and in the metastatic brain tumor treated twice. In surgical specimens, vascular changes were prominent in and around the tumor. Fibrinoid necrosis and fibrous thickening of the vascular wall were usually noted. Moreover, vascular proliferative changes were often seen around the tumor. Immunohistochemical staining revealed vascular proliferative changes consisting of endothelial and/or pericytic proliferation. An electron microscopic study of an acoustic schwannoma showed stratification of the endothelial cells in the vascular wall.

One of the critical tissues in radiosurgery is the endothelial cell. In experimental studies on the radiobiological effects of radiosurgery, proliferative changes were found in endothelial and media cells and in subendothelial connective tissue, in response to vascular injury. Fibroblastic activity increased and reparative proliferation of surviving endothelial cells occurred with increased deposition of collagen in the media of the vessel walls. These changes caused progressive reparative endothelial and medial thickening leading to fibrosis and occlusion of small vessels [4]. Our findings might be related to these repair processes. Furthermore, our study revealed that vascular proliferation was rather complex and dynamic, and included pericytes as well as endothelial cells. Remarkable pericyte proliferation was found in the area of vascular proliferation. In glial neoplasms, although the origin of the cells contributing to microvascular proliferation is not yet established, the proliferation is due in large measure to hypertrophy of smooth muscle cells rather than to changes in endothelial cells [14, 15].

As it has been suggested that endothelial proliferation may play an important role in suppressing tumor growth, we must reconsider the mechanisms and role of vascular changes from that standpoint. In addition to the mechanisms outlined above, degradation of the basement membrane of the vascular wall was observed in some regions. Moreover, electron microscopy on an acoustic schwannoma showed fenestration of vessel walls. These changes might increase vascular permeability causing peritumoral edema or enlargement of a tumor cyst. Study of the radiobiological behavior of normal brain or brain tumor tissue in vivo is just beginning [10–13]. To date, the mechanisms which suppress tumor growth remain obscure. However, from our study, the combination of central necrotic changes with increased fibrous stroma and peripheral vascular changes may well be important. Further histological studies in humans after radiosurgery, together with experimental studies in animals, are required.

Acknowledgments

The authors thank Mrs. M. Yokota and Mr. K. Isoda at the Department of Pathology, Gunma University School of Medicine, for technical assistance in staining autopsy and surgical specimens and providing excellent photographs.

References

1 Leksell L: The stereotaxic method and radiosurgery of the brain. Acta Chir Scand 1951;102:316–319.

2 Leksell L: Cerebral radiosurgery. 1: Gammathalamotomy in two cases of intractable pain. Acta Chir Scand 1968;134:585–595.

3 Ostertag CB: Stereotactic radiation therapy and radiosurgery. Stereotact Funct Neurosurg 1994;63: 220–232.

4 Steiner L, Lindquist C, Steiner M: Radiosurgery; in Symon L, Calliauw L, Cohadon F, Lobo Antunes J, Loew F, Nornes H, Pasztor E, Pickard JD, Strong AJ, Yasargil MG (eds): Advances and Technical Standards in Neurosurgery. Berlin, Springer, 1992, vol 19, pp 19–102.

5 Flickinger JC, Lunsford LD, Kondziolka D, Maitz AH, Epstein AH, Simons SR, Wu A: Radiosurgery and brain tolerance: An analysis of neurodiagnostic imaging changes after Gamma Knife radiosurgery for arteriovenous malformations. Int J Radiat Oncol Biol Phys 1992;23:19–26.

6 Larson DA, Flickinger JC, Loeffler JS: The radiobiology of radiosurgery. Int J Radiat Oncol Biol Phys 1993;25:557–561.

7 Lo EH, Fabrikant JI: Delayed biologic reactions to stereotactic charged-particle radiosurgery in the human brain. Stereotact Funct Neurosurg 1991;56:197–212.

8 Steiner L, Forster D, Leksell L, Meyerson BA, Boethius J: Gamma-thalamotomy in intractable pain. Acta Neurochir (Wien) 1980;52:173–184.

9 Wennerstrand J, Ungerstedt U: Cerebral radiosurgery. 2: An anatomical study of gamma radiolesions. Acta Chir Scand 1970;136:133–137.

10 Blatt DR, Friedman WA, Bova FJ, Theele DP, Mickle JP: Temporal characteristics of radiosurgical lesions in an animal model. J Neurosurg 1994;80:1046–1055.

11 Inoue HK, Kohga H, Hirato M, Nakamura M, Ohye C: Neurobiologic effects of radiosurgery: Histologic, immunohistochemical and electron-microscopic studies of a rat model. Stereotact Funct Neurosurg 1994;63:280–285.

12 Linskey ME, Martinez AJ, Kondziolka D, Flickinger JC, Maitz AH, Whiteside T, Lunsford LD: The radiobiology of human acoustic schwannoma xenografts after stereotactic radiosurgery evaluated in the subrenal capsule of athymic mice. J Neurosurg 1993;78:645–653.

13 Lunsford LD, Altschuler EM, Flickinger JC, Wu A, Martinez AJ: In vivo biological effects of stereotactic radiosurgery: A primate model. Neurosurgery 1990;27:373–382.

14 Haddad SF, Moore SA, Schelper RL, Goeken JA: Vascular smooth muscle hyperplasia underlies the formation of glomeruloid vascular structures of glioblastoma multiforme. J Neuropathol Exp Neurol 1992;51:488–492.

15 Wesseling P, Vandersteenhoven JJ, Downey BT, Ruiter DJ, Burger PC: Cellular components of microvascular proliferation in human glial and metastatic brain neoplasms: A light microscopic and immunohistochemical study of formalin-fixed, routinely processed material. Acta Neuropathol 1993;85:508–514.

Proc 7th Int Meeting Leksell Gamma Knife® Society,
Island of Lana'i, Hawaii, November 1995
Stereotact Funct Neurosurg 1996;66(suppl 1):17–28

Stereotactic and Functional Neurosurgery

In vitro Contractility Studies of the Rat Middle Cerebral Artery after Stereotactic Gamma Knife Radiosurgery

O. Major, A.A. Kemeny, D.M.C. Forster, J. Jakubowski, A.H. Morice

National Centre of Stereotactic Radiosurgery and Department of Experimental Medicine, Royal Hallamshire Hospital, Sheffield, UK

Key Words

Radiobiology · Stereotactic radiosurgery · Contractility · Cerebral vessels · Middle cerebral artery · Radiation effects

Abstract

The middle cerebral artery (MCA) was irradiated in 94 rats using the Gamma Knife. The vessels receiving 20, 50, 80 and 200 Gy were removed 24 h later and mounted on a myograph. Contractility responses to potassium and prostaglandin (PG) F2α were tested. After precontraction with PGF2α, the relaxant effects of histamine, papaverine, *L*-arginine and sodium nitroprusside were examined. Other vessels were preincubated with ouabain or Nω-nitro-*L*-arginine methyl ester before testing with the relaxant agents. After irradiation, the contractile response to maximal potassium and PGF concentrations was diminished, suggesting dose-dependent radiation damage to the contractile mechanism. The normal MCA shows an initial relaxation in the presence of a low K^+ concentration, which is Na^+,K^+-ATPase dependent. According to this study, the endothelium-derived relaxation function was suppressed by radiation, suggesting that there is an early change in irradiated vessels, demonstrable by functional studies, which affects both the smooth muscle and endothelial layers.

Introduction

Since the introduction of stereotactic radiosurgery in the treatment of cerebral arteriovenous malformations [1], over 20,000 patients have been treated worldwide [2]. One of the most intriguing features of radiation-induced thrombo-

KARGER
E-Mail karger@karger.ch
Fax + 41 61 306 12 34
http://www.karger.ch

1011–6125/96/0665–0017$10.00/0

A.A. Kemeny, FRCS, MD
National Centre of Stereotactic Radiosurgery
Royal Hallamshire Hospital
Glossop Road
Sheffield S10 2JF (UK)

obliteration is the latent period following irradiation. During this period of several months, radiological investigations such as angiography or magnetic resonance angiography (MRA) do not demonstrate changes. Furthermore, experimental irradiation in laboratory animals results in alterations of vasoarchitecture only after large doses and a long latency [3–6]. The aim of this study was to examine the early changes in cerebral vessels following single-dose radiation.

To detect changes in vessel vasoreactivity following irradiation, we selected the middle cerebral artery (MCA) in the rat as our study target. This vessel is small (200–250 μm in diameter at the proximal segment) and is suitable for in vitro myograph studies. We examined the isometric contraction forces generated by the vessels and determined their response to vasodilators active on both endothelial and smooth muscle cells [7–9].

Materials and Methods

We used 94 pathogen-free 230- to 250-g male Wistar rats, of which 58 were used as controls, while stereotactic radiosurgery was performed in 36 (table 1).

Irradiation

The position of the proximal section of the MCA was calculated using a rat stereotactic atlas [10]. In view of the small head size in the rat (giving a shallow lesion depth), a wax radiography mask was fashioned and used for correction. An 8-mm collimator field was defined with the left MCA in the target (isocentre 8 mm anterior and 0.5 mm superior to the interaural line and 4 mm lateral from the midline). The vessel was in a consistent anatomical position in all animals, confirmed at the time of brain removal. The relatively large collimator was chosen in order to ensure some dose homogeneity throughout the examined section of the vessel. In addition, this allowed the opposite MCA to receive a radiosurgically relevant dose. Twenty-four animals were prescribed 50 Gy to the ipsilateral and 20 Gy to the contralateral MCA, and 12 received 200 Gy to the ipsilateral and 80 Gy to the contralateral vessel.

The animals were anaesthetised with intraperitoneal pentobarbitone, 30 mg/kg body weight, and placed in a small animal stereotactic frame (Kopf Laboratories). The base plate was modified to fit into the Leksell G frame and thus into the Gamma Knife. After irradiation, the animals were allowed to recover from the anaesthetic and were maintained under standard conditions until the myograph study 24 h or 6 weeks later.

Myograph Studies

The animals were sacrificed using a pentobarbitone overdose followed by exsanguination. The brain was immediately removed and both MCAs were dissected under an operating microscope using microinstruments. The most proximal 3-mm section of the MCA was cut and mounted into an automated small vessel myograph (Cambustion, Cambridge, UK). The active length was 2.3 mm. The mean normalised lumen diameter was calculated according to Mulvany and Halpern [8]. The resting wall tension/internal circumference curve was established and a 0.9 × 100 mm Hg transmural pressure was emulated.

Table 1. Grouping of rat MCA specimens by treatment and timing of myograph study after the intervention

Group	Treatment	Time after treatment	Number of viable vessels
Normal	none	–	68
L-NAME	100 μ*M* *L*-NAME	10 min	12
Ouabain	100 μ*M* ouabain	10 min	12
Noradrenaline	100 μ*M* noradrenaline	10 min	12
Denuded	removal of endothelium	–	12
24h20Gy	20 Gy	24 h	12
24h50Gy	50 Gy	24 h	12
24h80Gy	80 Gy	24 h	11
24h200Gy	200 Gy	24 h	11
6w20Gy	20 Gy	6 weeks	8
6w50Gy	50 Gy	6 weeks	12

After mounting, the myograph was warmed to 37 °C and the chamber fluid aerated with 95% oxygen and 5% carbon dioxide. The vessels were equilibrated for 1 h in a physiological solution (PBS, composition in m*M*: sodium chloride 119, sodium bicarbonate 25, potassium chloride 4.7, calcium chloride 1.5, potassium dihydrogen orthophosphate 1.18, magnesium sulphate 1.17, diaminoethanetetraacetic acid 0.026 and glucose 11).

The maximal contraction response to 124 m*M* KCl was elicited three times to establish vessel viability. After 30 min rest concentration-response curves were obtained by adding KCl solution (5–165 m*M*) to the bath in a stepwise cumulative manner. Similar curves were obtained using prostaglandin F2α (PGF; 0.1–100 μ*M*, Prostin F2 Alpha, Upjohn). The maximal contraction after PGF for each vessel was also recorded.

Following the maximum PGF contraction, vasodilatation to endothelial- and non-endothelial-dependent agents was examined. After preconstriction with 50 μ*M* PGF, solutions of *L*-arginine (*L*-Arg; 0.01–200 μ*M*), histamine (His; 0.1–150 μ*M*), sodium nitroprusside (SNP; 0.01–200 μ*M*) or papaverine (PAP; 0.01–100 μ*M*) were added to the bath in a cumulative fashion to record relaxation concentration-response curves.

Three groups of normal vessels (n = 12) were incubated with 100 μ*M* ouabain, noradrenaline or the nitric oxide (NO) blocker Nω-nitro-*L*-arginine methyl ester (*L*-NAME) (all Sigma). Incubation continued for 10 min and then potassium concentration-response curves were elicited.

Endothelial Lesion

The endothelial layer of the MCA was mechanically traumatised in 12 of the non-irradiated vessels by gently rubbing the lumen with a human hair ('denuded' vessels). These vessels underwent the same protocol as outlined above.

Pathological Investigations

At the end of the experiments, all vessels were fixed in formaldehyde for pathological studies. After paraffin embedding, haematoxylin-eosin staining was carried out for light microscopy. Electron microscopy was also performed to investigate ultrastructural changes.

Data Processing

The analysed vessels were grouped according to their treatment before the myograph studies (table 1). Standard personal computer software (Microsoft Excel-5.0) was used for data storage and analysis. The half-maximal response values (EC_{50}) were determined graphically. All data are expressed as the mean ± SD. The differences between the various treatment groups were analysed using ANOVA and Student's t test, as appropriate.

Results

The general behaviour of the animals remained normal throughout the post-irradiation period without overt signs of neurological deficit. At dissection, no macroscopic alterations of the brain or vessels were seen. The normalised vessel diameter was similar in normal (205 ± 21 μm) and irradiated (206 ± 15 μm) vessels after 24 h ($p = 0.64$).

Contractility Studies

After 24 h there was no significant difference between normal and irradiated vessels in the maximal contractile response to potassium, except with the 200-Gy dose which gave a value of 0.99 ± 0.2 mN/mm as opposed to the normal value of 1.38 ± 0.5 mN/mm ($p < 0.05$; table 2). After 6 weeks, the response was reduced even with lower doses: there was a 37% reduction with 20 Gy and a 55% reduction with 50 Gy ($p < 0.01$; table 2). The maximal potassium response was increased after incubation with *L*-NAME by 50%. A mechanical endothelial lesion had a similar effect (40% increase; table 2).

The maximal PGF response was unchanged 24 h after small doses of radiation, whereas after 200 Gy, the reduction was about 30% to 1.58 ± 0.9 mN/mm compared with the normal value of 2.29 ± 0.8 mN/mm ($p < 0.05$). Six weeks later, even low doses caused a decrease in contractility in a radiation-dose-dependent fashion. Thus, with 20 Gy, contractility was 1.57 ± 1.3 mN/mm ($p < 0.05$) and with 50 Gy it was 0.12 ± 0.2 mN/mm ($p < 0.001$). Contraction in the latter group was so small that subsequent relaxation studies were not possible. The PGF reaction in denuded vessels was 60% less than in controls ($p < 0.01$; table 2).

Table 2. Maximal contractile forces (mN/mm) measured following incubation in high-concentration KCl and PGF

Group	Potassium (124 m*M*)	PGF (50 μ*M*)
Normal	1.38±0.5	2.29±0.8
Denuded	1.95±0.7	0.94±0.6***
24h20Gy	1.40±0.9	2.53±0.9
24h50Gy	1.54±0.6	2.69±1
24h80Gy	1.43±0.5	2.17±0.5
24h200Gy	0.99±0.2*	1.58±0.9
6w20Gy	0.87±0.6**	1.57±1
6w50Gy	0.61±0.4***	0.12±0.2***
L-NAME	2.07±0.8**	
Ouabain	0.88±0.3***	
Noradrenaline	1.84±0.4**	

* $p < 0.05$, ** $p < 0.01$, *** $p < 0.001$, two-tailed t test, compared with normal.

Concentration-Response Curves

Potassium. A stepwise increase in concentration resulted in an initial relaxation of the normal MCA at 12 and 15 m*M* KCl followed by contraction at higher K^+ concentrations (fig. 1). After *L*-NAME incubation, this relaxation remained unchanged (table 3). Ouabain decreased the relaxation significantly at both of these potassium concentrations (75 and 97%, respectively, $p < 0.01$). A mechanical lesion of the endothelium abolished the relaxation. All irradiation doses diminished the low-K^+-induced relaxation by at least 78% ($p < 0.01$), but there was no difference between the irradiated groups (ANOVA $p < 0.1$). Noradrenaline incubation caused a very marked (more than 300%) increase in relaxation ($p < 0.001$; table 3). The contraction response seen at higher potassium concentrations was radiosensitive. Twenty-four hours after irradiation with higher doses, we observed reduced K^+ sensitivity as demonstrated by larger EC_{50} values. With 80 Gy, there was a 33% increase, while with 200 Gy there was a 42% increase ($p < 0.01$; table 4, fig. 1). By 6 weeks the changes were reversed, so that after 50 Gy, the EC_{50} was 25% lower ($p < 0.01$; table 4).

PGF. Mechanical removal of the endothelium shifted the PGF concentration-response curves to the right indicating a reduced sensitivity, as expressed by larger EC_{50} values (29 ± 11 μ*M* compared with a normal value of 11.9 ± 5 μ*M*).

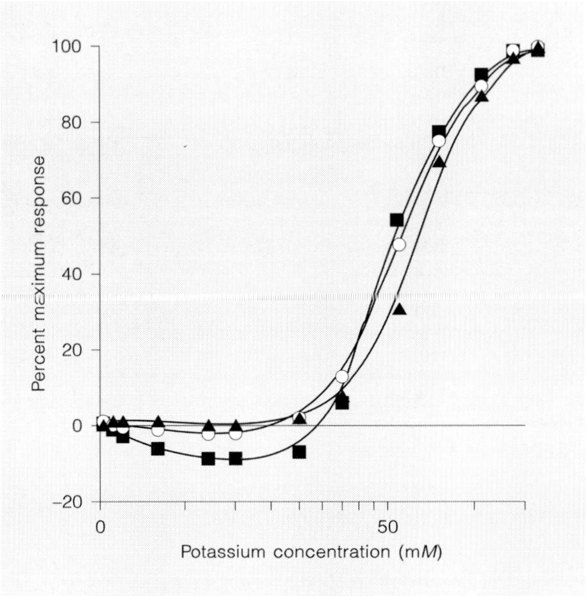

Fig. 1. Potassium concentration-response study of normal and irradiated rat MCA. Irradiation abolished the relaxation observed in normal vessels (■) at lower K^+ concentrations and after a larger radiation dose decreased the contraction sensitivity in the higher concentration range. The values are expressed as percentage of the maximal response to 165 m*M* KCl. ○ = 24h20Gy; ▲ = 24h200Gy (see table 1).

A similar effect was seen 24 h after irradiation with doses larger than 20 Gy. Even after this dose, a similar effect could be observed at 6 weeks (table 4).

Relaxation Studies

Mechanical damage to the endothelium greatly diminished *L*-Arg-induced relaxation. Radiation resulted in a downward shift of the concentration-response curves indicating enhanced relaxation, and a leftward shift (lower EC_{50} values, table 5), indicating increased sensitivity. The former was statistically significant at 80 Gy (83.7 ± 5 vs. 62.1 ± 14, $p < 0.001$). The latter effect was significant at all doses above 20 Gy (fig. 2). Similar increased sensitivity was observed using His SNP and PAP (table 5).

Pathological Investigations

Light and electron microscope studies failed to show changes in the vessels after irradiation with any dose at either 24 h or 6 weeks.

Table 3. Contractile forces in the rat MCA in low K^+

Group	12 m*M* K^+	15 m*M* K^+
Normal	−8.6±8	−9.2±7
Denuded	1.7±2**	2.3±3**
24h20Gy	−1.89±2*	−1.09±2**
24h50Gy	0.75±2**	−0.83±3***
24h80Gy	−2.21±2**	−1.22±3**
24h200Gy	0.22±3**	0.14±3**
6w20Gy	−0.35±4**	0.36±6**
6w50Gy	−1.12±5**	−0.14±6*
Ouabain	−2.1±2***	−0.2±3***
L-NAME	−7.23±3	−7.49±3
Noradrenaline	−41.6±19***	−39.8±19***

Values are expressed as the percentage of the maximal contractile force. Negative values indicate relaxation compared to the forces measured in physiologic solution.

* $p < 0.05$, ** $p < 0.01$, *** $p < 0.001$, two-tailed t test, compared with normal.

Table 4. EC_{50} values of concentration-response curves using KCl and PGF as contractile agents

Group	Potassium, m*M*	PGF, μ*M*
Normal	53.0±9	11.9±5
Denuded	57.7±12	29.0±11
24h20Gy	55.8±11	12.3±3
24h50Gy	48.7±9	24.3±9***
24h80Gy	70.5±10**	20.6±7**
24h200Gy	75.1±10**	17.9±8*
6w20Gy	52.9±12	21.2±12*
6w50Gy	39.3±7***	NM
L-NAME	43.3±3**	
Ouabain	53.3±9	
Noradrenaline	50.3±7	

NM = Not measurable.

* $p < 0.05$, ** $p < 0.01$, *** $p < 0.001$, two-tailed t test, compared with normal.

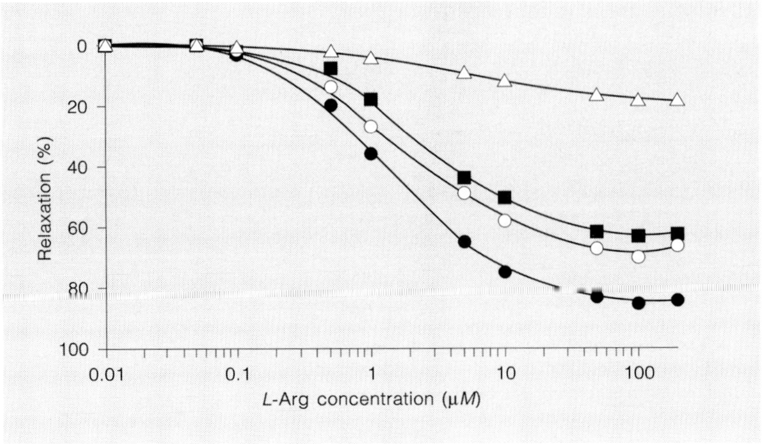

Fig. 2. Arginine relaxation study of the rat MCA after PGF preconstriction. An increased relaxation is observed after irradiation. Mechanical trauma of the endothelium ('denuded') diminished the response. The values are expressed as percentages of the maximally constricted state. ■ = Normal; △ = denuded; ○ = 24h50Gy; ● = 24h80Gy (see table 1).

Discussion

Since the introduction of stereotactic single-dose radiation in the treatment of various cerebral lesions, the study of radiation effects on cerebral tissue has taken on further relevance. Stereotactic radiosurgery is employed on a large scale worldwide in the management of cerebral arteriovenous malformations. In addition, due to close anatomical relationships between pathological targets of radiosurgery and major vascular structures, the latter are commonly exposed to large radiation doses. Thus, the effects of ionising radiation on cerebral vessels are of particular importance. Most studies in this field have concentrated on histological appearances, and only a few authors have analysed the functional changes in irradiated vessels [11–13].

The design of animal models for radiosurgery is fraught with difficulties. One of the problems is the apparent relative radio-resistance of cerebral vessels in experimental animals. In their rat model, Kondziolka et al. [3] found no vascular, or for that matter glial, changes even with a dose of 70 Gy. At 80 Gy mild arteriolar thickening, and at 100 Gy endothelial degeneration, was observed after 90 days. Nakagaki et al. [5] reported occasional vascular endothelial proliferation 6 months after 6,000 rad orthovolt whole-brain irradiation. We aimed in our study to employ doses between 20 and 200 Gy, which covers the dose range used in

Table 5. Relaxation response of rat MCA (expressed as percent of contractile force measured after preconstriction with PGF) to *L*-Arg, His, SNP and PAP

Group	*L*-Arg	His	SNP	PAP
Normal	62.1±14 (3.4±1)	88.9±10 (7.8±4)	85.8±11 (2.6±1)	107.8±17 (3.6±2)
Denuded	20.1±10** (5.2±4)	87.8±13 (10.5±10)	66.9±18*** (1.2±0.3**)	96.2±7 (3.1±1)
24h20Gy	62.5±22 (3.4±1)	104.1±10 (7.5±2)	83.9±9 (2.3±1)	95.5±7 (2.4±2)
24h50Gy	65.5±17 (2.6±2*)	100±5 (7.1±4)	86.5±13 (1.6±1)	94.5±11 (1.3±0.8***)
24h80Gy	83.7±5** (1.8±0.9**)	117.8±11* (7.3±3)	92.2±8 (1.5±1)	107.8±17 (1.9±1*)
24h200Gy	70.6±15 (1.9±1*)	95.4±5 (6.0±2)	89.1±8 (1.1±0.8**)	95.2±5 (0.95±0.6***)
6w20Gy	72.5±27 (1.9±1)	143.4±41** (12.2±8*)	80.1±19 (2.6±1)	102.8±20 (2.5±3)

Values in parentheses are the EC_{50} values (μ*M*).
* $p<0.05$, ** $p<0.01$, *** $p<0.001$, two-tailed t test, compared with normal.

clinical setting and also includes doses that are known to eventually lead to histopathological alterations [3, 5, 6, 12, 14, 15].

The ability to relax and contract using a complex smooth muscle and endothelial mechanism is arguably the most important feature of cerebral vessels. This function can be conveniently examined using the Mulvany myograph employed in this study [8, 16]. We chose the rat MCA as a target for both anatomical and technical reasons. The vessels are easy to dissect and are similar in size to human pial vessels (200–250 μm diameter). The rat MCA is in a fixed anatomical position which enables accurate irradiation, without imaging, based on atlas coordinates. We performed similar pilot studies on the anterior cerebral and basilar arteries. These vessels exhibit a very different pharmacological reactivity to MCA both in our experience and in previous studies [17], and thus the results are not included here.

The radiosensitivity of vessels, particularly the endothelium, has been established previously [18]. Thrombomodulin was suggested as a marker of endothelial injury induced by a low (up to 50 Gy) dose [19]. Lung vessel changes were demonstrated after a single dose of therapeutic irradiation [20]. It has been postulated that the primary site of radiation damage to the kidney is in the endothelium, and that progressive mesangial sclerosis leads to reduced renal function in radiation nephropathy [21]. Neointimal hyperplasia after endothelial injury was inhibited by gamma radiation [22]. At the biochemical level, 20–40 Gy α particle irradiation inhibited angiotensin-converting enzyme activity [23]. Radiation-induced alkaline phosphatase loss started 25 days after 20 Gy irradiation [24].

The endothelial cell layer is an active structure with several functions, including control of vascular tone. Locally synthesised PG-E2 and the endothelium-derived relaxing factor, which was identified as NO, reduce vessel tone [25]. The endothelins, peptides released from the endothelium, are potent agents with a mainly vasoconstrictor action [18]. These functions are potentially radiosensitive, and it was our aim to detect changes within these physiologic systems after stereotactic irradiation.

The integrity of the contractile apparatus was tested using the maximal potassium response. K^+ solution depolarizes the cell membranes, opening voltage-dependent Ca^{2+} channels. This mechanism bypasses the receptor-operated systems and is relatively insensitive to changes in intracellular enzyme systems [26, 27]. In the present study we found that the maximal potassium response was increased when the endothelium was mechanically damaged or when NO synthesis was blocked by *L*-NAME, suggesting the presence of a relaxing endothelial control. In contrast, the maximal potassium response was diminished by 6 weeks after 50 Gy irradiation, and the larger 200 Gy radiation dose had a similar effect after just 24 h, suggesting that irradiation has a direct effect on the contractile mechanism or on the mechanical properties of the vessels.

During the potassium concentration-response experiments, reproducible relaxation was observed between 12 and 15 m*M*. Endothelium-denuded vessels did not show this relaxation, it was also inhibited by incubation with 100 μ*M* ouabain. On the other hand, inhibition of NO synthesis with *L*-NAME did not alter this phenomenon, suggesting that the relaxation is endothelium-related, but not due to activation of the NO system. Previous studies have suggested that potassium-induced relaxation is a marker of Na^+,K^+-ATPase activity [28, 29]. Radiosensitivity of this enzyme has been shown before [30–32]. In our study, irradiation with even the lower doses employed abolished relaxation, indicating that radiation acts via the endothelium. The concentration-response curves were significantly shifted to the right, resulting in higher EC_{50} values 24 h after 80 and 200 Gy, indicating reduced potassium sensitivity.

L-Arg causes relaxation via enhancement of NO synthesis. Mechanical damage to the endothelium reduced the relaxation response to 18% of normal. Any remaining relaxation may be due either to incomplete removal of the endothelium by the method used or may represent NO synthesis in the smooth muscle layers [25]. In the context of the previously described pharmacological responses, it appeared paradoxical to find significantly smaller EC_{50} values and a larger degree of relaxation after radiation. This might suggest an enhanced sensitivity and response to *L*-Arg at 24 h with higher (80 and 200 Gy) radiation doses and at 6 weeks even with a 20-Gy dose. One may speculate that radiation-induced damage to the control mechanism tips the balance towards relaxation. We found a similar shift using SNP, His and PAP as the relaxing agent. Our data are in concordance with those of Lobanok and Luksha [33], who found decreased constriction responses in rat aorta, while the endothelium-dependent relaxation was enhanced. Maynard et al. [12] reported decreased relaxation after 45 Gy irradiation with unchanged constriction in an ear artery of the rabbit. These differences could be explained by interspecies differences.

In conclusion, the data presented in this report show that a single dose of ionising radiation leads to functional changes in cerebral vessels as early as 24 h following irradiation. Some of the changes are dose and time dependent. Further analysis of these changes are in progress, including similar investigations of vessels following a longer interval after irradiation. These studies may provide a basis for pharmacological manipulation of the radiosensitivity of cerebral vessels.

References

1 Steiner L, Leksell L, Greitz T: Stereotactic radiosurgery for cerebral arteriovenous malformation: Report of a case. Acta Chir Scand 1972;138:459–464.

2 Lunsford LD: Stereotactic radiosurgery: At the threshold or at the crossroads? Neurosurgery 1993; 32:799–804.

3 Kondziolka D, Lunsford LD, Claassen D: Radiobiology of radiosurgery. I: The normal rat brain model. Neurosurgery 1992;31:271–279.

4 Lunsford LD, Altschuler EM, Flickinger JF: In vivo biological effects of stereotactic radiosurgery: A primate model. Neurosurgery 1990;27:373–382.

5 Nakagaki H, Brunhart G, Kemper TL: Monkey brain damage from radiation in the therapeutic range. Neurosurgery 1976;44:3–11.

6 Nilsson A, Wennerstrand J, Leksell D: Stereotactic gamma irradiation of basilar artery in cat. Acta Radiol Oncol 1978;17:150–160.

7 Laing RJ, Jakubowski J, Morice AH: An in vitro study of the pharmacological responses of rat middle cerebral artery: Effect of overnight storage. J Vasc Res 1995;32:230–236.

8 Mulvany MJ, Halpern W: Mechanical properties of vascular smooth muscle cells in situ. Nature 1976;260:616–619.

9 Rogers TK, Stewart AG, Morice AH: Effect of chronic hypoxia on rat pulmonary resistance vessels: Vasodilatation by atrial natriuretic peptide. Clin Sci 1992;83:723–729.

10 Paxinos G, Watson CH: The Rat Brain in Stereotactic Coordinates. London, Academic Press, 1986.

11 Kantak SS, Diglio CA, Onoda JM: Low dose radiation-induced endothelial cell retraction. Int J Radiat Biol 1993;64:319–328.

12 Maynard KI, Stewart-Lee AL, Milner P: X-irradiation attenuating relaxant responses in the rabbit ear artery. Br J Pharmacol 1992;105:126–128.

13 Wiedermann JG, Leavy JA, Amols H: Effect of high-dose intracoronary irradiation on vasomotor function and smooth muscle histopathology. Am J Physiol 1994;267:H125–H132.
14 Reinhold HS: Late changes in the architecture of blood vessels of the rat brain after irradiation. Br J Radiol 1980;53:693–696.
15 Spiegelmann R, Friedman WA, Bova FJ: LINAC radiosurgery: An animal model. J Neurosurg 1993;78:638–644.
16 Mulvany MJ, Hansen PK, Aalkjaer C: Direct evidence that the greater contractility of resistance vessels in spontaneously hypertensive rats is associated with narrowed lumen, a thicker media and an increased number of smooth muscle cell layers. Circ Res 1978;43:854–864.
17 Mügge A, Barton MR, Cremer J: Different vascular reactivity of human internal mammary and inferior epigastric arteries in vitro. Ann Thorac Surg 1993;56:1085–1089.
18 Pearson JD: Endothelial cell biology. Radiology 1991;179:9–14.
19 Zhou Q, Zhao Y, Li P: Thrombomodulin as a marker of radiation-induced endothelial cell injury. Radiat Res 1992;131:285–289.
20 Kwock L, Davenport WC, Clark RL: The effect of ionising radiation on the pulmonary vasculature of intact rats and isolated pulmonary endothelium. Radiat Res 1987;111:276–291.
21 Jaenke RS, Robbins ME, Bywaters T: Capillary endothelium: Target site of renal radiation injury. Lab Invest 1993;68:396–405.
22 Shimotakahara S, Mayberg MR: Gamma irradiation inhibits neointimal hyperplasia in rats after arterial injury. Stroke 1994;25:424–428.
23 Speidel MT, Holquist B, Kassis AI: Morphological, biochemical and molecular changes in endothelial cells after alpha-particle irradiation. Radiat Res 1993;36:373–381.
24 Schultz-Hector S, Balz K: Radiation-induced loss of endothelial alkaline phosphatase activity and development of myocardial degeneration: An ultrastructural study. Lab Invest 1994;1:252–260.
25 Stoclet JC: The *L*-arginine-NO pathway and cyclic GMP in the vessel wall. Z Kardiol 1991; 80(suppl):87–90.
26 Baron C, Cunningham M, Strauss J: Pharmacomechanical coupling in smooth muscle may involve phosphatidyl inositol metabolism. Proc Natl Acad Sci USA 1984;81:6899–6903.
27 Ignarro L, Kadowitz P: The pharmacological and physiological role of cyclic GMP in vascular smooth muscle relaxation. Annu Rev Pharmacol Toxicol 1985;25:171–191.
28 Lockette WE, Webb RC, Bohr DF: Prostaglandins and potassium relaxation in vascular smooth muscle of the rat: The role of Na-K ATPase. Circ Res 1980;46:714–720.
29 Nguyen DH, Voss U, Brecht K: Effect of potassium in isolated bovine facial and human saphenous veins. Experientia 1980;36:975–976.
30 Dvoretskii AI, Shainskaia AM, Ananteva TV: Postradiation changes of active ion transport systems of the CNS: The effect of superlethal doses of ionising radiation on the Na-K pump in surviving brain slices. Radiobiologia 1989;29:477–480.
31 Karlish SJ, Kempner ES: Minimal functional unit for transport and enzyme activities of Na^{+}+K^{+}-ATPase as determined by radiation inactivation. Biochim Biophys Acta 1984;776:288–298.
32 Shainskaia AM, Dvoretskii AI: Mechanism of radiation injury in the ion transport system of nervous tissue. Acta Physiol Hung 1990;75:295–299.
33 Lobanok LM, Luksha LS: The contractile reactions of aortic segments to noradrenaline in the immediate and late postradiation periods. Radiat Biol Radioecol 1995;35:269–273.

Proc 7th Int Meeting Leksell Gamma Knife® Society,
Island of Lana'i, Hawaii, November 1995
Stereotact Funct Neurosurg 1996;66(suppl 1):29–38

Stereotactic and Functional Neurosurgery

First Biochemical Evidence of Differential Functional Effects following Gamma Knife Surgery

J. Régis[a], *L. Kerkerian-Legoff*[b], *M. Rey*[c], *M. Vial*[c], *D. Porcheron*[a], *A. Nieoullon*[b], *J.C. Peragut*[a]

[a] Stereotactic and Functional Neurosurgery Department,
[b] Functional Cellular Neurobiology Laboratory, and
[c] Neurophysiology Department, Timone Hospital, Marseille, France

Key Words

Epilepsy · Functional neurosurgery · Stereotactic radiosurgery · Radiobiology · Rat brain · Excitatory amino acids · Catecholamine · Acetylcholine · Striatum · γ-Aminobutyric acid

Abstract

Clinical experience with radiosurgery for epilepsy on lesions located in highly functional areas has suggested the possibility of Gamma-Knife-induced functional effects without deterioration of the underlying cerebral cortex. To investigate these hypothetical functional changes, we have developed a special frame dedicated to small-animal radiosurgical experimental models, allowing purely atlas-guided protocols. The left striatum of the first series of rats was targeted with high doses (200 Gy maximum) for validation of this new device. The same target was used with lower doses (50 Gy at the 50% isodose) in the second series to evaluate the biochemical changes and their chronology. The main biochemical changes occurred between 59 and 90 days after Gamma Knife irradiation, with different amplitudes depending on the biochemical parameter observed. Differential effects were first observed between glutamate decarboxylase and choline acetyltransferase, and secondarily between excitatory amino acids (AAs) and non-excitatory AAs, particularly γ-aminobutyric acid. These preliminary results need to be confirmed and completed by further experimental studies. However, Gamma-Knife-induced differential biochemical effects provide the basis for a promising new concept for functional radiosurgery and particularly the Gamma Knife surgery of epilepsy.

KARGER

E-Mail karger@karger.ch
Fax + 41 61 306 12 34
http://www.karger.ch

1011–6125/96/0665–0029$10.00/0

Dr Jean Régis
Service de Neurochirurgie Stéréotaxique
Hôpital la Timone
F–13385 Marseille Cedex 5 (France)

Introduction

Despite extensive clinical experience with Gamma Knife surgery, the radiobiology of single-fraction, small- to moderate-volume irradiation remains largely unknown. Radiosurgical animal experiments focus mainly on high-dose effects on a very small volume [1–6]. Data derived from such experiments are relevant for functional radiosurgery in the field of pain, parkinsonism, and psychosurgery [7–9]. Nonetheless, clinical and experimental data remain limited, and further experimental data from animal models are required.

Our involvement in functional radiosurgery (in particular the radiosurgery of epilepsy without a space-occupying lesion) led us to study biochemical and histological changes in normal brain related to the volume, dose and observation time.

There are some basic questions to be answered if we are to understand radiosurgical effects.

(1) What is the relationship between volume, dose and time in the development of a necrotic histological effect?

(2) What brings about the early effects of 'lesional' irradiation, such as the immediate cessation of seizures with radiosurgical entorhino-amygdalo-hippocampotomy? This effect occurs soon after irradiation, while images indicating necrosis appear only 10 months after the Gamma Knife procedure.

(3) When the dose and volume to a lesion are insufficient to produce histological necrosis, is there some kind of neuronal or astrocytic loss? (a) If it occurs, does it differ among cell populations (cell-type-dependent sensitivity)? (b) Do cell functions change concomitantly with cellular loss? What kind of astrocytic changes are induced? (c) Can these changes modify the functional status of the irradiated central nervous system (CNS) structure?

(4) What is the significance of computed tomography (CT) and magnetic resonance imaging (MRI) changes surrounding the target area? (a) Are these changes induced by low doses delivered outside the target volume? We have previously reported some evidence against this hypothesis [10]. (b) If these changes are induced by phenomena occurring in the target area, what is the mechanism? (c) What are these surrounding tissue changes: vasogenic edema, demyelination or astrocytosis?

Material and Methods

A special stereotactic frame (fig. 1) has been developed (derived from a Kopf system) for small animals [11]. This system allows us to use stereotactic atlases (Degroot) for guidance to reach intracerebral structures precisely, without any kind of imaging. The radiosurgical dose planning was calculated using a microVAX II computer. Coordinates of the target

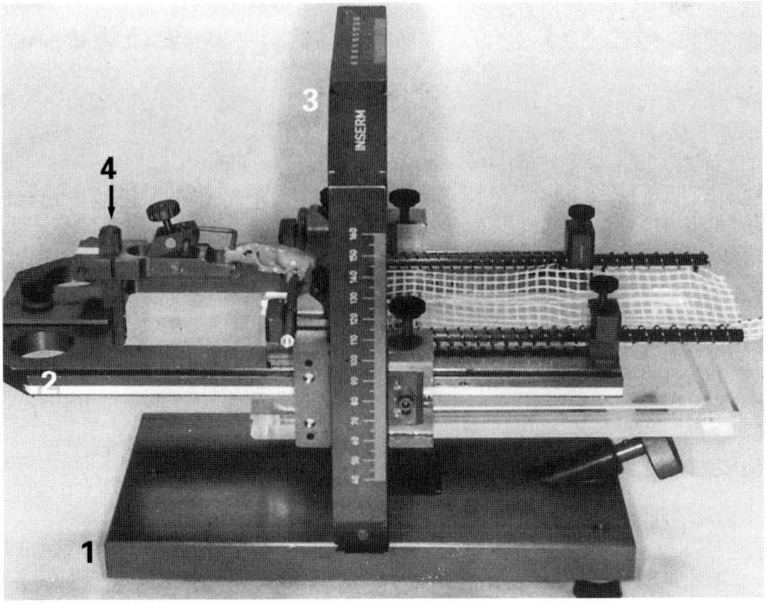

Fig. 1. View of the small-animal device for Gamma Knife radiosurgery with its removable platform (1), vertical and horizontal sliding platform (2), Leksell's stereotactic frame modified for small-animal radiosurgery (3) and adjustment of the head tilt according to stereotactic atlases (4). A laser emitter is fixed to the Gamma Knife for zero checking.

were determined directly on the Degroot atlas without the aid of individual images. The accuracy of this system has been demonstrated by the performance in high-dose irradiation (200 Gy, 4 mm collimator) to the left striatum of six rats (fig. 2). The results of this first series were evaluated 21, 34, and 47 days after irradiation. At 34 and 47 days, necrotic lesions were located exactly as targeted.

We studied biochemical changes in a second series of 32 rats at 7, 15, 24, 31, 45, 59, 72 and 90 days after irradiation to the left striatum using 100 Gy with the 4-mm collimator to a volume of 33.5 mm^3.

Choline acetyltransferase (CAT) and glutamate decarboxylase (GAD) were studied by radioenzymology techniques. The levels of these enzymes were compared between irradiated animal striatum and non-irradiated animal striatum at 7, 15, 24, 31, 45, 59, 72 and 90 days.

The concentrations of amines [dopamine (DA) and serotonin (5-HT)], their metabolites [dihydroxyphenylacetic acid (DOPAC), homovanillic acid (HVA) and 5-hydroxyindoleacetic acid (5-HIAA)], and aspartic acid (Asp), glutamic acid (Glu), Serine (Ser), glutamine (Gln), glycine (Gly), taurine (Tau), Tyrosine (Tyr) and γ-aminobutyric acid (GABA) were measured by high-pressure liquid chromatography at 31, 45, 59, 72 and 90 days.

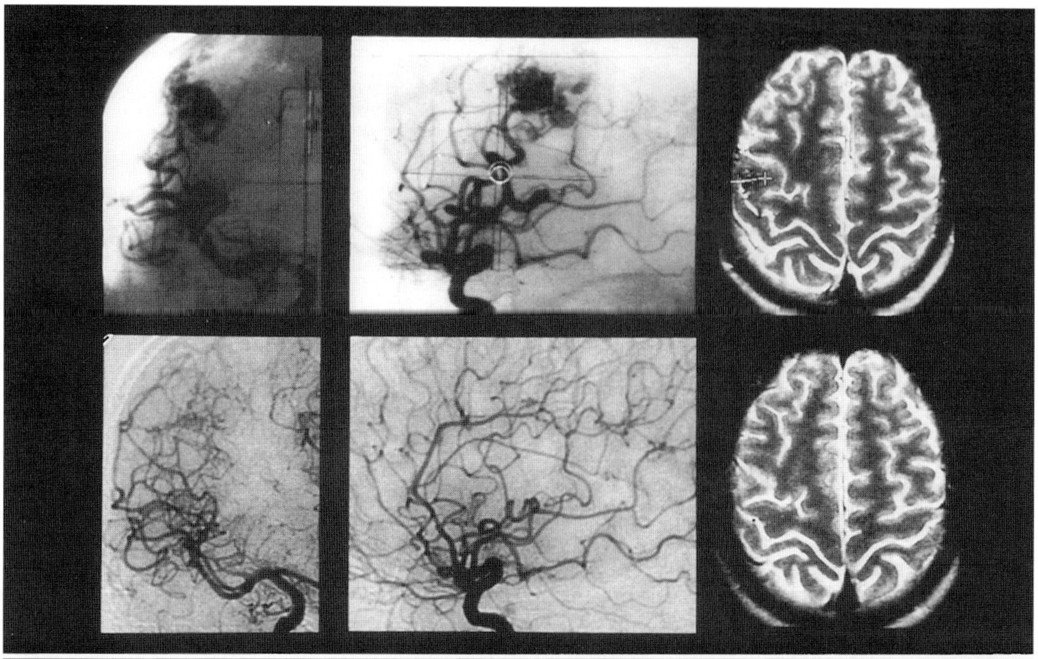

a

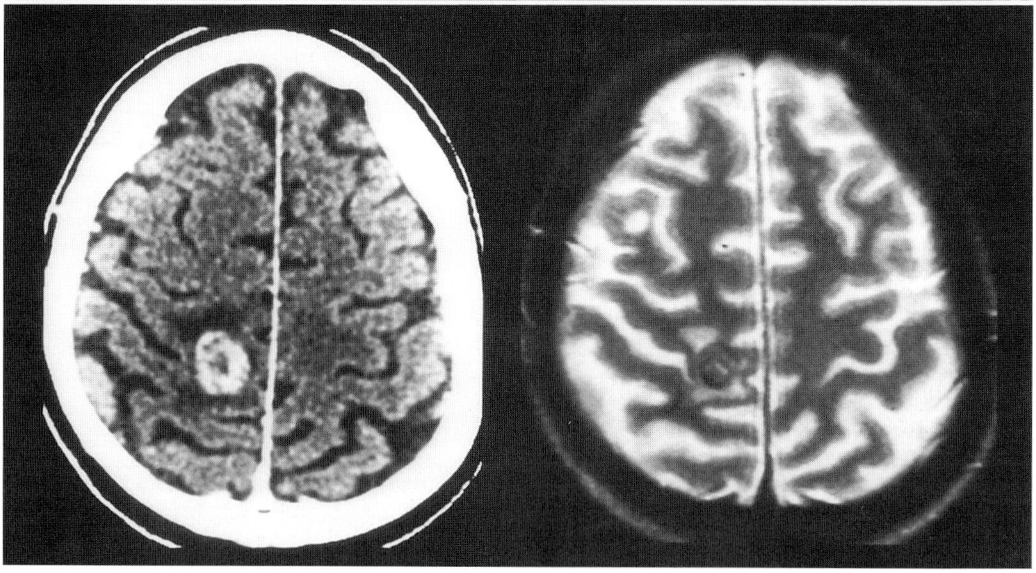

b

Fig. 2. Clinical evidence for differential Gamma Knife effects. **a** M1 angioma. The only clinical expression were frequent partial somatomotor seizures. Early cessation of seizures, 6 weeks after Gamma Knife surgery (top), was observed, with no motor function deterioration. The occlusion is complete on the 15th-month control (bottom). **b** M1 cerebral

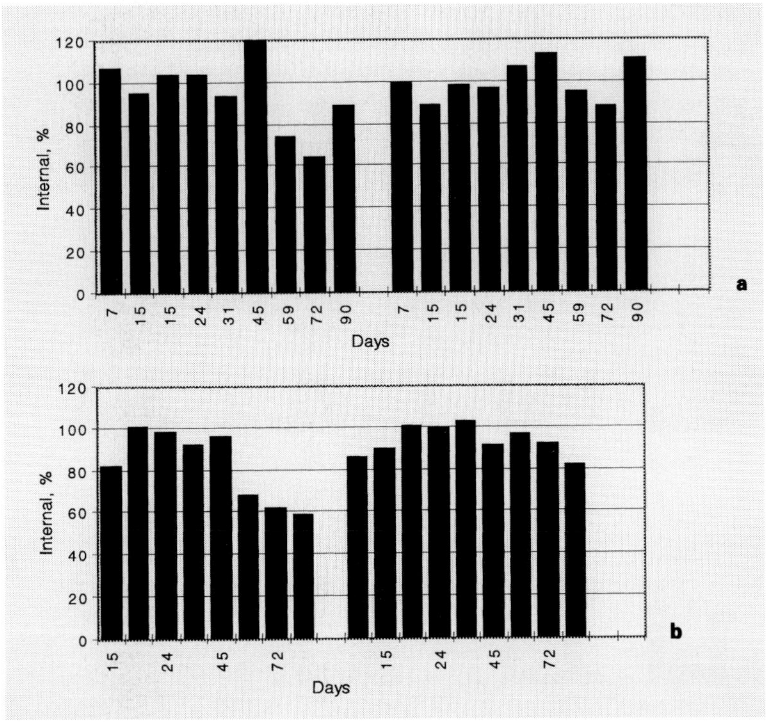

Fig. 3. GAD (**a**) and CAT (**b**) studied by radioenzyme techniques. Levels of both were decreased at 59 days (treatment side on the left, contralateral side on the right). Ninety days after Gamma Knife surgery, GAD levels had returned to baseline, but CAT levels remained low.

Results

The detailed results of these experiments are depicted in figures 3–5. Our preliminary results (fig. 3) clearly demonstrated a differential effect of single-fraction gamma irradiation on cholinergic and GABAergic systems in the striatum. GAD and CAT were decreased at day 59 (maximally at day 72). After day 90, only GAD returned to higher values (normalization).

---

metastasis (melanoma) with partial somatomotor seizures and a slight hemiparesis. Seizures ceased immediately after radiosurgery. Hemiparesis improved gradually after the third post-Gamma Knife surgery month (left). At 15 months, the control MR scan demonstrated reduction in both the lesion and oedema (right).

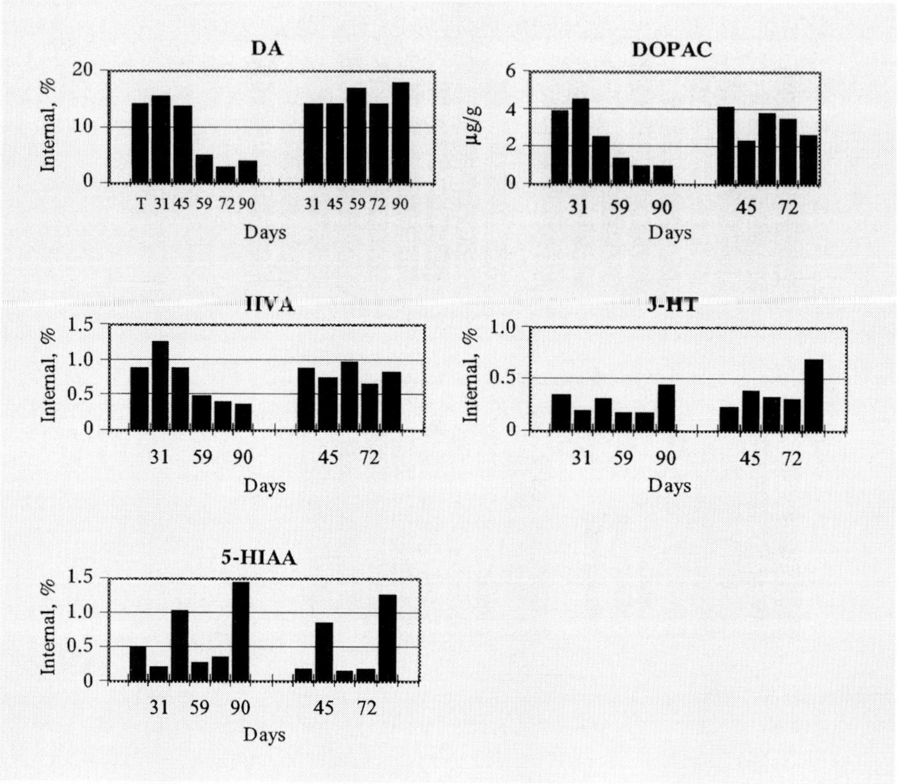

Fig. 4. Amine levels after Gamma Knife surgery.

A second differential effect of radiation was observed on amino acid (AA) concentrations. Excitatory AAs (EAAs) demonstrated dramatic decreases after day 59, while GABA remained stable and glycine even showed a pronounced increase (fig. 5).

Discussion

This is the first study demonstrating differential effects of Gamma Knife irradiation at the biochemical level. Cessation of seizures after Gamma Knife surgery of visible lesions, such as arteriovenous malformations or cerebral metastases in highly functional areas like the primary motor cortex, had alrady been observed. This phenomenon, which occurs without postradiosurgery functional

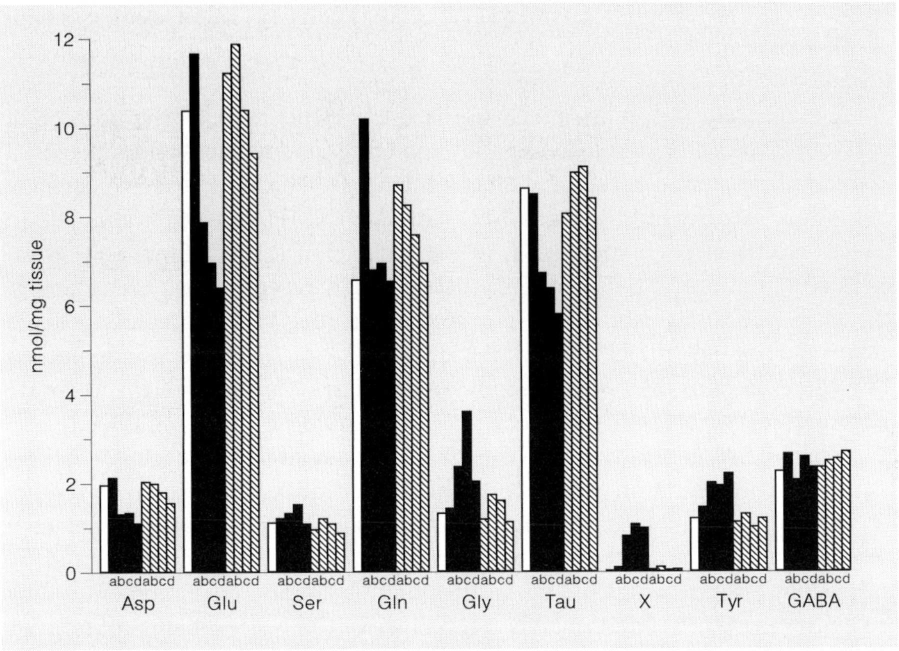

Fig. 5. Amino acid concentrations 45 (a), 59 (b), 72 (c) and 90 (d) days after Gamma Knife surgery. Filled bars = ipsilateral measurement; hatched bars = contralateral measurements; open bar = control; X = unidentified element.

deterioration (fig. 1), led us to the hypothesis that direct cellular and biochemical changes induced by Gamma Knife radiation should reduce epileptogenicity of the cortex while preserving its functional capability.

To validate this hypothesis, we developed an experimental animal model, beginning with the rat striatum, because of the existing knowledge of its biochemistry and its appropriate size and shape. The apparatus was dedicated to small-animal Gamma Knife surgery experimental models. It permits precise and repeatable Gamma Knife irradiation of normal brain anatomical targets without the necessity for expensive and time-consuming imaging techniques, providing a rapid means to examine the effects of radiosurgery on the CNS.

Today, a biochemical explanation for focal epileptogenesis should involve a decrease in GABAergic inhibition, EAA, and ion movement abnormalities. The role of the GABAergic system is indicated by the ability to induce epileptic phenomena by administration of biochemical substances which either modify GABA synthesis (GABA dehydrogenase inhibition by allylglycine) or which block GABA receptors. The reduction in GABA [12] and GAD activity [13] in lesional epileptogenic foci is further evidence that these substances play a role in the epileptic process.

A major role is also attributed to the EAAs (Glu, Asp). Their presence in postsynaptic receptor sites increases Na^+ and Ca^{2+} conductance (action potential production). Systemic injection of Glu or analogues like kainic acid or quisqualic acid induce seizures [14]. N-methyl-*D*-asparatate (NMDA) receptor stimulation induces electrical phenomena and, in particular, long-term administration induces potentiation [15]. The role of these NMDA receptors has been demonstrated in a kindling model [16, 17]. Activation of NMDA receptors induces bursts of action potentials when inhibition GABAergic mechanisms are blocked [18]. More recently MR spectroscopy studies have shown N-acetyl aspartate abnormalities within epileptic foci [19–21]. Our observation of a dramatic decrease in EAAs contrasting with GABA stability in an epileptic focus would be associated with inhibition of seizure production, according to the above hypothesis. The last major biochemical mechanism proposed today focuses on the ionic environment and the properties of ion channels [22]. Ca^{2+} channel modulation by magnesium, the action of Ca^{2+} on calmodulin [23, 24] and regulation of Ca^{2+} by protein kinase C [25] underline the importance of Ca^{2+} in regulation of NMDA burst activity.

These sorts of changes have not been followed in this first study. Our next experimental series with rats focuses on changes in ion channels induced by Gamma Knife irradiation of the hippocampus region. The results are not yet available. Some recent evidence such as the efficiency of felbamate against epilepsy has suggested that the Gly sites of the NMDA receptor may play an important role in focal epileptogenicity.

Another limit of the present study is the delay in the biochemical changes observed. We suggest that changes after Gamma Knife surgery can be separated into early changes (prelesional effects from a neuroradiological point of view) and late (postlesional) effects. Some data from the literature and our own data concerning epilepsy Gamma Knife surgery (without a space-occupying lesion) indicate that functional clinical changes occur very early; even immediately after radiosurgery, long before MRI changes can be demonstrated.

We recently reported subjective paresthesia during Gamma Knife surgery of a fifth nerve neurinoma [26]. Linskey et al. [27] have reported early facial palsy after Gamma Knife surgery of an acoustic neurinoma. Our first case of Gamma Knife entorhino-amygdalo-hippocampotomy experienced an immediate cessation of seizures after the treatment, 9–10 months before the appearance of the MRI changes [9]. It seems reasonable to speculate that functional changes occurring during or immediately after the Gamma Knife treatments have a different mechanism to the changes observed later.

In our model, the biochemical changes occurred at the same time as the histological changes (59 days after Gamma Knife irradiation). Our biochemical observations do not explain very early functional changes. A future goal remains to investigate earlier, slight functional changes. It must be significant that the target volume used in this study (33.5 mm^3) is smaller than that necessary for epilepsy Gamma Knife surgery (6,440 mm^3 for temporomesial epilepsy in our experience). In the future we need to reproduce these experimental conditions in a primate model with volumes comparable to those we use in Gamma Knife epilepsy surgery. Functional radiosurgery has always used high doses per volume with an ablative aim. The differential biochemical effects obtained by radiosurgery as described in this study suggest a possibly new way to use the Gamma Knife in the treatment of functional disorders. The aim would be greater selective action on the neuronal network.

In conclusion, this report is the first to show that the Gamma Knife can induce differential biochemical effects. These preliminary results must be confirmed and extended by further studies. More precise knowledge of these kinds of differential effects in relation to dose and volume will be of major interest for functional Gamma Knife surgery, in particular that for epilepsy.

References

1 Altschuler E, Lunsford LD, Kondziolka D, Wu A, Maitz AH, Sclabassi R, Martinez AJ: Radiobiologic models for radiosurgery. Neurosurg Clin N Am 1992;3:61–77.

2 Inoue HK, Kohga H, Hirato M, Nakamura M, Ohye C: Neurobiologic effects of radiosurgery: Histologic, immunohistochemical and electon-microscopic studies of a rat model. Stereotact Funct Neurosurg 1994;63:280–285.

3 Kihlström L, Lindquist C, Asler J, Collins P, Karlsson B: Histological studies of Gamma Knife lesions in normal and hypercholesterolemic rabbits; in Stiner L, Backlund EO, Forster DVC (eds): Radiosurgery: Baseline and Trends. NewYork, Raven Press, 1992, pp 111–119.

4 Kondziolka D, Lunsford LD, Claasen D, Maitz AH, Flickinger JC: Radiobiology of radiosurgery. 1: The normal rat brain model. Neurosurgery 1992;31:271–288.

5 Lo EH, Frankel KA, Poljak A, DeLaPaz RL, Phillips MH, Woodruff KH, Brennan KM, Valk PH, Fabrikant JI: Focal heavy-charged particle irradiation of the mammalian cortex: Temporal pattern of changes followed by magnetic resonance imaging and positron emission tomography; in Steiner L, Baclund EO, Forster DVC (eds): Radiosurgery: Baseline and Trends. New York, Raven Press, 1992, pp 129–138.

6 Lunsford LD, Altschuler EM, Flickinger JC, Wu A, Martinez AJ: In vivo biological effects of stereotactic radiosurgery: A primate model. Neurosurgery 1990;27:373–382.

7 Lindquist C, Steiner L, Hindmarsh T: Gamma Knife thalamotomy for tremor. Report of two cases: Topography; in Steiner L, Backlund EO, Forster DVC (eds): Radiosurgery: Baseline and Trends. New York, Raven Press, 1992, pp 237–243.

8 Steiner L, Forster D, Leksell L, Meyerson BA, Boethius J: Gamma-thalamotomy in intractable pain. Acta Neurochir (Wien) 1980;52:173–184.

9 Kihlström L, Guo WY, Lindquist C, Mindus P: Radiobiology of radiosurgery for refractory anxiety disorders. Neurosurgery 1995;36:294–302.

10 Régis J, Peragut JC, Rey M, Samson Y, Levrier O, Porcheron D, Régis H, Sedan R: First selective amygdalohippocampal radiosurgery for 'mesial temporal lobe epilepsy'. Stereotact Funct Neurosurg 1995;64(suppl 1):193–201.
11 Rey M, Valliccioni P, Viale M, Porcheron D, Régis J, Nieouillon A, Millet Y, Peragut J: Technical description of a stereotactic device for experimental Gamma Knife radiosurgery in rats. Neurochirurgie, in press.
12 Koyana: Amino acids in the cobalt-induced epileptogenic and nonepileptogenic cat's cortex. Can J Physiol Pharmacol 1972;50:740–752.
13 Ribak CE, Harris CB, Vaughan JE, Roberts E: Inhibitory GABAergic nerve terminals decrease at site of focal epilepsy. Science 1979;205:210–214.
14 Johnston G: Convulsions induced in 10-day old rats by intraperitoneal injection of monosodium glutamate and related excitant amino acids. Biochem Pharmacol 1973;22:137.
15 Fagg GE, Foster AC, Ganong AH: Excitatory amino acids: Synaptic mechanisms and neurological function. Trends Neurosci 1986;9:357–363.
16 Stelzer A, Slater N: Activation of NMDA receptor clocks GABAergic inhibition in an in vitro model for epilepsy. Nature 1987;326:698–701.
17 Mody I, Heinemann U: NMDA receptors of dentate gyrus granule cells participate in synaptic transmission following kindling. Nature 1987;326:701–704.
18 Dingledine R: NMDA receptors: What do they do? Trends Neurosci 1986;9:47–49.
19 Nowychy MC, Fow AP, Tsien RW: Three types of neuronal calcium channel with different calcium agonist sensitivity. Nature 1985;326:440–443.
20 Delorenzo RJ, Freedman SD, Yohe WB, Maurer S: Stimulation of Ca^{++} dependent neurotransmitter release and presynaptic nerve terminal protein phosphorylation by calmodulin and calmodulin-like protein isolated from synaptic vesicles. Proc Natl Acad Sci USA 1979;76:1838–1842.
21 Klee CB, Crouch TH, Richmand PG: Calmodulin. Rev Biochem 1980;49:489–515.
22 Connelly A, Jackson GD, Duncan JS, King MD, Gadian DG: Magnetic resonance spectroscopy in temporal lobe epilepsy. Neurology 1994;44:1612–1617.
23 Hugg LW, Laxed KD, Matson GB, Maudsley AA, Weiner MW: Neuron loss localizes human temporal lobe epilepsy by in vivo proton magnetic resonance spectroscopic imaging. Ann Neurol 1993;34:788–794.
24 Peeling JP, Sutherland G: ^{1}H-Magnetic resonance spectroscopy of extracts of human epileptic neocortex and hippocampus. Neurology 1993;43:589–594.
25 Rasmussen H: The calcium messenger system. N Engl J Med 1986;314:1094–1101.
26 Régis J, Manera L, Dufour H, Porcheron D, Sedan R, Peragut JC: Effect of the Gamma Knife on trigeminal neuralgia. Stereotact Funct Neurosurg 1995;64(suppl 1):182–192.
27 Linskey ME, Lunsford LD, Flickinger JC, Kondziolka D: Stereotactic radiosurgery for acoustic tumors. Neurosurg Clin N Am 1992;3:191–205.

Proc 7th Int Meeting Leksell Gamma Knife® Society,
Island of Lana'i, Hawaii, November 1995
Stereotact Funct Neurosurg 1996;66(suppl 1):39–48

Stereotactic and Functional Neurosurgery

Tumor Cell Proliferation and Apoptosis Associated with the Gamma Knife Effect

T. Tsuzuki[a], *S. Tsunoda*[c], *T. Sakaki*[a], *N. Konishi*[b], *Y. Hiasa*[b], *M. Nakamura*[b], *E. Yoshino*[d]

[a] Department of Neurosurgery, and
[b] 2nd Department of Pathology, Nara Medical University, Nara,
[c] Department of Integrated Science, Osaka Prefecture University, Osaka, and
[d] Department of Neurosurgery, Kyoto Prefecture University of Medicine, Kyoto, Japan

Key Words

Cell proliferation · Apoptosis · Gamma Knife · Bcl-2 · Proliferating-cell nuclear antigen

Abstract

In this study, the expression of proliferating-cell nuclear antigen (PCNA) and Bcl-2 protein was examined in neurinomas, meningiomas, pituitary adenomas, and malignant lymphomas before treatment with Gamma Knife radiosurgery. Tumor volume was rapidly reduced by radiosurgery in all malignant lymphomas and in some benign tumors. The latter had been characterized by strong positive immunohistochemical staining for PCNA and Bcl-2. Radiation-induced apoptosis is thought to contribute to the low-dose effects of Gamma Knife radiosurgery. A population with a large proportion of proliferating cells may be susceptible to the induction of apoptosis, and the presence of Bcl-2 may not suppress this Gamma Knife effect.

Introduction

Apoptosis was first described as a morphological pattern of cell death, initially characterized by cell shrinkage, membrane bleeding, and chromatin condensation [1]. In the final stage of apoptosis, the dying cells become segmented into

KARGER

E-Mail karger@karger.ch
Fax + 41 61 306 12 34
http://www.karger.ch

1011–6125/96/0665–0039$10.00/0

Toshihide Tsuzuki, MD
Department of Neurosurgery
Nara Medical University
840 Shijo-cho Kashihara, Nara 634 (Japan)

apoptotic bodies and are phagocytosed by neighboring cells and macrophages, so that no overt inflammatory reaction occurs. One of the characteristic biochemical hallmarks of the early stage of apoptosis is internucleosomal DNA cleavage. The morphological nuclear changes are associated with activation of a specific endogenous endonuclease that breaks the double-stranded DNA of the chromatin at the internucleosomal linkers [2]. Apoptosis is an active physiological process which plays a significant role in embryonic development and tissue homeostasis [3]. It also occurs spontaneously in various types of tumors [4, 5]. Furthermore, it has been established in many in vitro systems that apoptosis can be induced by appropriate stimuli, such as hyperthermia, radiation or exposure to glucocorticoids. It can also be induced by the removal of stimuli, such as deprivation of serum or interleukin-2 [6–8]. Recent investigations have begun to reveal the molecular mechanisms underlying programmed cell death. Some known oncogenes and suppressor genes such as c-*myc* and p53 have been shown to be important in apoptosis [9–11], and several candidate controlling genes have been found. The *bcl*-2 gene was first identified at the site of a t(14;18)(q21;q32) chromosomal translocation in human follicular B cell lymphomas [12–14]. Initial studies indicated that the Bcl-2 protein is located at the inner mitochondrial membrane [15]. However, recent reports have documented that it associates with the nuclear envelope and endoplasmic reticulum membrane, as well as with mitochondria [16]. Previous studies demonstrated that Bcl-2 protein overexpression prolongs cell survival by suppressing apoptosis in response to a wide variety of stress and cytotoxic agents, such as ionizing radiation. The Bcl-2 protein is thought to function as an antioxidant and free radical scavenger [5, 17, 18].

The induction of apoptosis by ionizing radiation has been studied in many different types of cells, and its mechanism and time course appear to be somewhat variable. In thymocytes, loss of cell viability after radiation exposure occurs within hours and has been described as rapid interphase cell death [19, 20]. On the other hand, lymphocyte-derived leukemias and lymphomas show variable degrees of radiation-induced apoptosis in vitro. Unlike thymocytes, many malignant lymphoblast cell lines apparently require longer intervals after radiation exposure before cell viability is lost. In these cells, the onset of DNA fragmentation appears to be preceded by a period of radiation-induced G_2/M block (delayed interphase cell death) [21]. Thus, the radiation-inducible processes of apoptosis and G_2/M block would seem to have a temporal relationship in some cell types. Furthermore, some cell lines appear to progress to apoptosis after the first postirradiation mitosis (mitotoc death), whilst others are able to complete several mitoses (delayed mitotic death) before dying [22]. Therefore, radiation-induced apoptosis must be associated with the tumor cell cycle.

The effects of Gamma Knife radiosurgery are believed to be partly brought about by radiation-induced apoptosis, especially in treatments with low irradiation doses [23]. In this study, we examined the expression of proliferating-cell nuclear antigen (PCNA) and Bcl-2 protein in benign tumors and malignant lymphomas before low-dose Gamma Knife radiosurgery, and analyzed their effects on the outcome of treatment.

Materials and Methods

Tumors

A total of 22 brain tumor specimens were obtained by surgical operations at the Departments of Neurosurgery at Nara Medical University and Kyoto Prefecture University of Medicine. Included were 6 cases of neurinoma, 7 cases of meningioma, 6 cases of pituitary adenoma, and 3 cases of malignant lymphoma. Specimens were fixed in 10% neutral formalin for paraffin embedding. Serial sections of representative blocks were cut at 4–6 μm. One section was routinely stained with hematoxylin and eosin for histopathological evaluation and the others were used for immunohistochemical studies. All the patients had residual or recurrent lesions after surgery, and were tested with Gamma Knife radiosurgery with 20–40 Gy as a maximum and 8–16 Gy as a minimum dose. The subsequent course was followed with computed tomography (CT) or magnetic resonance imaging (MRI) examinations.

Immunohistochemical Studies

Sections were deparaffinized and hydrated through graded alcohols. Antigen activation for staining Bcl-2 protein was carried out by boiling at 120 °C for 15 min. Endogenous peroxidase activity was blocked by immersion in 1% hydrogen peroxide in methanol at room temperature for 30 min followed by rinsing in neutral phosphate-buffered saline (PBS) and exposure to normal horse serum for an additional 10 min. Mouse monoclonal antibodies raised against PCNA (PC 10, Dako, Glostrup, Denmark) and human Bcl-2 protein (124, Dako) were diluted 1:40 in PBS at pH 7.4 (neutral PBS). The sections were then incubated with these overnight at 4 °C. The next morning, sections were again rinsed with neutral PBS and exposed to the biotinylated secondary antibodies. Visualization of binding was achieved using the streptavidin-biotin method and a Histofine SAB-PO(M) Kit (Nichirei, Tokyo, Japan). Excess secondary antibody was removed in a neutral PBS rinse, and sections were incubated with the chromogen diaminobenzidine for 30 s. Following a final rinse in tap water, the sections were lightly counterstained with hematoxylin and evaluated. Sections of human tonsil served as positive controls for PCNA and Bcl-2 protein staining.

Results

Malignant Lymphomas

All cases of malignant lymphoma had more than 30% of cells positive for PCNA and Bcl-2 protein staining, and showed a remarkably rapid remission of tumor volume on CT or MRI after Gamma Knife radiosurgery (fig. 1, 2).

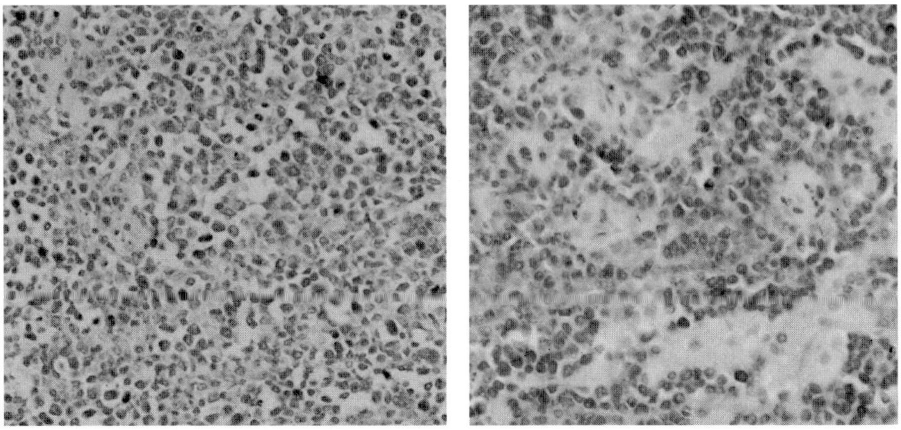

1a 1b

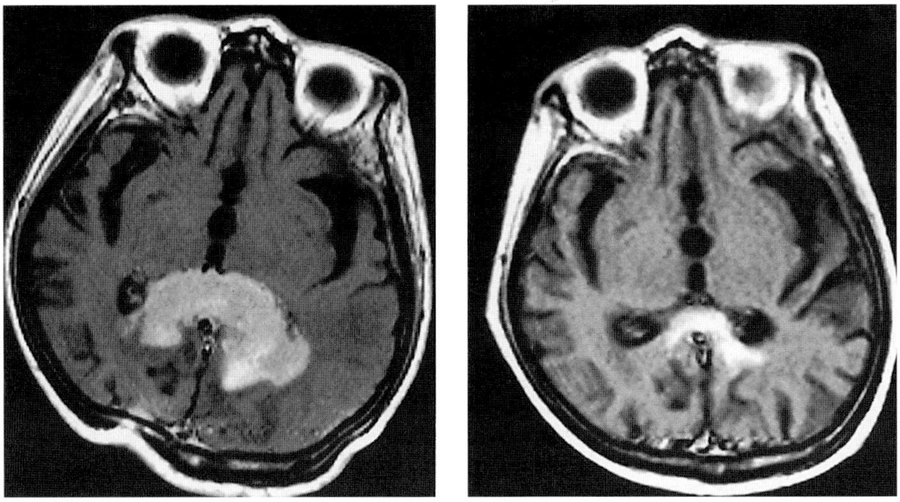

2a 2b

Fig. 1. A case of malignant lymphoma showing more than 30% of cells staining positively for PCNA (**a**) and Bcl-2 protein (**b**).

Fig. 2. MRI image with Gd-DTPA at Gamma Knife radiosurgery shows a large malignant lymphoma (**a**) whose volume is remarkably reduced 1 month after radiosurgery with a maximum dose of 20 Gy and a marginal dose of 8 Gy (**b**).

Benign Tumors

Cells staining positively for PCNA were found in 5 of 19 cases (26%) of benign tumors, including 2 cases of neurinoma, 2 cases of meningioma and 1 case of pituitary adenoma. The average staining index was about 14%. Of 19 cases, 4 (21%) stained positively for Bcl-2 protein with an average staining index of about 12%. Except for 1 case of pituitary adenoma, all the tumors positive for PCNA

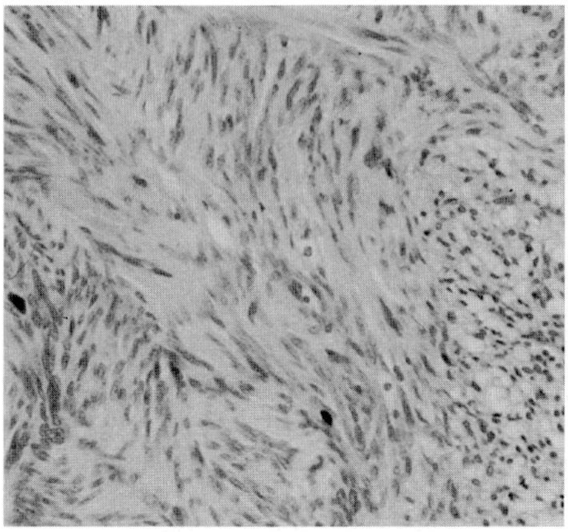

3a

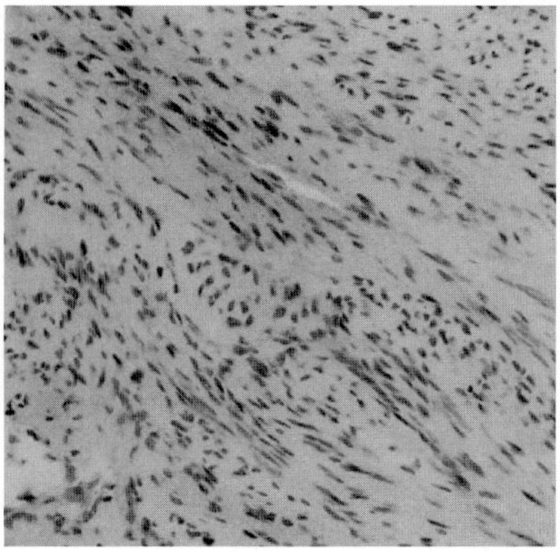

3b

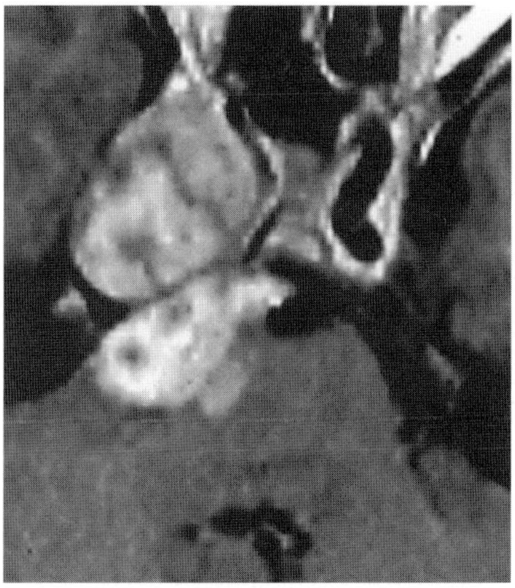

4a

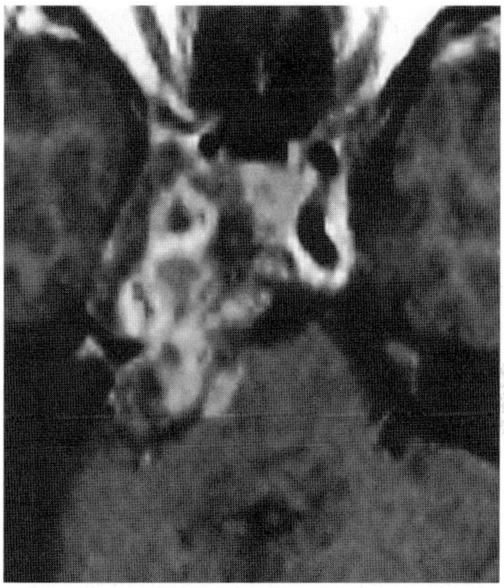

4b

Fig. 3. A case of neurinoma showing an average of 16% of cells positive for PCNA (**a**) and an average of 18% positive for Bcl-2 protein (**b**).

Fig. 4. MRI image with Gd-DTPA at Gamma Knife radiosurgery showing a large trigeminal neurinoma which grew rapidly after surgery (**a**), and whose volume decreased 12 months after radiosurgery with a maximum dose of 20 Gy and a marginal dose of 8 Gy (**b**).

also demonstrated Bcl-2 protein. Little remission was identified on CT or MRI in many cases of benign tumors, though the average follow-up period of about 12 months was not adequate to judge the full effect of Gamma Knife therapy. However, 3 of 5 cases with PCNA-positive staining showed remarkable changes on radiological examinations (fig. 3–6).

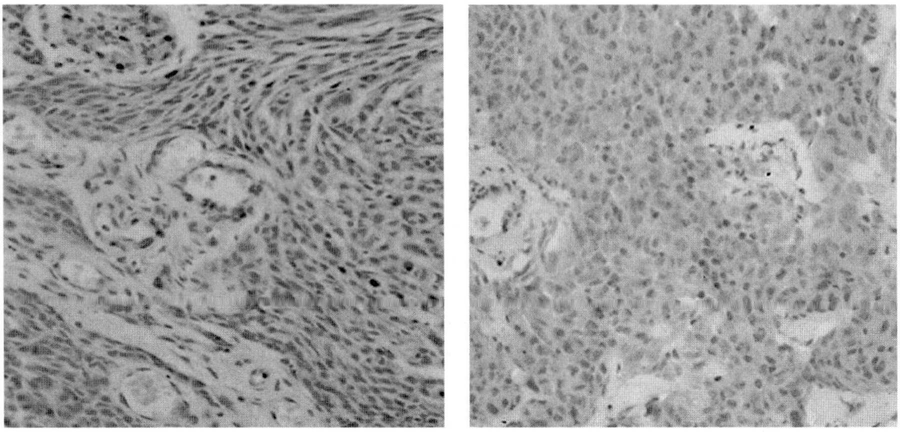

5a 5b

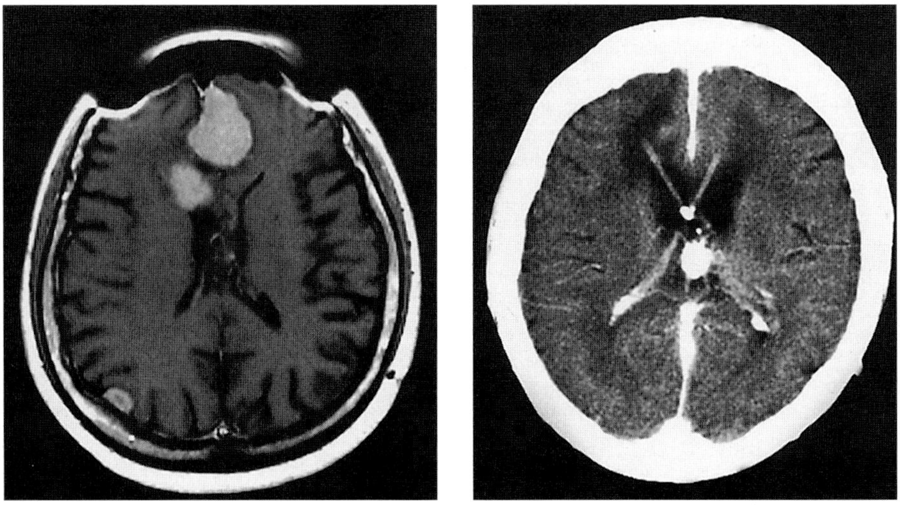

6a 6b

Fig. 5. A case of meningioma showing an average of 8% of cells positive for PCNA (**a**) and an average of 5% positive for Bcl-2 protein (**b**).

Fig. 6. a MRI image with Gd-DTPA at Gamma Knife radiosurgery showing multiple meningiomas which include a new growing lesion at the frontal falx after surgery. **b** Enhanced CT showed that the lesion at the frontal falx was reduced most markedly 4 months after radiosurgery with a maximum dose of 24 Gy and a marginal dose of 12 Gy.

Discussion

Apoptosis generally occurs after a delay in the progression of cells through the cell cycle. However, the inhibition of cell proliferation and onset of apoptosis may take place at different points in the cycle. Physiological changes, such as withdrawal of growth factors, may inhibit cell proliferation at the G_0/G_1 phase boundary, initiating apoptosis at some point prior to entry into the S phase. Exposure to radiation induces a more pronounced G_2/M block, and in this case apoptosis appears to be manifested at the time of cell release from the block or during the subsequent G_1 phase [7, 21, 24, 25]. Furthermore, it was observed in irradiated hematopoietic cell lines that radiation induced mitotic/delayed mitotic death as well as interphase death [21, 22]. These findings suggest that different signals and pathways can lead to apoptotic death. For cells undergoing fast interphase death the rapidity of their response suggests direct signaling due to a DNA disturbance. On the other hand, cells undergoing delayed interphase or mitotic/delayed mitotic death have presumably responded to the presence of chromosomal aberrations [26]. The signal that triggers apoptosis is dependent upon the cell line and the radiation dose used [21]. In this study, all cases of malignant lymphoma showed strongly positive staining for PCNA, and rapid remission after low-dose Gamma Knife radiosurgery. These results lead us to suspect that malignant lymphoma cells with DNA damaged by gamma beams rapidly enter the cell cycle and subsequently undergo rapid and/or delayed interphase death by apoptosis. In contrast, many benign tumors treated by low-dose radiosurgery showed negative staining for PCNA and little remission. This suggests that in these cases, apoptosis could not be triggered because cells with damaged DNA or chromosomes were not programmed to go into the cell cycle. Thus, such cells remained alive for a long time in the G_0 phase. However, a few benign cases with positive PCNA findings did show remarkable remission several months after radiosurgery, providing further evidence for a link between proliferation and susceptibility to induction of apoptosis.

Recent investigations have revealed that apoptosis may be due to programmable molecular mechanisms, and the existence of positive and negative regulators has been documented. Cell death is a normal homeostatic mechanism that occurs in essentially all tissues with the capacity for self-renewal and helps to ensure that the rate of new-cell production is balanced by a proportional rate of old-cell death. Thus, it stands to reason that *bcl*-2 and other genes that regulate the cell death side of the equation are at least as important as classical oncogenes, which primarily exert their effect by accelerating the rate of cell proliferation [27]. In this study, all malignant lymphomas showed strong expression of Bcl-2 protein as well as PCNA, and expression of Bcl-2 protein may endow cells with a greater growth potential. Even in the benign tumors, 4 of 5 cases with positive PCNA staining showed positive findings for Bcl-2 protein. These tumors demonstrated rapid regrowth after surgery. Combined expression of PCNA and Bcl-2 protein suggests that Bcl-2 protein may suppress spontaneous apoptosis during accelerated tumor cell proliferation. Several studies have shown that overexpression of Bcl-2 protein in pre-B lymphocytes inhibits apoptosis when cells are exposed to certain environmental conditions. These include the withdrawal of cytokines or growth factors, and treatment with a glucocorticoid, ionizing radiation, heat shock, or a variety of cancer therapeutic agents [2, 6–8]. However, the present study showed that all malignant lymphomas and some benign tumors with positive expression of Bcl-2 protein also showed rapid remission after Gamma Knife radiosurgery, even with low-dose radiation. Therefore, the expression of Bcl-2 protein cannot be equated with resistance to radiation-induced apoptosis by Gamma Knife radiosurgery. Recent studies have proposed that tumor necrotic factor-α (TNF-α) and ionizing radiation induce apoptosis by activating hydrolysis of sphingomyelin to ceramide [28–30], with apoptotic DNA fragmentation. The radiation-induced apoptosis is accompanied by concomitant decreases in *bcl*-2 mRNA levels in human leukemia cells. Moreover, after exposure to TNF-α and C2-ceramide, apoptosis is also associated with down-regulation of *bcl*-2 mRNA. These results suggested that modulation of *bcl*-2 gene expression may be a target for ceramide-mediated apoptosis following exposure to ionizing radiation and TNF-α [31]. Another important factor is the role of other members of the *bcl*-2 gene family. Bcl-2 forms a heterodimer with a related protein, Bax, and when the Bcl-2:Bax ratio is disturbed, especially in favor of an increase in Bax, apoptosis is blocked [32, 33]. However, the exact mechanisms by which the Bcl-2:Bax ratio enhances or blocks apoptosis are as yet unknown. Furthermore, *bcl*-X, a gene related to *bcl*-2, has been identified. Alternative splicing of *bcl*-X produces two mRNA species: *bcl*-XL, and *bcl*-XS. Bcl-XL, a functional analogue of Bcl-2, inhibits apoptosis upon growth factor withdrawal or after irradiation, whereas overexpression of Bcl-XS counteracts the effect of Bcl-2 prevention of apoptosis [18, 34]. The susceptibility of cells to apoptosis may then be determined by regulation of both the expression and splicing of *bcl*-X as well as *bcl*-2 and/or *bax*.

It should also be borne in mind that there may be different mechanisms of cell killing at different radiation dose levels. Moreover, one of the prevailing theories in radiobiology is that relatively low and high doses of radiation act in different ways [21]. Such data may be explained by differential expression of *bcl*-2 family members resulting in differential cellular susceptibility to apoptosis. Recently, Gamma Knife radiosurgery has tended to use lower doses for benign tumors such as neurinomas, meningiomas, and pituitary adenomas in order to minimize damage to normal brain tissue and cranial nerves. However, low-dose radiosurgery may also be advantageous from the perspective of the effects on tumor cells, because some pathways of radiation-induced apoptosis may be activated by low-dose irradiation. Understanding the molecular mechanisms of apoptosis should provide an appropriate background for introducing new and effective therapeutic strategies.

References

1 Wyllie AH, Kerr JFR, Currie AR: Cell death: The significance of apoptosis. Int Rev Cytol 1980;68: 251–306.
2 Wyllie AH: Glucocorticoid-induced thymocyte apoptosis is associated with endogenous endonuclease activation. Nature 1980;284:555–556.
3 Kerr JFR, Wyllie AH, Currie AR: Apoptosis: A basic biological phenomenon with wide-ranging implications in tissue kinetics. Br J Cancer 1972;26:239–257.
4 Kerr JFR, Searle J: A suggested explanation for the paradoxically slow rate of growth of basal carcinomas that contain numerous mitotic figures. J Pathol 1972;107:41–45.
5 Kyprianou N, English HF, Isaacs JT: Programmed cell death during regression of PC-82 human prostate cancer following androgen ablation. Cancer Res 1990;50:3748–3753.
6 Sellins KS, Cohen JJ: Hyperthermia induces apoptosis in thymocytes. Radiat Res 1991;126:88–95.
7 Warters RL: Radiation-induced apoptosis in a murine T-cell hybridoma. Cancer 1992;126:88–95.
8 Duke RC, Cohen JJ: IL-2 addiction: Withdrawal of growth factor activates a suicide program in dependent T cells. Lymphokine Res 1986;5:289–299.
9 Shi Y, Glynn M, Guilbert LJ, Cotter TG, Bissonnette RP, Green DR: Role for c-*myc* activation-induced apoptotic cell death in T cell hybridomas. Science 1992;257:212–214.
10 Lowe SW, Schmitt EM, Smith SW, Osborne BA, Jacks T: p53 is required for radiation-induced apoptosis in mouse thymocytes. Nature 1993;362:847–849.
11 Clarke AR, Purdie CA, Harrison DJ, Morris RG, Bird CC, Hooper ML, Wyllie AH: Thymocyte apoptosis induced by p53-dependent pathways. Nature 1993;362:849–852.
12 Tsujimoto Y, Finger LR, Yunis J, Nowell PC, Croce CM: Cloning of the chromosome breakpoint of neoplastic B-cell with the t(14;18) chromosome translocation. Science 1984;226:1097–1099.
13 Tsujimoto Y, Gorham J, Cossmen J, Jaffe E, Croce CM: The t(14;18) chromosome translocations involved in B-cell neoplasms result from mistakes in VDJ joining. Science 1985;229:1390–1393.
14 Cleary M, Smith S, Sklar J: Cloning and structural analysis of cDNAs for bcl-2 and a hybrid bcl-2/immunoglobulin transcript resulting from the t(14;18) translocation. Cell 1986;47:19–28.
15 Hockenbery D, Nunez G, Millian C, Schieiber RD, Korsmeyer SJ: Bcl-2 is an inner mitochondria membrane protein that blocks programmed cell death. Nature 1990;348:344–346.
16 Chen-Levy Z, Nourse J, Cleary ML: The Bcl-2 candidate proto-oncogene product is a 24-kilodalton integral-membrane protein highly expressed in lymphoid cell lines and lymphomas carrying the t(14;18) translocation. Mol Cell Biol 1989;9:701–710.
17 Stasser A, Harris AW, Cory S: *bcl*-2 transgene inhibits T cell death and perturbs thymic self-censorship. Cell 1991;67:889–899.
18 Hockenbery DM, Oltvai ZN, Yin SM, Milliman CL, Korsmeyer SJ: Bcl-2 function in an antioxidant pathway to prevent apoptosis. Cell 1993;75:241–251.
19 Sellins KS, Cohen JJ: Gene induction by γ-irradiation leads to DNA fragmentation in lymphocytes. J Immunol 1987;139:3199–3206.
20 Yamada T, Ohyama H: Radiation-induced interphase cell death of rat thymocytes is internally programmed (apoptosis). Int J Radiat Biol 1988;53:65–75.
21 Radford IR, Murphy TK: Radiation response of mouse lymphoid and myeloid cell lines: Different signals can lead to apoptosis and may influence sensitivity to killing by DNA double-strand breakage. Int J Radiat Biol 1994;65:229–239.
22 Maruyama Y, Feola JM: Relative radio-sensitivities of the thymus, spleen, and lymphohemopoietic systems. Adv Radiat Biol 1987;12:1–82.
23 Ganz JC, Aanderud S, Mork SJ, Smievoll AI: Tumor volume reduction following Gamma Knife radiosurgery: The relationship between X-ray and histological findings. Acta Neurochir 1994;62: 39–42.
24 Barry MA, Behnke CA, Eastman A: Activation of programmed cell death (apoptosis) by cisplatin, other anticancer drugs, toxins and hyperthermia. Biochem Pharmacol 1990;40:2353–2362.
25 Kruman IA, Matylevich NP, Beletsky IP, Afanasyev VN, Umansky SR: Apoptosis of murine BW 5147 thymoma cells induced by dexamethasone and γ-irradiation. J Cell Physiol 1991;148:267–273.

26 Radford IR: Mouse lymphoma cells that undergo interphase death show markedly increased sensitivity to radiation-induced DNA double-strand breakage as compared with cells that undergo mitotic death. Int J Radiat Biol 1991;59:1353–1369.
27 Reed JC: Bcl-2 and regulation of programmed cell death. J Cell Biol 1994;124:1–6.
28 Dressler KA, Mathias S, Kolesnick RN: Tumor necrosis factor-α activates the sphingomyelin signal transduction pathway in a cell free system. Science 1992;255:1715–1718.
29 Jarvis WD, Kolesnick RN, Fornari FA, Taylor RS, Gewirtz DA, Grant S: Induction of apoptotic cell death by sphingomyelinase and ceramide in a variety of mammalian cells. Proc Natl Acad Sci USA 1990;91:73–77.
30 Kolesnick RN, Golde DW: The sphingomyelin pathway in tumor necrosis factor and interleukin-1 signalling. Cell 1994;77:325–328.
31 Mei C, Quintans J, Fuks Z, Thompson C, Kufe DW, Weichselbaum RR: Suppression of *bcl*-2 messenger RNA production may mediate apoptosis after ionizing radiation, tumor necrosis factor α, and ceramide. Cancer Res 1995;55:991–994.
32 Oltvai ZN, Milliman CL, Korsmeyer SJ: Bcl-2 heterodimerizes in vivo with a conserved homology Bax that accelerates programmed cell death. Cell 1993;74:609–619.
33 Yin XM, Oltvai ZN, Korsmeyer SJ: BH1 and BH2 domains of Bcl-2 are required for inhibition of apoptosis and heterodimerization with Bax. Nature 1994;369:321–323.
34 Boise LH, Gonzalez GM, Postema CE, Ding LY, Lindsten T, Turka LA, Mao XH, Nunez G, Thompson CB: *bcl*-X, a *bcl*-2 related gene that functions as a dominant regulator of apoptotic cell death. Cell 1993;74:597–608.

Proc 7th Int Meeting Leksell Gamma Knife® Society,
Island of Lana'i, Hawaii, November 1995
Stereotact Funct Neurosurg 1996;66(suppl 1):49–56

Stereotactic and Functional Neurosurgery

Accuracy of Stereotactic Localisation Using Magnetic Resonance Imaging: A Comparison between Two- and Three-Dimensional Studies

L. Walton[a], *A. Hampshire*[a], *D.M.C. Forster*[b], *A.A. Kemeny*[b]

[a] National Centre For Stereotactic Radiosurgery, Royal Hallamshire Hospital, and
[b] Department of Medical Physics and Clinical Engineering, Weston Park Hospital, Sheffield, UK

Key Words

Stereotactic · Magnetic resonance · Localisation · Radiosurgery

Abstract

The accuracy of stereotactic localisation using magnetic resonance (MR) imaging has been assessed in a phantom study. Parallel studies compared the accuracy obtained. First, a series of two-dimensional (2D) MR slices (transverse, coronal, and sagittal) was acquired sequentially to image the three-dimensional (3D) volume of the phantom. Then, the same volume was imaged in a 3D MR study in which the entire volume was excited simultaneously and 2D slices in transverse, coronal, and sagittal planes were then reconstructed from the 3D data set. The results showed that the 3D acquisition gave superior results in all three planes, and overall it was found that only 1% of the phantom volume was affected by an error greater than 2 mm, compared with 11% for the 2D study. New facilities for image quality assurance provided in GammaPlan version 3.0 have been tested against images from the 2D study with known distortion and consequent localisation errors and successfully identified all images in which the localisation errors were likely to be greater than 3.7 mm.

KARGER

E-Mail karger@karger.ch
Fax + 41 61 306 12 34
http://www.karger.ch

1011–6125/96/0665–0049$10.00/0

Mr. Lee Walton
Department of Medical Physics and Clinical Engineering
Weston Park Hospital
Whitham Road
Sheffield S10 2SJ (UK)

Introduction

At the 6th Leksell Gamma Knife Society Meeting in May 1994 (Kyoto, Japan), we related our experience with inaccuracies in stereotactic localisation using magnetic resonance imaging (MRI) [1, 2]. In a phantom study, we identified errors in stereotactic localisation which could be as large as ± 10 mm, but noted that there was considerable spatial variation in the accuracy obtained. Particularly affected were the Y coordinates in transverse sections and the Z coordinates in coronal and sagittal sections.

More recently, Sumanaweera et al. [3] have published a theoretical appraisal of the factors affecting spatial distortion in MR images, with particular emphasis on the relevance of such distortion to stereotactic localisation. This group maintains that the principle causes of distortion are non-linearities in the gradient fields and resonance offsets (which encompass inhomogeneities in the main magnetic field and object-induced chemical shifts). These causes have different effects in each direction of the image, depending on whether the spatial information is encoded in the frequency or the phase of the RF signals. To some extent this could explain why the preponderance of the errors is identified in one direction only.

Sumanaweera et al. [3] stated that some of the causes of image distortion are eliminated if the MR images are acquired in a three-dimensional (3D) study, in which the entire imaged volume is simultaneously excited, and only weak slice selection is used. The purpose of the current study was to compare the accuracy of stereotactic localisation using two-dimensional (2D) study (in which individual slices are selectively excited – as in the previously reported study) with the results from a 3D acquisition.

Materials and Methods

Two phantoms were used, to facilitate the assessment of accuracy. Both consisted of a Perspex box, 150 × 150 × 180 mm, with an array of 5-mm diameter Perspex rods spaced 20 mm apart within the body of the phantom. In the first phantom, the rods were parallel to one of the 150-mm-length sides, and this could be used in two orientations to assess the accuracy in transverse and sagittal images. The second phantom had rods parallel to the longest side and was used for coronal images. Both were filled with a dilute copper sulphate solution.

The phantoms were mounted on a thick plate of Perspex which could be secured to the base of the Leksell stereotactic 'G' frame (Elekta Instruments, Stockholm, Sweden). To reproduce the patient procedure as closely as possible, the four skull fixation posts were also included. However, the phantom prevented them from being placed in their usual location, and so they were positioned as near to their normal position as could be reasonably achieved. The stereotactic coordinates of five of the Perspex rods were measured physically using a vernier height gauge, with the frame and the phantom positioned on a surface plate.

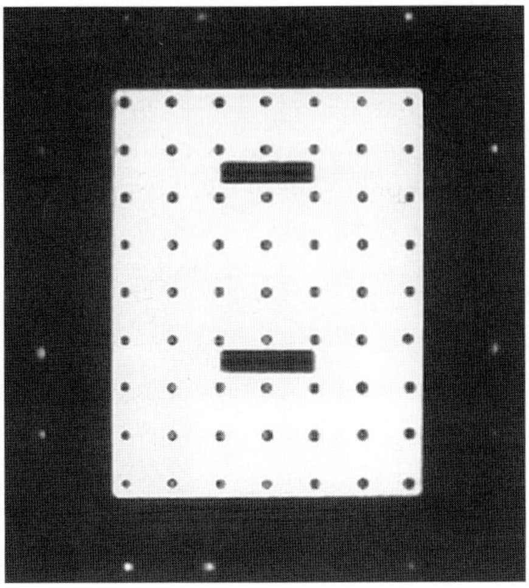

Fig. 1. A typical transverse section image.

The measurement of the position of these rods was achieved accurately, without parallax error, since these rods protruded through the outer surface of the phantom. The positions of the remaining rods could then be determined from the known positions.

The MRI localiser box (fiducial system) was attached to the base frame, and the phantoms were scanned within the head coils of a Siemens 1.5 T Magnetom within the Academic Department of Radiology, University of Sheffield, UK. This scanner had been carefully shimmed at installation, resulting in a high specification for the homogeneity of magnetic field strength within the magnet bore. Care was taken to ensure that the planes of the localiser box were square with the planes of the head coils, and then a 2D study was performed, consisting of a series of T_1-weighted images covering the phantom, parallel to the principal planes of the coils. Immediately following the 2D study and without moving the phantom, a further 3D study was performed to image the same volume. The pulse sequence used is referred to as an MPRage, an abbreviation for magnetisation prepared rapid gradient recalled echo sequence [4]. The resultant 3D data set consisted of a set of thin sagittal slices from which images in the principal planes of interest were reconstructed.

At the time of investigation, no direct mechanism existed for the transfer of the MR data to our radiosurgery dose-planning workstation. All images were therefore transferred to film and then imported into our planning system (GammaPlan, Elekta Instruments) using a flat-bed image scanner. This had been previously checked to ensure a linear spatial response in both directions and thus could be relied upon to faithfully reproduce the original images. The 'image definition' section of this software has facilities for the scaling of images with stereotactic fiducials into Leksell stereotactic space, and each image was appropriately calibrated. Figure 1 shows a typical transverse section image of the phantom, revealing the twelve fiducials and the volume of copper sulphate, with circular signal voids representing the positions of the Perspex rods.

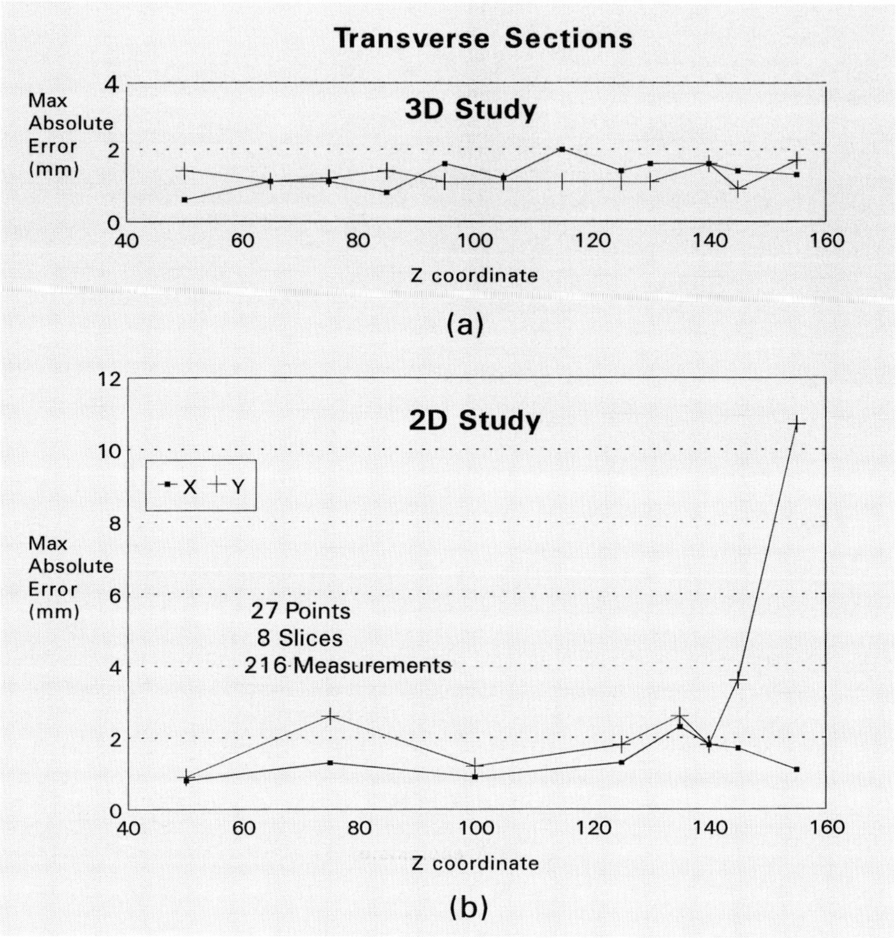

Fig. 2. Plot showing the variation with slice level of the error in the computed X and Y coordinates for transverse sections. **a** 3D study. **b** 2D study.

The stereotactic coordinates of a number of points were measured in each image in the 2D and 3D series. First, the calculated stereotactic coordinates of the fixed fiducial markers were measured using the 'point' measurement facility. These fiducials, by definition, are at fixed and known positions with respect to the frame. The stereotactic coordinates of about 20 of the rods were then measured, the centre of the rods being determined by positioning the eye lens marker (a circle of adjustable diameter) to achieve the best outline of the image of each rod. The error associated with each of the 20 or so measurement points in each slice was determined, and the maximum absolute error for each slice in the series was recorded.

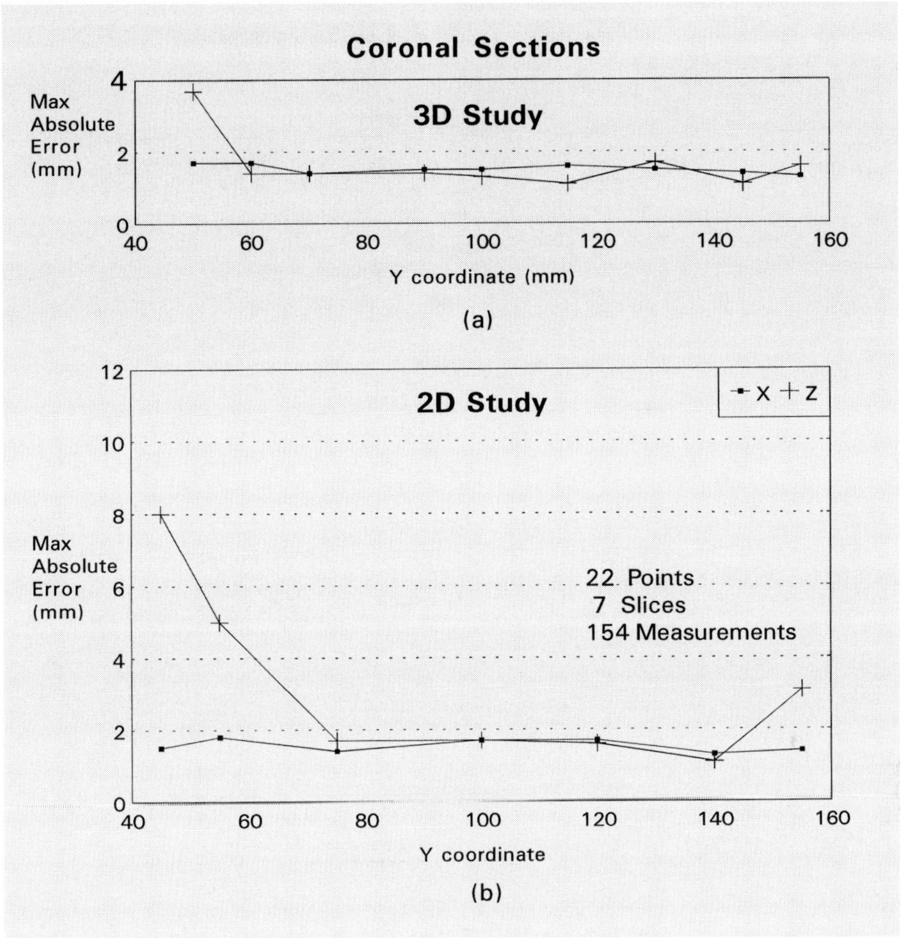

Fig. 3. Plot showing the variation with slice position of the error in the computed X and Z coordinates for coronal sections. **a** 3D study. **b** 2D study.

Results and Discussion

Figure 2 shows the variation with the Z coordinate of the maximum absolute error in the X and Y coordinates. Each pair of points represents the maximum error experienced in the slice at the indicated level. In figure 2a, the errors in the 3D study for both X and Y coordinates can be seen to be below 2 mm throughout the range of slices. They are obviously better than those obtained in the 2D study (fig. 2b), where errors as large as 10.7 mm were identified.

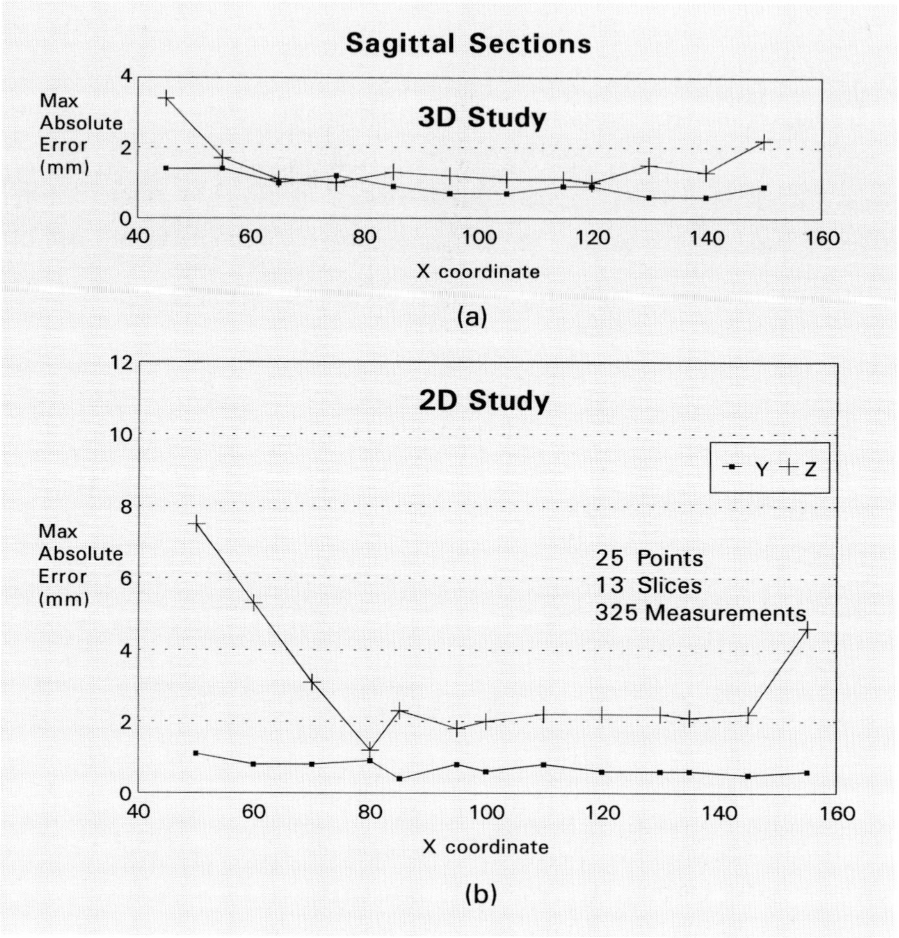

Fig. 4. Plot showing the variation with slice position of the error in the computed Y and Z coordinates for sagittal sections. **a** 3D study. **b** 2D study.

Figure 3 shows the variation with the Y coordinate of the maximum absolute error in the X and Z coordinates. Again the results from the 3D study (fig. 3a), with a maximum error of 3.7 mm, are superior to those obtained in the 2D study (maximum error 8 mm). Figure 4 shows similar improvement in accuracy levels for the sagittal plane (maximum error: 3D study, 2.6 mm; 2D study, 7.8 mm). The improved accuracy levels obtained with the 3D study suggest that gradient field non-linearities were indeed contributing to the errors experienced in the 2D study. However, the fact that the errors are not completely resolved suggests that

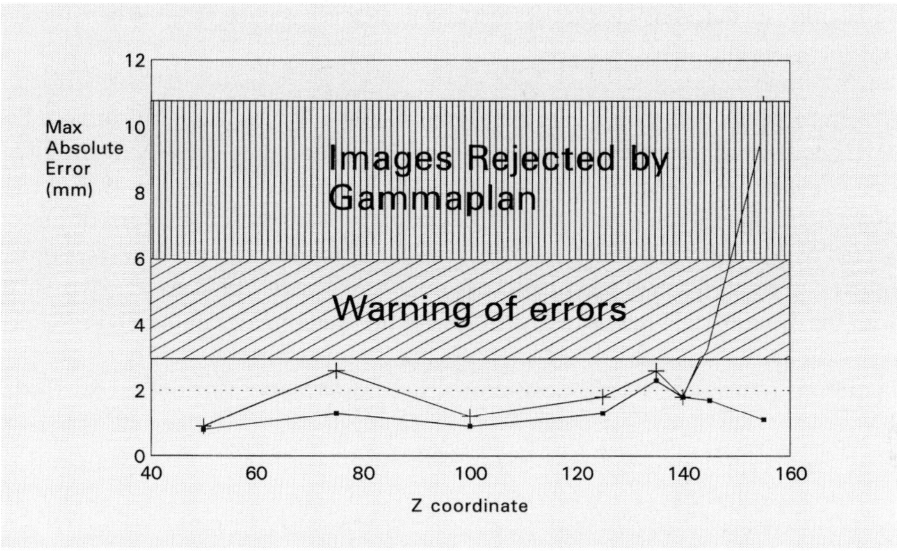

Fig. 5. Plot showing the level at which the GammaPlan 3.0 image quality assurance routines first warn of large errors in image calibration and, second, reject images as unsuitable for accurate localisation.

resonance offsets may be responsible for some of the distortion. Overall, in the 3D study, 1% of the phantom volume was affected by an error greater than 2 mm compared with 11% for the 2D study.

We completed this study some months ago and have now used the 3D acquisition in more than 60 stereotactic radiosurgery cases. The images obtained have been consistently superior, and we have been able to plan our radiosurgery treatments with confidence. Targets defined in one plane (for example transverse) now superimpose on the coronal and sagittal planes with good agreement, and we no longer see alarming discrepancies between image planes. The results of our image quality assurance (measurement of known fiducial positions) have been consistently good except for inaccuracy on one occasion, which was due to an MR scanner fault, when the RF was said to be 'flapping about'. This experience highlighted the need for continued vigilance with image quality assurance. GammaPlan version 3.0 (Elekta Instruments) introduced new facilities for automated image quality assurance, following image definition. Figure 5 shows the results following the testing of this software against images from the 2D study with known distortion and localisation errors. Images are accepted by the defintion algorithms provided the errors are below about 3.7 mm; thereafter, a warning is issued. Any images exhibiting errors in the fixed fiducial positions of more than 7.0 mm are rejected and cannot be defined. This software has significantly reduced the burden of routine image quality assurance.

In conclusion, there appears to be a significant advantage in performing a 3D MRI acquisition for stereotactic localisation. We found that stereotactic localisation could be performed with an accuracy level of below ± 2 mm in 99% of the imaged volume. Some image quality assurance is still advised, to warn of unexpected MR scanner malfunction. However, GammaPlan version 3.0 has significantly helped with its built-in quality assurance processes. Our clinical experience with the 3D study has led us to dispense with the stereotactic computed tomography scan on the same day. We previously felt that this was mandatory for confirmation of radiosurgery field positioning, but now reserve this option for those occasions when the image quality assurance results indicate that one is necessary.

Acknowledgements

We would like to express our thanks to the staff of the Instrument Workshop for their help constructing the phantoms, and also to the Academic Department of Radiology, University of Sheffield, for their patience and assistance in performing the study reported here.

References

1 Walton L, Hampshire A, Forster DMC, Kemeny AA: Accuracy of stereotactic localization using magnetic resonance imaging. Stereotact Funct Neurosurg 1995;64(suppl 1):155–163.

2 Walton L, Hampshire A, Forster DMC, Kemeny AA: A phantom study to assess the accuracy of stereotactic localisation using T1 weighted magnetic resonance imaging with the Leksell stereotactic system. Neurosurgery 1996;38:170–178.

3 Sumanaweera TS, Adler JR, Napel S, Glover GH: Characterization of spatial distortion in magnetic resonance imaging and its implications for stereotactic surgery. Neurosurgery 1994;35:696–704.

4 Brant-Zawadski M, Gillan GD, Nitz WR: MP-RAGE: A three-dimensional, T1-weighted, gradient-echo sequence – Initial experience in the brain. Radiology 1992;182:769–775.

Proc 7th Int Meeting Leksell Gamma Knife® Society,
Island of Lana'i, Hawaii, November 1995
Stereotact Funct Neurosurg 1996;66(suppl 1):57–62

Stereotactic and Functional Neurosurgery

Digital Subtraction Angiography for Arteriovenous Malformations in Stereotactic Radiosurgery

E. Piovan[a], *M. Dal Sasso*[b], *G.P. Urbani*[b], *R. Sartori*[b], *R. Foroni*[a], *A. Benati*[a]

[a] Verona University Hospital, Verona, and
[b] PROGRAM S.r.l., Vicenza, Italy

Key Words
Gamma Knife · Stereotactic radiosurgery · Arteriovenous malformation · Digital subtraction angiography

Abstract
Images coming from digital subtraction angiography (DSA) are affected by a perspective distortion due to the use of image intensifiers. As a result, DSA cannot be used for the accurate definition of stereotactic coordinates. A correction method has been developed to enable the use of DSA for the radiosurgery of arteriovenous malformations. A software program and a special phantom tool were employed. The phantom is made by a computer-controlled drilling machine which makes holes in a Plexiglas plate. It has 865 calibration steel spheres with coordinates determined with a precision of 0.01 mm. A calibration image is acquired by a personal computer, and the software calculates the transformation algorithm to superimpose the image on the known positions of the phantom. This algorithm is saved and then recalled to transform the diagnostic images.

Introduction

Digital subtraction angiography (DSA) simplifies angiographic procedures and has significant advantages over conventional angiography: the examination time is shorter, the catheters are smaller, the dose of contrast medium is lower and

KARGER
E-Mail karger@karger.ch
Fax + 41 61 306 12 34
http://www.karger.ch

1011–6125/96/0665–0057$10.00/0

Enrico Piovan, MD
Department of Neuroradiology
University Hospital
P. le Stefani 1
I–37126 Verona (Italy)

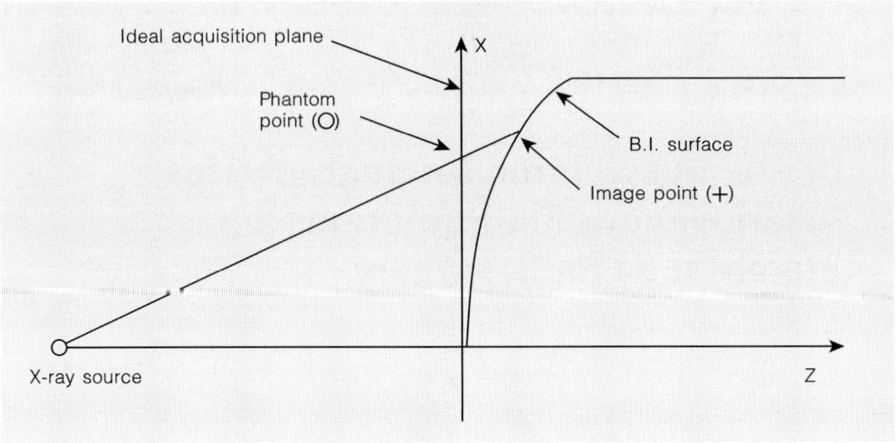

Fig. 1. Acquisition geometry in the image intensifier. The distortion progressively increases from the center of the image intensifier to the border for its surface curvature. BI = Brillance intensifier.

the procedure is more cost-effective. However, the images coming from DSA are affected by a perspective distortion due to the use of image intensifiers. The distortion originates from the curvature of the acquisition surface in the image intensifier and from the electron-focusing system. Thus, DSA cannot assure the spatial accuracy necessary for the determination of stereotactic coordinates. The aim of our work was to develop a correction method so that DSA can be used for arteriovenous malformation (AVM) radiosurgery.

Material and Methods

Film-screen combinations have a simple flat geometry. On the other hand, image intensifiers are large vacuum bottles containing a complex arrangement of an X-ray-absorbing, light-emitting phosphor and a specially shaped photocathode and electrodes which electronically focus the electron beam. The two-dimensional distribution of this beam carries the image information to the output phosphor. Thus, the image quality available at the output of image intensifiers depends greatly upon electron optics. Since electron lenses are governed by many of the same principles governing classical light optical elements, the same possibilities for lens aberrations in light optics apply to electron optics [1].

The first three Seidel aberrations (spherical aberration, coma and astigmatism) directly affect spatial resolution by causing blurred focusing, but they do not cause a geometrical distortion of the image. Each of these aberrations is applicable to image intensifiers. Astigmatism is caused by deviations from cylindrical symmetry of the focusing electrodes, which causes curvature of the field. Other blurring can be minimized by carefully computer-

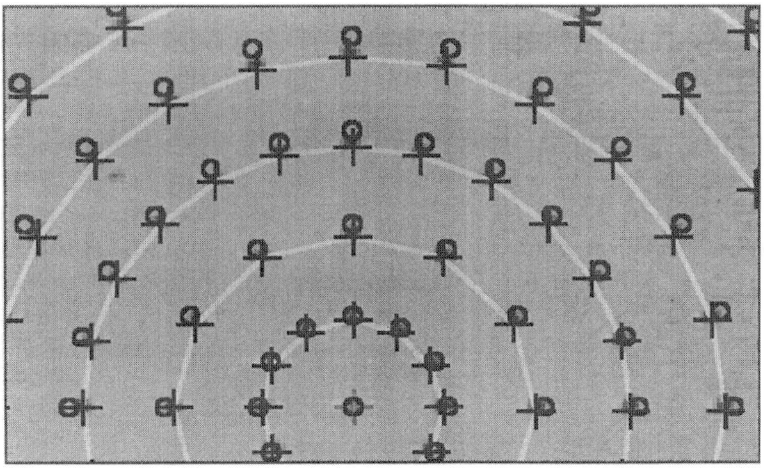

Fig. 2. Position of the calibration points on the image and on the phantom surface. The software program superimposes the points of the image on those known positions on the phantom using a 'local transformation' algorithm. + = Sampling points measured on the surface of the image intensifier (image); o = position of the sampling points on the phantom surface.

designed electron lens structures. However, even after correcting the first three Seidel aberrations, image intensifier images differ from the real object they represent, due to curvature distortion (the fourth Seidel aberration) [2, 3]. This image distortion depends on the surface curvature of the image intensifier (fig. 1). It increases progressively from the center of the image intensifier to the border. The maximum error is approximately 1 cm in a 27-cm image intensifier. Consequently, it is not possible to apply a constant magnification factor to calculate the real object dimensions at all points of an image, as in the X-ray plain film. This artifact leads to anatomical distortion. Thus, DSA cannot assure the spatial accuracy necessary for stereotactic localization.

We developed a correction method to avoid this problem, enabling DSA to be employed for the radiosurgery of AVMs. We used a software program and a special phantom tool. The phantom is made by a computer-controlled drilling machine and a Plexiglas plate. It has 865 calibration holes with coordinates determined with a precision of 0.01 mm. A high-precision steel sphere is placed inside every hole. The phantom can then be used with any type of image intensifier. Calibration images are acquired by a personal computer (PC Pentium 66/100 MHz, 32 Mb RAM, 1 Gb hard disk) and connected to the video system of the DSA (resolution 1,088 × 1,024). The software program automatically detects the calibration point position, and then calculates the necessary transformation to superimpose the calibration points of the image on the known positions of the phantom, with an accuracy of 0.1 mm. The transformation function is calculated using a 'local transformation' algorithm (fig. 2), based on the singular decomposition value, which is saved and then recalled to transform diagnostic images automatically (fig. 3). The center of the acquisition matrix may change position during angiographic arch rotation. To compensate, the position of the cen-

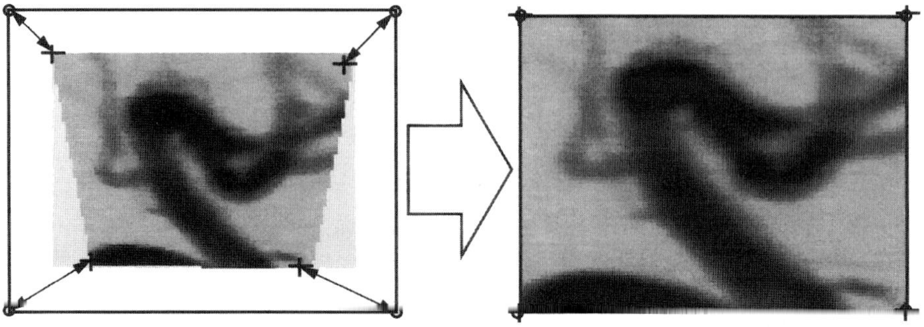

Fig. 3. Diagnostic images are stretched to make the sampling points of the image [+] coincident with the phantom points [o].

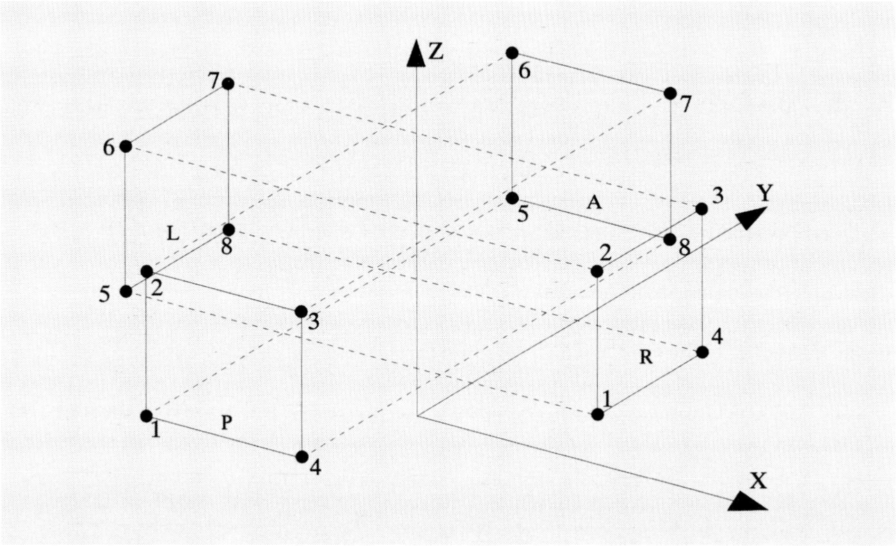

Fig. 4. Geometry of stereotactic indicator for DSA, with four steel spheres on each side.

ter is automatically detected at the beginning of every acquisition series by means of a Plexiglas plate, containing a central steel sphere, which is fixed to the image intensifier [4].

Using a special stereotactic indicator with four steel spheres on each side (fig. 4), the software program calculates the stereotactic coordinates and the magnification factor for both posteroanterior and laterolateral projections. When we began using DSA for AVM stereotactic localization, we always tested the computer program, calculating the stereotactic coordinates of the fixation screw points, both for DSA and computed tomography (CT).

The software enables performance of the following additional functions.

(a) Image postprocession functions, such as rotation, inversion, mirroring, detail extraction, detail increase or decrease, contrast control through the window/level interactive setting.

(b) Measurement of distances, areas and angles in the diagnostic images.

(c) Notes, symbols and free text insertion on the images.

(d) Patient information database management.

(e) Creation of a patient folder with information from the examinations.

(f) Examination selection and visualization with different extraction criteria (such as date, patient name, code, diagnosis).

(g) Use of key words for image identification and retrieval.

(h) Data and images can be imported into any standard word processor or presentation program.

(i) Image printing for laser paper printing or laser radiological printing.

Results

Images of the calibration phantom were acquired with a Siemens Angiotron CMP DSA for two different angiographic arch rotations (posteroanterior and laterolateral). The transformation function was calculated for each of the two different projections. It is possible that the earth's magnetic field could have an effect on the electrons in the image intensifier when it rotates from one orthogonal projection to the other. However, in reality we did not find a significant difference between the two transformation functions, so it is possible to work using only one calibration image.

The transformation algorithm was tested with more than 1,500 measurements before it was used with patients. In addition, we performed about 100 tests comparing conventional angiography and CT to DSA stereotactic coordinate determination. Finally, we calculated the distance between two or more points of a known phantom using DSA stereotactic coordinates and fixing the phantom in the center and at the border of the system. The program accuracy was defined as equal to 0.1 mm. However, the maximum error in a transformed diagnostic image was equal to the pixel size (from 0.3 to 0.5 mm depending on field of view and matrix size).

Discussion

The distortion of an image intensifier is absent in the center of the acquisition matrix but it increases as the cube of the image intensifier surface radius according to the function:

$$r' = r + Dr^3,$$

where r′ is the radial distance of an object from the center of the image intensifier field with distortion, r is the radial distance of the feature without distortion, and D is the distortion parameter adjusted to the geometrical characteristics of the image intensifier.

Therefore, the undistorted central region dimension is a function of the image intensifier radius. There are two possible solutions to this problem. A larger image intensifier may be used or a correction system is needed. The first solution is very expensive, while the second solution has already been described. In particular, some authors have proposed applying a grid to the image intensifier. By comparing the position of the calibration straight line on the grid and on the images it is possible to define a polynomial function to solve the problem [5].

In our method we use a plate with 865 calibration points instead of a grid. This permits an automatic acquisition of the points with more precision and in less time. Morevoer, the software program uses a stable numerical algorithm as the singular decomposition value and is independent of the kind of image intensifier used [6].

In conclusion, this study describes the precision of a 'transformation' technique, which enables DSA to be used for angiographic stereotactic localization. Moreover, this method uses computer techniques to reduce the time of the procedure and to check the normal and pathological structures in the two radiological projections. With this technique, DSA may be used for angiographic stereotactic localization with sufficient accuracy.

References

1 Hawkes PW, Kasper E: Principles of Electron Optics. London, Academic Press, 1989, vol 1, pp 306–338.
2 Casperson LW, Speigler P, Grollman JH: Characterization of aberrations in image-intensified fluoroscopy. Med Phys 1976;3:103–106.
3 Rudin S, Bednarek DR, Wong R: Accurate characterization of image intensifier distortion. Med Phys 1991;18:1145–1151.
4 Bernardi L, Colombo F, Francescon P, Cora S, Dal Sasso M, Puzzuoli A, Pinna V, Marchi M, Castellan L: Sistema di correlazione della distorsione di immagine in angiografia digitale; in Pero G (ed): Neuroradiologia 1994. Udine, Centauro, 1994, pp 173–176.
5 Chakraborty DP: Image intensifier distortion correction. Med Phys 1987;14:249–252.
6 Press WH, Flannery BP: Numerical Recipes in C: The Art of Scientific Computing. Cambridge, Cambridge University Press, 1986.

Proc 7th Int Meeting Leksell Gamma Knife® Society,
Island of Lana'i, Hawaii, November 1995
Stereotact Funct Neurosurg 1996;66(suppl 1):63–70

Stereotactic and Functional Neurosurgery

Clinical Experience with Stereotactic Digital Subtraction Angiography with Distortion Correction Software

K. Ericson[a], *M. Söderman*[a], *E. Maurincomme*[c], *C. Lindquist*[b]

Departments of
[a] Neuroradiology and
[b] Neurosurgery, Karolinska Hospital, Stockholm, Sweden;
[c] Advanced Applications Department, General Electric Medical Systems, Buc, France

Key Words
Stereotactic angiography · Image distortion · Arteriovenous malformation · Radiosurgery · Digital subtraction angiography

Abstract

Recently developed software for correction of the geometric distortion in digital subtraction angiography was tested clinically. Localization and subsequent radiosurgical treatment of intracranial arteriovenous malformations was undertaken in 60 patients. During each angiographic series, a series of grid images was also acquired. All images were transferred to a workstation where the grid images were compared to a previously stored ideal image of the grid. A distortion correction was then performed on the grid images. The same pixel-by-pixel correction was applied to the respective angiographic images. The target was outlined on corrected subtracted images on the monitor. The outlined regions of interest and reference points were transferred to another workstation for dose planning, and the treatment was subsequently executed in the Gamma Knife unit. The clinical applicability of the distortion correction program was tested and possible sources of error examined. The experience gained is being used for further development of the software and for smoother data management and reduction of the processing time.

KARGER

E-Mail karger@karger.ch
Fax + 41 61 306 12 34
http://www.karger.ch

1011-6125/96/0665-0063$10.00/0

Kaj Ericson, MD, PhD
Department of Neuroradiology
Karolinska Hospital
S-171 76 Stockholm (Sweden)

Introduction

Stereotactic angiography is performed at the Karolinska Hospital to delineate arteriovenous malformations (AVMs) for stereotactic irradiation with the Gamma Knife (Elekta, Stockholm, Sweden). The requirements for conventional stereotactic angiography have been described in detail elsewhere [1–3]. The aim has been to acquire films with as little distortion as possible to ensure the highest possible accuracy. Digital subtraction angiography (DSA) has certain advantages over cut film angiography. However, it is also associated with complex and partly unstable, non-linear geometric distortions. The 'pincushion' distortion is caused by the curvature of the image intensifier (II) screen, and the S-distortion by the earth's magnetic field. There are also geometric distortions caused by other magnetic fields and by the optical quality of the video chain. Efforts have been made to correct for these distortions [4–8]. However, so far there has been no commercially available software for distortion correction. This has certain implications for centers working with stereotactic procedures including angiography. It has been recommended that DSA should not be used for stereotactic applications without a well-validated correction method. This study reports the initial clinical experience with a previously described correction program [8] in which a pixel-by-pixel correction is made, based on the image of a grid with a well-defined configuration.

Patients, Equipment and Methods

Sixty consecutive patients with AVMs scheduled for stereotactic irradiation with the Gamma Knife were included in this study. The patients ranged in age from 3 to 73 years (mean, 36). Angiography was performed selectively after transfemoral catheterization. A non-ionic contrast medium (Omnipaque-300, Nycomed, Norway) was used. The amount of contrast injected depended on the size and arteriovenous shunting of the malformation: 7 ml/s with a total volume of 8 ml was a common contrast dose injected into the internal carotid artery.

Distortion correction was applied in the examination of several vascular territories in each patient. Thus, 135 angiographic series were corrected in these patients (mean, 2.25/patient).

The angiographic equipment consisted of a biplane Advantx DLX unit with biplane interventional digital fluoroscopy (General Electric Medical Systems, France). A matrix of 1,024 was used. To reduce radiation exposure and, to some extent, improve image quality, the standard antiscatter grids were permanently removed. Moreover, the IIs were positioned a far away from the X-ray tubes as possible. This allowed an air gap of 30 cm in the lateral projection and 34 cm in the posteroanterior (PA) projection. The FOV was permanently reduced from 23 to 22 cm, so that the head of a patient completely filled the FOV, allowing optimal utilization of the matrix and yielding the best spatial resolution possible. During the arterial phase, it was usual for 3 images/s to be exposed with a focal spot of 0.6 mm. The input dose on the II was 500 μR/image. In the lateral projection, typical exposure parameters were 80 kV, 200 mA and 50 ms.

There were specially designed collision protection devices in front of each II, where removable mesh grids could easily be mounted. When the examination was finished, all images were stored on Exabyte (Exabyte Corporation, USA) tape for transfer to the Advantage Windows workstation (General Electric Medical Systems, France). An Ethernet connection between the angiography suite and the workstation is at present lacking. The workstation is a Hewlett-Packard 715/100 equipped with a platform for further development of the standard Advantage Windows software. Hard copies of the corrected images were obtained on a standard laser camera (Matrix Laser Camera, Agfa, Germany).

Methods

A stereotactic frame was fixed to the head of the patient before starting the angiography. The frame was then fixed to the examination couch, and a localizing box specially designed for stereotaxic DSA (Elekta, Sweden) was mounted onto the frame. The appropriate vessel was catheterized and the patient was centred for biplane angiography. The positions of the gantry, II, X-ray tubes and patient table were stored. After acquisition of one biplane series, the patient table was withdrawn from the FOV. No other change in the position of the equipment was permitted. The grids were placed in position in front of each II and the exposure parameters adjusted before acquisition of the grid series (one for each projection). This procedure was repeated for each set of angiographic images. When several vessels were examined, care was taken to return the table top to exactly the same position to enable a full appreciation of the AVM by overlay of the different series. After transferring the images to the workstation, each selected angiographic series was linked to its corresponding grid series. When every series had been correctly identified and linked, correction of the grid images was started, using a previously published correction program based on a pixel-by-pixel transformation of the distorted grid image back to its original, known, shape [8]. The corrected grid images were then reviewed to ensure that a proper correction had been performed (fig. 1, 2). The parameters used to create a distortion-free grid image were stored and then applied to the respective images in the angiographic series.

The corrected angiographic images were reviewed and the target was outlined on the screen. The final outline of the AVM and a reference point in the PA and lateral view were documented on subtracted and non-subtracted images (fig. 3). Subtracted and non-subtracted images with a region of interest outlining the AVM were then transferred over the network to the dose planning system. Initially, hard copies were obtained and scanned into the dose planning system.

The stereotactic coordinates of the reference point were initially determined by the neurosurgeon and the neuroradiologist independently and compared, as a safety measure. The former used the fiducials and the dose planning system (Leksell GammaPlan). The latter employed a previously described graphic method [9], using the scales of the stereotactic box. The manual, graphic coordinate determination was later abandoned, and we are now relying only on the computerized dose planning system for coordinate determination.

1 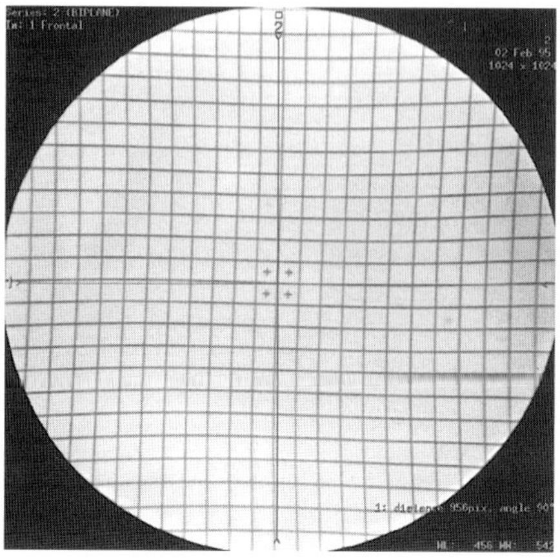 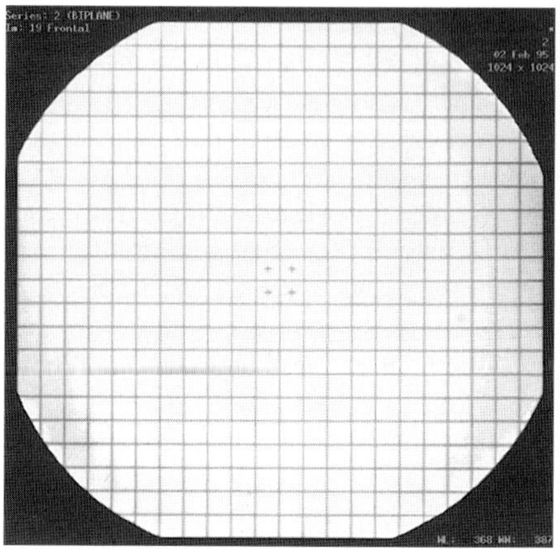 2

Fig. 1. Uncorrected grid image. Both the pincushion distortions and the S-distortions are clearly seen.

Fig. 2. Corrected grid image. No distortions are seen.

Results

The whole procedure still has the characteristics of a prototype set-up. Nevertheless, it has not once been aborted, nor have we been forced to change to conventional cut film angiography. Minor incompatibility problems have been encountered, due to use of software in different stages of development. These problems have not resulted in errors in the correction procedure. Time was saved with the DSA procedure: the lengthy manual subtraction procedure could be omitted with the new technique. Considerable time was also saved by omitting the manual, graphic coordinate determination, which is no longer necessary. The image quality with the present set-up was judged sufficient for high-precision stereotactic angiography. However, a FOV of 22 cm was necessary to obtain the very high resolution needed.

In one examination, the grid images were overexposed, resulting in serious correction errors (fig. 4), caused by rapid image acquisition in combination with incorrect adjustment of the aperture of the video camera, inducing remaining fluorescence in the II. This added to the light intensity of the II input screen resulting in video overexposure after a number of examinations. The correction program is at present starting with the last grid image of the series. If an acceptable correction is not obtained, the program continues with the previous image in the series. When the program reaches a correctly exposed image, normal correction follows.

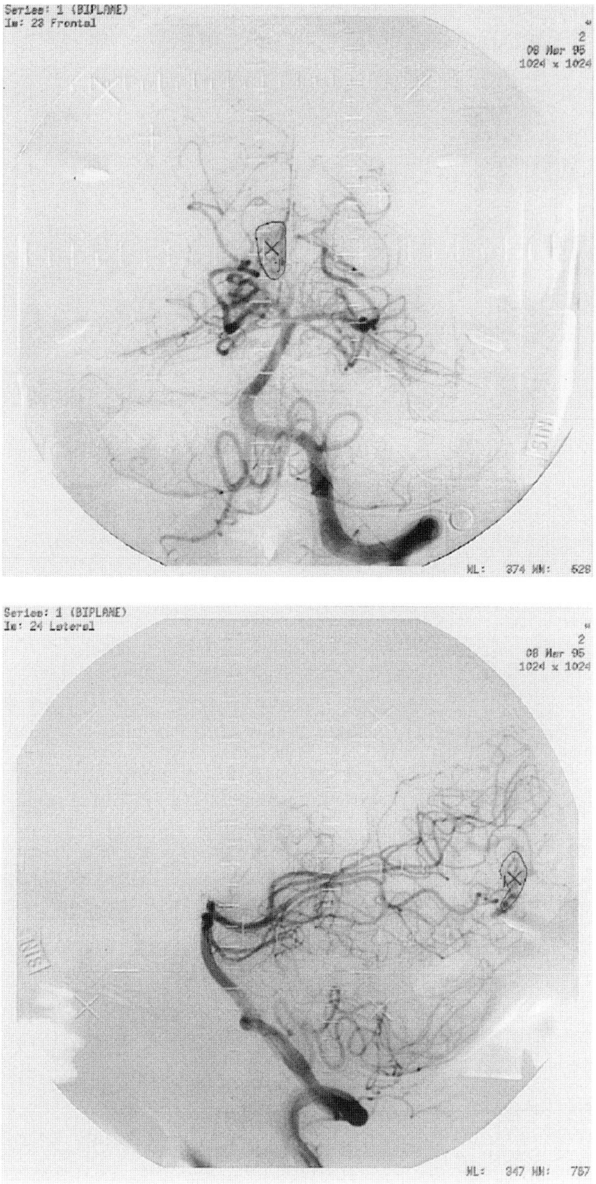

a b

Fig. 3. Corrected angiographic images in frontal (**a**) and lateral (**b**) views with the AVM outlined and a reference point marked.

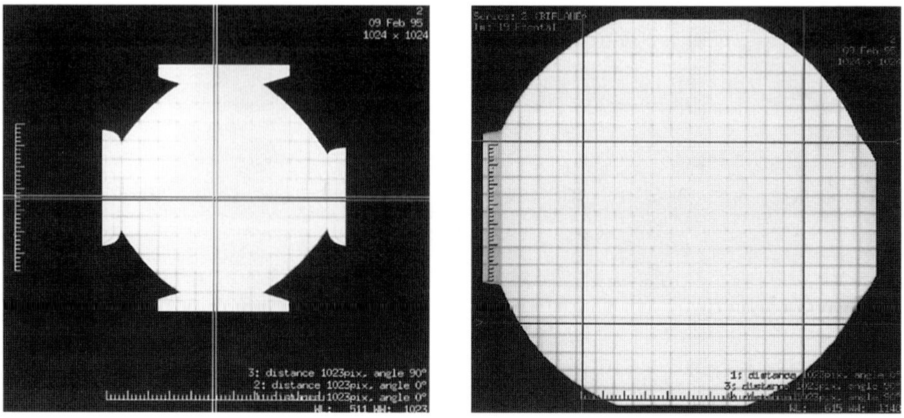

a b

Fig. 4. Error in correction of grid images due to overexposure. **a** Misinterpretation is obvious. **b** Note the excess of vertical lines appearing near the center of the image.

Discussion

The program used for correcting the distortion in DSA images is based on a classical non-parametric calibration/correction, where the amount of distortion for each pixel is directly measured on a grid image with known properties. The distortion field (i.e., the value of the distortion for each pixel) is estimated by bilinear interpolation. The angiographic images are resampled using the distortion field so that each pixel is relocated to the estimated, undistorted, position. The correction program has been presented previously [8] and found to be reliable.

The introduction of DSA into stereotactic angiography implies that there is no longer a need for conventional cut film changers in neuroradiology. Elimination of the geometric distortion in the DSA images also means that a digital technique can be employed for the whole procedure, including outlining, coordinate determination and dose planning. Furthermore, this development means that a full integration with other imaging techniques, such as magnetic resonance, computed tomography and positron emission tomography is now possible. This opens new perspectives for 3D target appreciation, targeting optimization, dose planning and at follow-up. This could help to improve treatment results and reduce undesired side-effects [1].

It is essential that the grid images are correctly exposed. Overexposure may result in difficulties running the correction program or in serious misinterpretation (fig. 4). Until more has been learned about the variations in the distortion it has been considered suitable and safe to keep the acquisition parameters as similar as possible between angiographic and grid series and to acquire one grid series for each angiographic series.

Improvements to the procedure are on the way. The transfer of images from the angiography unit to the workstation with Exabyte tape will be replaced by an Ethernet connection, which may speed up the transfer. The angiographic series should probably be linked with its corresponding grid series at an early stage. The correction procedure may be optimized and less time consuming.

It is easy to see that a correction has been made on the grid images, but it is not obvious on the angiographic images. Thus, it might be possible that the program claims to have performed a correction that has actually not been done. Addition of peripheral straight lines on the localizing box might aid as a marker. If no deviation of these lines can be seen, it is likely that a correction has not been performed. In the first prototype stereotactic box, the standard fiducials and the added engraved scales were located centrally and thereby close to the target, minimizing any measurement error. The scales and other straight objects in the image were used to check that a correction had actually taken place. In later versions of the stereotactic box, the scales for manual coordinate determination have been omitted.

Further development is planned with regard to outlining and integration of the outlined regions and volumes of interest with other imaging modalities and with other applications, such as the dose-planning program or the therapeutic unit itself.

Angiographic equipment from General Electric has been used for all examinations in this study. In a previous paper describing the correction algorithm [8], a Siemens angiographic unit with an ADAC add-on DSA system was used in the same way. The correction software may in principle be used on any type of image from any manufacturer, provided a corresponding grid image is also acquired. The image format can be adequately handled if the necessary procedures are followed meticulously.

In conclusion, stereotactic DSA can be performed rapidly and safely with existing software for the correction of geometric distortion. A transition to a fully digital technique makes it possible to improve stereotactic procedures on a number of levels.

Acknowledgment

We would like to extend our gratitude to Catherine Picard, PhD, Advanced Applications Department, General Electric Medical Systems, Buc, France, for her efforts before devoting her skills and intelligence to other fields of radiology.

References

1 Guo WY: Radiological aspects of Gamma Knife radiosurgery for arteriovenous malformations and other non-tumoural disorders of the brain. Acta Radiol 1993;34(suppl No 388).
2 Guo WY, Lindqvist M, Lindquist C, Ericson K, Nordell B, Karlsson B, Kihlström L: Stereotaxic angiography in Gamma Knife radiosurgery of intracranial arteriovenous malformations. Am J Neuroradiol 1992;13:1107–1114.
3 Steiner L, Lindquist C, Adler J, Torner J, Alves W, Steiner M: Clinical outcome of radiosurgery for cerebral arteriovenous malformations. J Neurosurg 1992;77:1–8.
4 Chakraborty DP: Image intensifier distortion correction. Med Phys 1987;14:249–252.
5 Coste E, Rousseau J, Gibon D, Deleume J, Blond S, Marchandise X: Frameless method of stereotaxic localization with DSA. Radiology 1993;189:829–834.
6 Graumann R, Bertram C, Hildebrand T, Hentschel D, Plets P, Sindel C, Zourlides V, Petersen D, Ruder H, Gybels J, Suetens P: Neurovision, a multimodality image fusion package for neuroradiological diagnosis and neurosurgical planning; in Lemke HU, Inamura K, Jaffe CC, Felix R (eds): Computer Assisted Radiology. Heidelberg, Springer, 1993, pp 315–320.
7 Rudin S, Bednarek D, Wong R: Accurate characterization of image intensifier distortion. Med Phys 1991;18:1145–1151.
8 Söderman M, Picard C, Ericson K: An algorithm for correction of the distortion in stereotaxic digital subtraction angiography. Neuroradiology, in press.
9 Bergström M, Greitz T, Ribbe T: A method of stereotaxic localization adopted for conventional and digital radiography. Neuroradiology 1986;28:100–104.

Proc 7th Int Meeting Leksell Gamma Knife® Society,
Island of Lana'i, Hawaii, November 1995
Stereotact Funct Neurosurg 1996;66(suppl 1):71–84

Stereotactic and Functional Neurosurgery

Do We Need Conventional Angiography?

The Role of Magnetic Resonance Imaging in Verifying Obliteration of Arteriovenous Malformations after Gamma Knife Surgery

W.Y. Guo[a], *H.C. Pan*[b], *W.Y. Chung*[b], *L.W. Wang*[c], *M.M.H. Teng*[a]

[a] Department of Radiology, [b] Neurological Institute, and [c] Cancer Center,
Veterans General Hospital-Taipei, and National Yang Ming University, Taiwan

Key Words

Magnetic resonance · Stereotaxy · Gamma Knife radiosurgery · Angiography · Arteriovenous malformation

Abstract

Sixteen cerebral arteriovenous malformations (AVMs) were examined to determine the role of magnetic resonance (MR) imaging in verifying obliteration. The AVMs (mean volume 7.5 cm^3, range 2–17 cm^3) were treated with Gamma Knife surgery between March 1993 and May 1994. Integration of stereotactic MR and stereotactic conventional X-ray angiography (XRA) was used for targeting in the Gamma Knife surgery. All MR examinations, both for targeting and follow-up, were performed on a 1.5-Tesla superconductive MR scanner (Signa). Multiple pulse sequences (spin echo T_1- and T_2-weighted MR imaging, and three-dimensional time-of-flight MR angiography) were used. The mean maximum target dose was 37.4 Gy (range 25.0–44.0 Gy). The mean minimum target dose was 20.1 Gy (range 17.5–25.2 Gy). Follow-up imaging was performed about every 6 months or when clinically warranted. XRA was performed when the AVM was no longer seen on MR images. The time from the last MR image to the XRA was within 1 month in nine patients, and longer in seven. MR imaging demonstrated regressing AVMs in all patients as early as 3 months after Gamma Knife surgery. For seven of the nine patients total obliteration on MR was confirmed on XRA within 1 month. In the other two, previous hemorrhage and adverse radiation effects probably caused overestimation of AVM obliteration. In the remaining seven patients, XRA confirmed the MR observation although the time intervals were longer. It is concluded that, for medium- to large-volume AVMs, MR can demonstrate not only the regressing AVMs but also verify total obliteration. However, verification has to be based on an integration of MR imgaging and MR angiography. The use of MR reduces the invasiveness of Gamma Knife surgery for cerebral AVMs.

KARGER

E-Mail karger@karger.ch
Fax + 41 61 306 12 34
http://www.karger.ch

1011–6125/96/0665–0071$10.00/0

W.Y. Guo, MD, PhD
Department of Radiology
Veterans General Hospital-Taipei
Shih-pai, 11217 Taipei (Taiwan)

Table 1. Patient data, treatment parameters, volume estimation, follow-up and results

Patient No.	Age/sex	Initial clinical presentation of the AVMs	Location	Target dose (max/min) Gy	Estimated nidus volume cm^3	Imaging follow-up months	Treatment result		Adverse radiation effects on MR[a]
							clinical	radiological	
1	49/F	headache, facial numbness	basal ganglion	36/18	3.0	6, 13, 19, 20[b]	improved	CO	+
2	15/F	seizures	temporal lobe	40/20	7.0	7, 12, 19, 22[b]	improved	CO	+[c]
3	20/F	ICH	parietal lobe	40/24	3.0	6, 11, 18, 21[b]	improved	CO	+
4	32/F	seizures	temporoparietal lobe	37/18.5	12.0	3, 6, 12, 21, 22[b]	improved	CO	+[c]
5	44/M	headache, seizures	paraventricular	44/22	7.0	7, 4, 19, 28[b]	improved	CO	+
6	25/M	ICH	frontal lobe	36/25.2	3.0	5, 14, 25[b]	improved	CO	+
7	34/M	seizures	parietal lobe	36/18	18.0	6, 12, 19, 19[b]	improved	CO	+
8	39/M	ICH + SAH	parietal lobe	26/18	8.0	6, 12, 20, 21[b]	improved	CO	+[c]
9	27/M	ICH	pons	25/17.5	2.0	6, 15, 16[b]	improved	CO	+
10	36/M	ICH	corpus callosum	40/20	11.0	7, 13, 20, 20[b]	improved	CO	+
11	23/M	ICH	corpus callosum	40/20	3.0	7, 14, 19[b]	improved	CO	–
12	10/M	IVH	temporo-occipital lobe	40/20	3.0	6, 12, 13[b]	improved	CO	+
13	38/M	ICH	basal ganglion	40/20	3.0	6, 12[b]	improved	CO	+
14	9/F	ICH	thalamus	36/18	17.0	6, 12, 18, 19[b]	improved	minute remnant	+[c]
15	26/M	ICH + IVH	temporal	36/18	14.0	6, 12, 16, 16[b]	improved	ST	–
16	14/F	ICH	temporal	36/25	2.0	7, 13[b]	improved	CO	+

CO = Complete obliteration; ST = subtotal obliteration; IVH = intraventricular hemorrhage; ICH = intracerebral hemorrhage; SAH = subarachnoid hemorrhage.
[a] Observed as high signals on T_2-weighted images.
[b] Followed up with conventional XRA.
[c] Neurological symptoms relevant to the adverse radiation effects were observed in the patients; only one patient had permanent neurological deficits (No. 14).

Introduction

Magnetic resonance imaging (MRI) is a powerful imaging technique to detect intracranial pathology and a reliable imaging modality for targeting in Gamma Knife surgery. For this special clinical application, it is superior to other imaging modalities in many respects. In Gamma Knife surgery for cerebral arteriovenous malformations (AVMs), MRI is complementary to conventional X-ray angiography (XRA). Integration of these two imaging techniques can improve the distinction between the AVM and normal brain and may render large AVMs treatable by Gamma Knife surgery [1–5]. After Gamma Knife surgery, use of nonionizing, noninvasive and high-sensitivity MRI facilitates longitudinal evaluation of Gamma Knife treatments [6–10].

Protection from rebleeding in partially obliterated AVMs is controversial. However, AVMs with *only* an early draining vein and without residual nidus probably represent radiosurgical cure and are free from the risk of rebleeding [11, 12]. Nevertheless, rebleeding occurs if even the smallest remnants of a nidus remain [13]. The goal of Gamma Knife surgery for AVMs is total obliteration, which is usually confirmed by XRA or high-quality digital subtractive angiography. These are invasive procedures, and sometimes the risk of angiographic complications causes patients to resist follow-up. To develop a reliable noninvasive method to verify obliteration of AVMs will not only improve our understanding of Gamma Knife treatment for AVMs but will also enhance the essence of a noninvasive Gamma Knife surgery. A prospective study was conducted to compare MR with XRA as a means of verifying total AVM obliteration.

Patients and Methods

Patient Selection and Imaging Protocol

Sixteen medium- to large-volume AVMs (mean volume 7.5 cm^3, range 2–17 cm^3) were treated between March 1993 and May 1994 by Gamma Knife surgery and were totally obliterated after latent periods in 14 patients (table 1). The AVM volumes were estimated by measuring irradiation volume confirmed within the best-fit isodose shell on dose planning [9]. Total obliteration of AVMs was defined in the study by the total absence of AVM signs on a cerebral angiogram, viewed from the arterial to the venous phases. Inclusion criteria of the patients were (1) AVMs which had been regularly followed using MR about every 6 months after Gamma Knife surgery or when clinically warranted, and (2) when MR did not show a residual nidus, XRA had been performed to verify the MR observation. General data on the AVMs are summarized in table 1. Integration of stereotactic MRI and stereotactic XRA was used for targeting at radiosurgery. All MRI, both for targeting and follow-up, was performed on a 1.5-Tesla superconductive MR scanner (Signa). In the first year, version 5.3 was used; thereafter, version 5.4. Pulse sequences including spin echo (SE) T_1- and T_2-weighted MRI, three-dimensional time-of-flight MR angiography (3D TOF MRA) were

Table 2. Pulse sequences and imaging parameters used in the study

	Pulse sequences repetition time/ echo time, ms	Image	Approximate scanning time	Remarks
2D SE[a] (0.5 NEX)	500/11	T1WI[b] (transaxial)	0 min 47 s	only for positioning checkup in stereotactic MR
2D SE[a] (2 NEX)	500/11	T1WI (coronal)	3 min 41 s	for targeting and follow-up
2D SE[a] (2 NEX)	500/11	T1WI (sagittal)	3 min 41 s	for targeting and follow-up
2D SE[a] (4 NEX)	500/11	T1WI (transaxial)	7 min 30 s	for targeting and follow-up
2D FSE[a] (2 NEX)	2,700/80	T2WI (transaxial)	2 min 30 s	for targeting and follow-up
3D TOF[d] (1 NEX)	50/3.1	MR angiography[c]	7 min 0 s	for targeting and follow-up
Total		Six pulse sequences	25 min 9 s	total scanning time is less than 60 min (including preparation, positioning and prescan)

Field of view = 260 × 260 mm. 2D = Two-dimensional; 3D = three-dimensional; SE = spin echo; FSE = fast spin echo; NEX = number of acquisitions; TOF = time-of-flight (in version 5.3, 3D TOF capable of magnetization transfer was available, while in version 5.4, 3D/TOF/SPGR was used); T1WI = T_1-weighted image; T2WI = T_2-weighted image.

[a] For 2D SE images, slice thickness/interslice space = 3/0 mm, matrix = 512 × 256.

[b] Slice thickness/interslice space = 3/17 mm.

[c] For MR angiography, the flip angle is 15°, slice thickness is between 0.7 and 1.5 mm, depending on the size of the AVMs.

[d] Matrix is 512 × 256.

used. To maximize inflow enhancement involved in the scanned volume, the volume of 3D TOF MRA was oriented in the transaxial plane. The total scanning time, including preparation, positioning and prescan, did not exceed 60 min (table 2). SE images, source and collapsed images of the 3D TOF MRA were used to evaluate the detailed vasculature of the AVMs (table 2).

Irradiation and Criteria of Obliteration on MR

The mean maximum target dose ws 37.4 Gy (range 25.0–44.0 Gy). The mean minimum target dose was 20.1 Gy (range 11.5–25.2 Gy).

AVMs were observed as flow void on the SE MR images, that is to say, low signals. In flow-sensitive pulse sequences (3D TOF MRA), the flow voids become high signals. Total obliteration on MR was indicated when both the low signals on SE and the high signals on 3D TOF MRA were no longer observed (fig. 1).

XRA was performed after AVMs were no longer visualized by MR. Time intervals between the last MR and the XRA were less than 1 month in nine patients. For the other seven patients, the last MR displayed a minute nidus remnant. For logistic reasons, the time lags were longer than 1 month in these patients.

Results

After Gamma Knife surgery, MR demonstrated early AVM regression in all patients, from as early as 3 months. For seven of the nine patients with shorter time intervals from the last MR to XRA, total obliteration observed on MR was confirmed by XRA. Confirmation of AVM obliteration occured 13–22 months after Gamma Knife surgery. One of the patients rebled before total obliteration (patient No. 7). On 3D TOF MRA, products of hemoglobin appeared as bright signals next to the AVM and could be confused with a residual nidus, which was, however, excluded, because they were also bright on SE MRI (fig. 2).

Of the other two patients, one had a minute remnant and the other had no nidus but early opacification of a draining vein. These changes were demonstrated on XRA even though MR had shown 'total obliteration.' In the former case (patient No. 14), the minute remnant was erroneously missed on the MR, which may be related to some superimposed signal aberration derived from adverse radiation effects (fig. 3). In the later case (patient No. 15), the 'microscopic' AV shunting was beyond the spatial resolution of the current computerized imaging techniques. The problems in this case were compounded by changes due to previous hemorrhage in the region of interest. In the other seven patients whose time lags between the last MR and XRA were longer than 1 month, XRA confirmed the MR observation 12–28 months after Gamma Knife surgery.

Discussion

Characteristics of the Study and Imaging Techniques

Total cover of an AVM nidus with an adequate radiation dose is essential for successful Gamma Knife treatment. In the current series, based on integration of stereotactic XRA and MR, coverage of the nidi had been considered optimal. Moreover, both in targeting and in the follow-up, the MR scanner and the pulse sequences used were the same. This homogeneous material made the longitudinal study of treatment results feasible and reliable.

Total obliteration on MR was based on the integration of multiple pulse sequences. It is one of our concerns to keep total scanning time within 1 h both in stereotactic and follow-up MR. Thus, we had to modify the imaging protocol as follows. Demonstration of all fiducial markers requires expansion of the field of view (FOV) to a minimum of 26 cm. To compensate for the concomitant depreciation in spatial resolution, the imaging matrix had to increase, in this study to 256 × 512. The scanning time was, consequently, increased. Larger lesions also take more time to scan. However, our latest MR software (version 5.4) can perform multislab 3D TOF MRA. In the multislab technique, the advantages of the

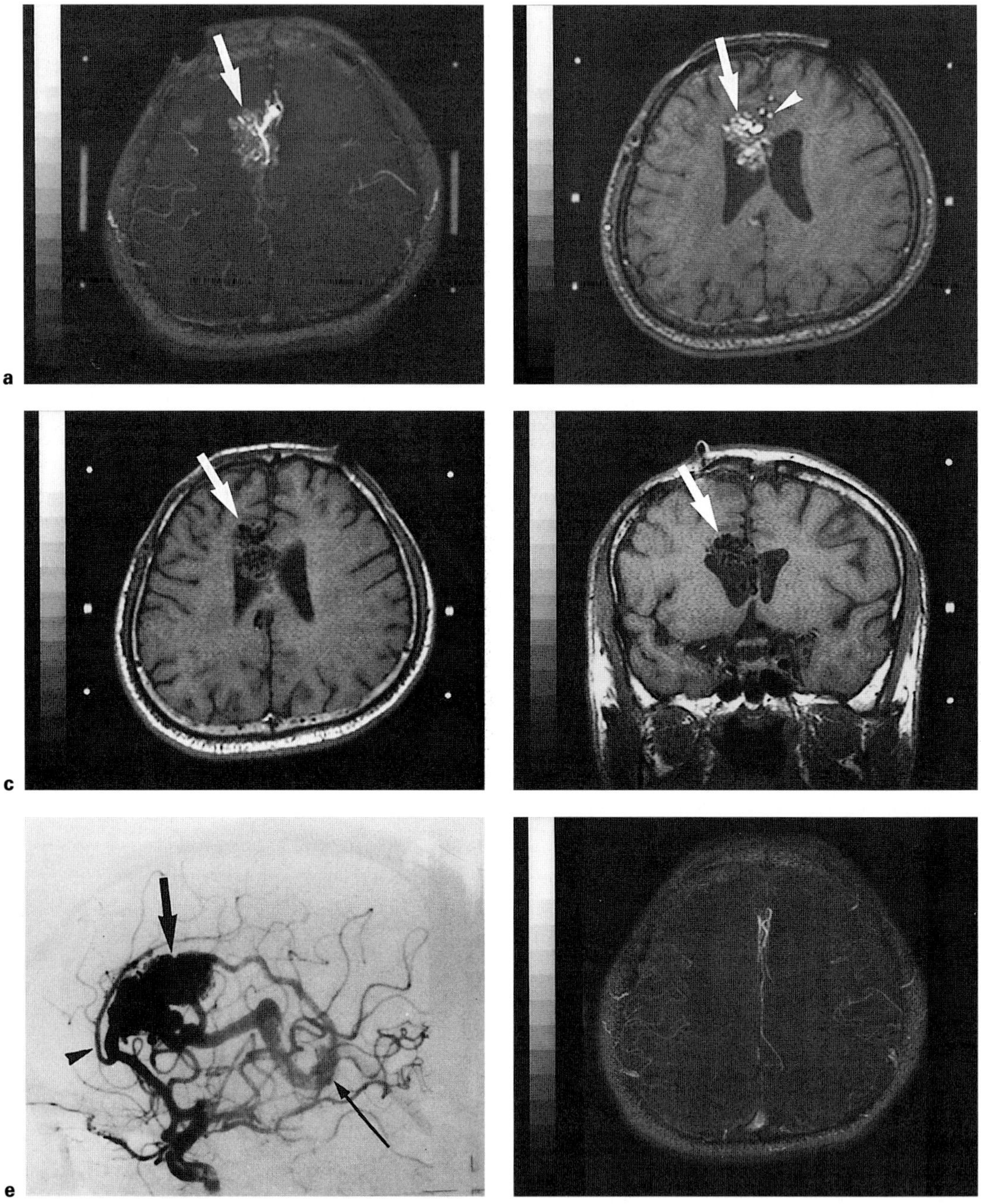
a
b
c
d
e
f

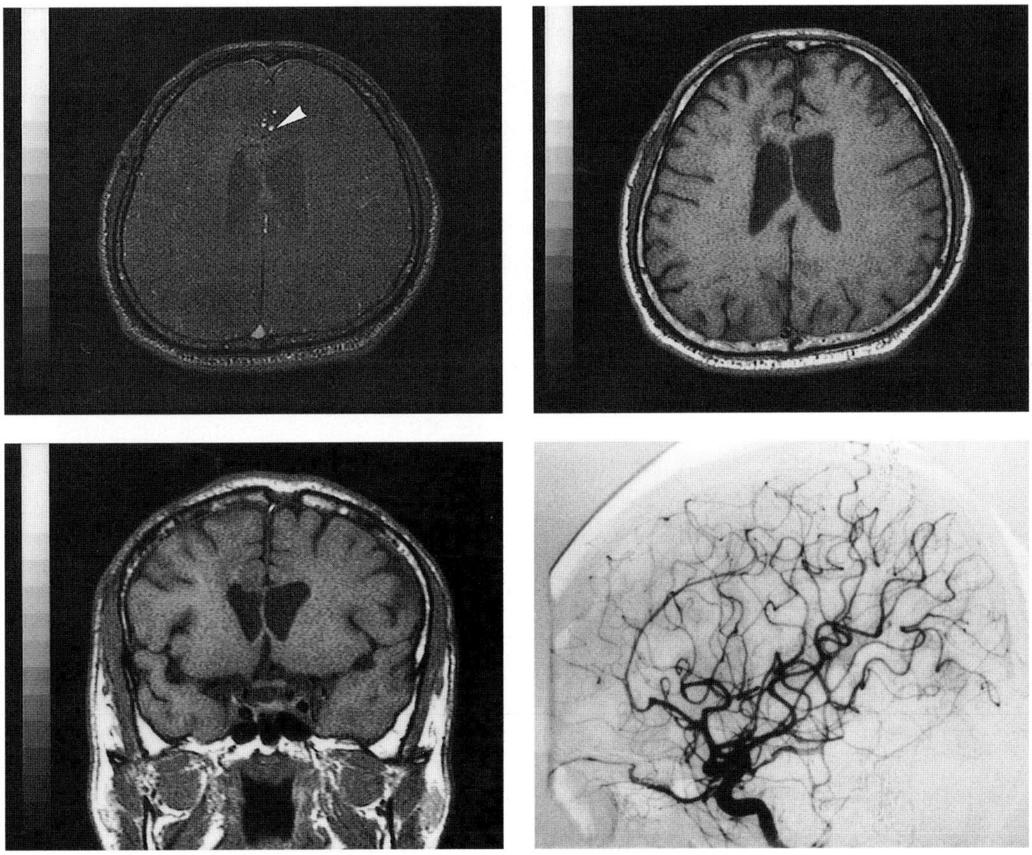

g h i j

Fig. 1. Corpus callosum AVM (patient No. 10). **a–e** Before Gamma Knife surgery. **a** 3D TOR MRA collapsed view showed the AVM as high signals (arrow). **b** One of the source images of the MRA showed the flowing blood in the AVM nidus (arrow) and its feeding artery (arrow head) as high signals. **c, d** 2D SE transaxial (**c**) and coronal (**d**) MR images showed the AVM nidus as flow voids (arrow). **e** Lateral view of stereotactic angiogram, used for treatment planning, showing the engorged feeders (arrow head), pericallosal artery, the nidus (arrow), and the deep venous drainage of the AVM (long arrow). **f–j** The AVM was treated by Gamma Knife surgery with a mxaimum target dose of 40 Gy and a minimum target dose of 20 Gy. Nidus volume was estimated to be 11 ml. Twenty months after surgery, on 3D TOF/SPGR MRA collapsed view (**f** and one of the source images (**g**), the AVM was no longer visualized, the feeding arteries (pericallosal artery) were patent and remain observed as high signals (arrow head). On 2D SE transaxial (**h**) and coronal (**i**) MR images no flow voids in the previous AVM region were observed. **j** Lateral view of the follow-up angiogram performed at 20 months after surgery showed total obliteration of the AVM and confirmed the MR observations.

high-spatial-resolution 3D technique were maintained while progressive saturation effects were reduced [14]. This enabled us to encompass larger AVMs or the entire intracranial vasculature with the same scanning time as for the repeated single-slab technique. For radiosurgery, we focused the volumes of interest only on the AVMs and ignored the remote structures. Special attention was paid to the vasculature detail of AVMs. The multislab 3D TOF was not used. These technical adaptations enabled us to optimize imaging techniques and improve the imaging, with increased spatial resolution and reduced intravoxel dephasing. This strategy is somewhat different from routine diagnostic procedures.

In the study, XRA was planned as soon as possible after MR showed total obliteration. A 1-month interval seemed to be clinically reasonable. In seven patients, for logistic reasons, the time intervals were longer. Nevertheless, total obliteration was confirmed in the 'late' XRA. This observation supported the notion that if the AVM nidus had been accurately covered with an adequate radiation dose, total obliteration should be expected at an appropriate time after Gamma Knife surgery.

To enhance the essence of the noninvasiveness of Gamma Knife surgery – a bladeless surgery – no MR contrast medium was administered in the study. In other words, 'needleless imaging' was prescribed. Contrast medium increases the signal-to-noise ratio by shortening the T_1 time of blood, and thus reducing the effects of saturation on slow flow components of AVMs [14]. Thus a minute AVM remnant may be more visible in a contrast-enhanced MR study. Unfortunately, not only signals from blood but also those from stationary tissues are enhanced. The background enhancement degrades the imaging quality and probably reduces the chance of verifying total obliteration. The situation is even worse if adverse radiation effects, such as blood-brain barrier breakdown, have occurred.

Pitfalls in the Imaging Study

Rebleeding before total obliteration is not uncommon [12, 13]. The hemorrhage and its degradation display various signals on MRI. In SE pulse sequences, hemosiderin and calcification resulting from an old hemorrhage or thrombus could have the same signals as flow voids, on both T_1- and T_2-weighted images. The similarity in signals confuses a differentiation using SE images. However, in flow-sensitive pulse sequences, e.g., TOF, the hemosiderin gives low signals in contrast to bright signals from flow. This confusion is resolved by integrating the different pulse sequences. Interestingly, for subacute hemorrhage, the breakdown products of hemoglobin (for example, methemoglobin) are bright on TOF, similar to flowing blood [15]. The high signals on TOF make comparison with SE images necessary, since the high methemoglobin signals on SE exclude the possibility of flow voids (fig. 2).

Adverse radiation effects are observed in AVM patients after Gamma Knife surgery, occuring in 30–40% of patients on MRI irrespective of clinical significance [16]. Adverse radiation effects can cause signal aberration on MR images, and misleading interpretations (fig. 3). For example, in patient No. 14, MR at 18 months was erroneously interpreted as 'total obliteration,' although reexamination indicated evidence of a minute remnant.

For subtotally obliterated AVMs, early opacification of draining veins on XRA is the only abnormality in terms of hemodynamics. The microscopic AV shunting which is probably involved is beyond the spatial resolution of current imaging modalities, both XRA and MRI. Total obliteration has been the only goal of treatment. However, AVMs with only an early draining vein and without residual nidus may represent radiosurgical cure and are free from the risk of rebleeding [12]. MRI could play some role in verifying treatment results.

Our conclusions based on the small series of this comparative study are as follows.

(1) MR is far superior to any other imaging modality in demonstrating regressing AVMs in a completely noninvasive manner.

(For fig. 2 see pages 80 and 81.)

Fig. 2. Right motor cortex AVM (patient No. 7). **a–e** Before Gamma Knife surgery. **a** 3D TOF MRA collapsed view showed the AVM as high signals (arrow). **b** One of the MRA source images showed the flowing blood of the AVM nidus (long arrow) in the brain parenchyma and its feeding arteries (short arrows) as high signals in the relevant cortical cerebrospinal fluid (CSF) space. **c, d** 2D SE transaxial (**c**) and coronal (**d**) MR images showed the AVM nidus as flow voids (long arrow) and the feeding arteries in the CSF space (short arrow). **e** Lateral view of the stereotactic angiogram, used for treatment planning, showed the engorged feeders-callosomarginal arteries (small arrowhead), and the nidus (long arrow) of the AVM. For Gamma Knife surgery, only the nidus of the AVM was outlined as a target. The engorged feeding arteries (short arrow) in the CSF space were considered secondary to the AVM and not covered by the effected irradiation dose level. The AVM was then treated with a maximum target dose of 36 Gy and a minimum target dose of 18 Gy. The volume of the nidus was estimated to be 18 ml. **f** Twelve months after surgery, one of the source images showed the conspicuously regressed AVM nidus (long arrow). **g–j** Nineteen months after Gamma Knife Surgery. On one of the source images of 3D TOF/SPGR MRA (**g**) the AVM was no longer visualized on the same area. However, on the collapsed view (**h**) and one of the source images (**i**) cranial to **g**, high signals were observed in the right high parietal region (large arrowhead). On the MRA images, a hemorrhage might have the same signals as flowing blood. On 2D SE transaxial (**j**) and coronal (**k**) MR images, no flow voids in the previous AVM region were observed, but there was a high-signal subacute hemorrhage (large arrowhead). Conventional angiography was then performed. **l** Lateral view of the follow-up angiogram showing the total obliteration and confirming the MR observation.

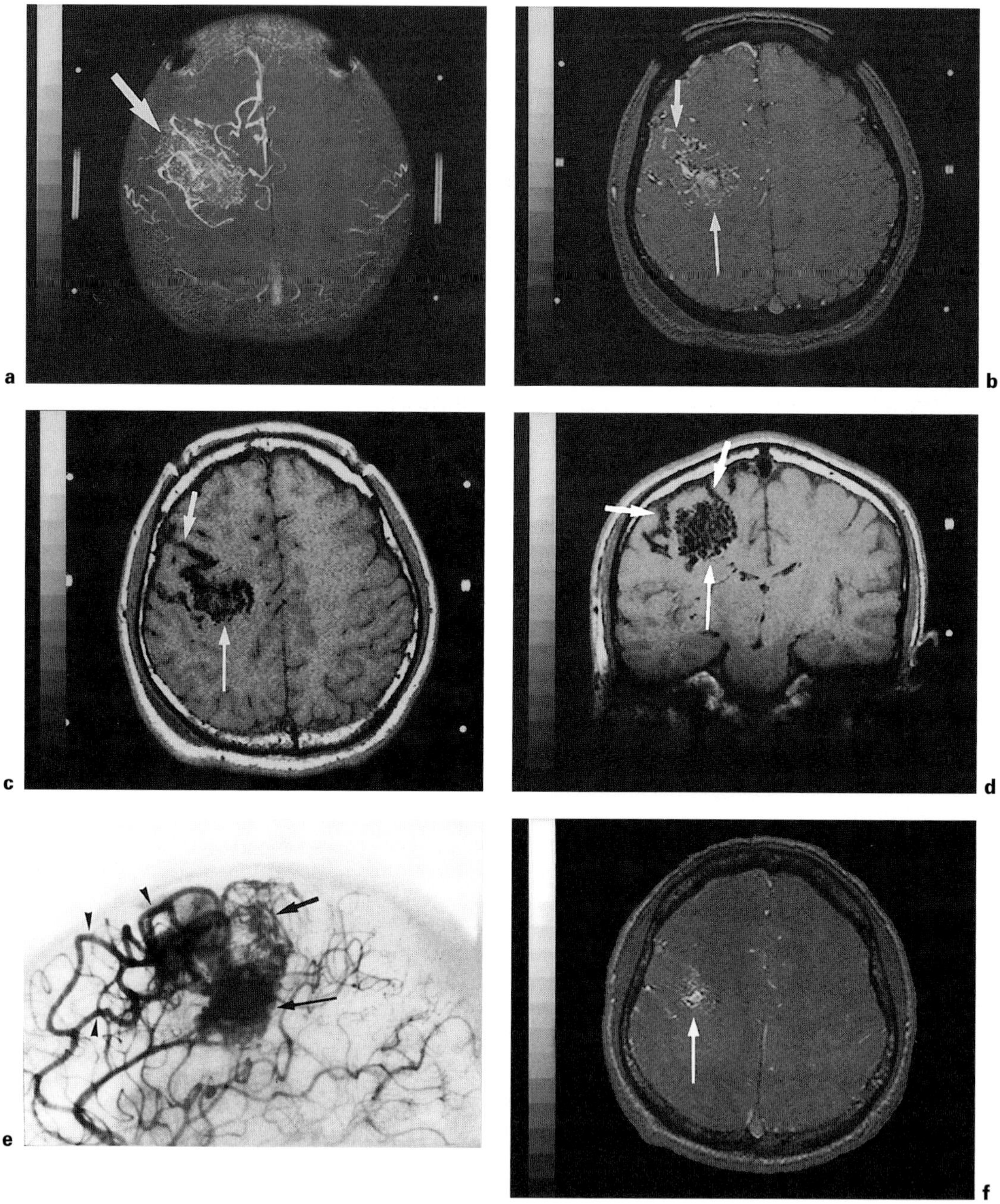

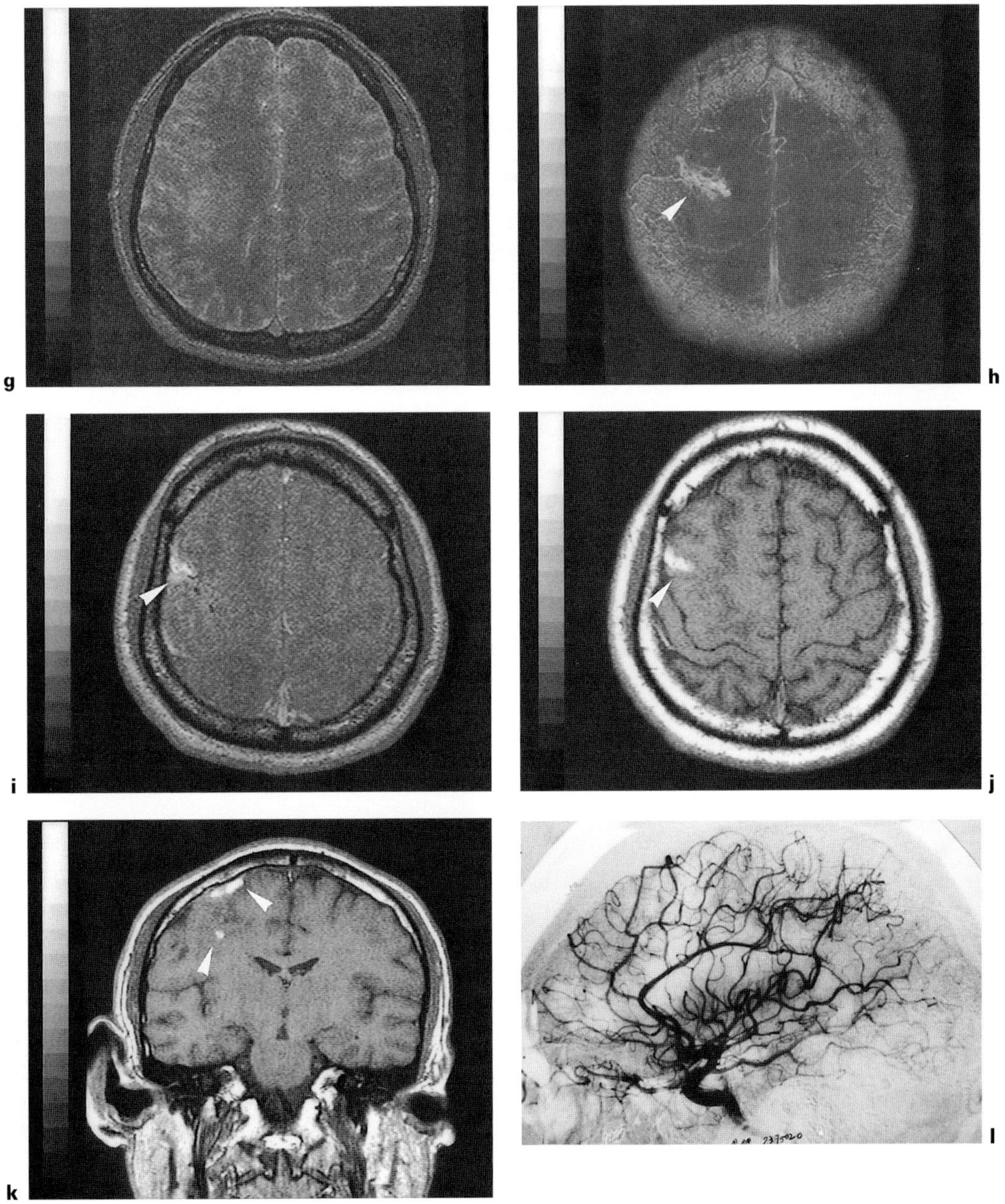

(For legend fig. 2 see page 79.)

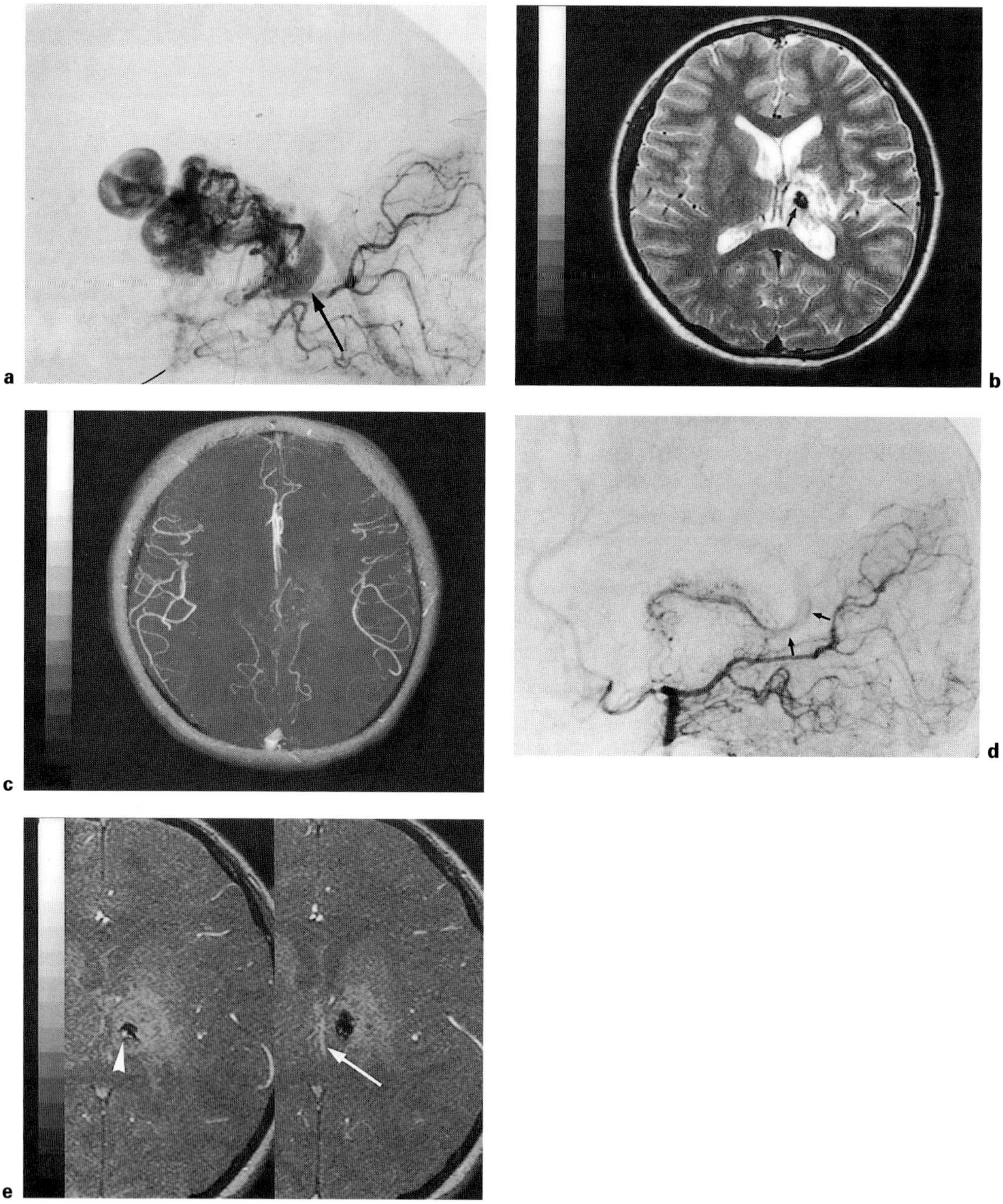

(2) With multiple sequences, MRI provides almost the same accuracy as conventional angiography in verifying totally obliterated AVMs. This is particularly true for medium- to large-volume AVMs without previous hemorrhage or adverse radiation effects.

(3) In the current development of MR technology, stereotactic XRA remains needed. Integration of stereotactic MRI and XRA is a guarantee of good results.

(4) If proper coverage of AVMs in Gamma Knife surgery is ensured, minute remnants can be observed on MR. Further MR follow-up some months later may demonstrate complete obliteration.

(5) Improving MR technology, i.e., providing better temporal and spatial resolution, will show the strength of MR in the near future. The application of MRI has further minimized the invasiveness of Gamma Knife surgery for AVMs.

Acknowledgment

The study was supported in part by research grant number NSC 85-2331-B-075-105, Veterans General Hospital-Taipei research grant number 333, 1996, and the Tjing-Ling Neurological Foundation.

Fig. 3. Patient with left thalamic AVM (No. 14). **a** Before Gamma Knife surgery on a lateral view of the stereotactic angiogram, the thalamic AVM was supplied by thalamoperforating arteries and a prominent posterior choroidal artery, and took the internal cerebral vein (ICV) and vein of Galen for drainage (long arrow). A venous aneurysmal dilatation was observed anterior to the AVM. The AVM was treated by Gamma Knife surgery with a maximum target dose of 36 Gy and a minimum target dose of 18 Gy. The nidus volume was estimated to be 17 ml. **b** Eighteen months after surgery, on one of the T_2-weighted (T2W) images, high-signal adverse radiation effects were observed. The low signal (short arrow) in the center was considered to be a calcification, old thrombus or hemosiderin after previous hemorrhage. However, no flow void on the T2W image was noted in the AVM region. **c** 3D TOF MRA collapsed view showed the minute high signal dots and prominent left ICV compared to the right side. These subtle findings were easily missed and the AVM was considered 'obliterated'. Conventional angiography was then performed at 19 months after Gamma Knife surgery. **d** Unfortunately, on a lateral view of the follow-up vertebral angiogram, minute remnants of the AVM with early opacification of the ICV remained (arrow). **e** On a composite image of two consecutive source images of the 3D TOF MRA, abnormal high signals were observed (arrowhead) and the left ICV (long arrow) was larger than on the right side. In summary, these high-signal dots and enlarged ICV may indicate that the AVM was not yet totally obliterated. The subtle AVM remnant can be easily missed, especially when adverse radiation effects occur and the signal aberration confuses the imaging observation.

References

1 Guo WY, Nordell B, Karlsson B, Soderman M, Lindquist M, Ericson K, Franck A, Lax I, Lindquist C: Target delineation in radiosurgery for cerebral arteriovenous malformations: Assessment of the value of stereotactic MR imaging and MR angiography. Acta Radiol 1993;34:457–463.

2 Kauczor HU, Engenhart R, Layer G, Gamroth AH, Wowra B: 3D TOF MR angiography of cerebral arteriovenous malformations after radiosurgery. J Comput Assist Tomogr 1993;17:184–190.

3 Petereit D, Mehta M, Turski P, Levin A, Strother C, Mistretta C, Mackie R, Gehring M, Kubsad S, Kinsella T: Treatment of arteriovenous malformations with stereotactic radiosurgery employing both magnetic resonance angiography and standard as a database. Int J Radiat Oncol Biol Phys 1993;25:309–313.

4 Phillips MH, Kessler M, Chuang FY, Frankel KA, Lyman JT, Fabrikant JI, Levy RP: Image correlation of MRI and CT in treatment for radiosurgery of intracranial vascular malformations. Int J Radiat Oncol Biol Phys 1991;20:881–889.

5 Ehricke HH, Schad LR, Gademann G, Wowra B, Engenhart R, Lorenz WJ: Use of MR angiography for stereotactic planning. J Comput Assist Tomogr 1992;16:35–40.

6 Guo WY, Lindquist C, Karlsson B, Kihlstrom L, Steiner L: Gamma Knife surgery of cerebral arteriovenous malformations: Serial MR imaging studies after radiosurgery. Int J Radiat Oncol Biol Phys 1993;25:315–323.

7 Kihlstrom L, Guo WY, Lindquist C, Mindus P: Radiobiology of radiosurgery for refractory anxiety disorders. Neurosurgery 1995;36:294–302.

8 Quisling RG, Peters KR, Friedman WA, Tart RP: Persistent nidus blood flow in cerebral arteriovenous malformation after stereotactic radiosurgery: MR imaging assessment. Radiology 1991;180:785–791.

9 Guo WY, Pan DHC, Liu RS, Chung WY, Shiau CY, Cheng SS, Chang CY, Chen KY, Yeh SH, Lee LS: Early irradiation effects observed on magnetic resonance imaging and angiography, and positron emission tomography for arteriovenous malformations treated by Gamma Knife radiosurgery. Stereotact Funct Neurosurg 1995;64(suppl 1):258–269.

10 Pan DHC, Guo WY, Chung WY, Shiau CY, Liu RS, Lee LS: Early effects of Gamma Knife surgery on malignant and benign intracranial tumors. Stereotact Funct Neurosurg 1995;64(suppl 1):19–31.

11 Steiner L, Lindquist C, Adler JR, Torner JC, Steiner M: Clinical outcome of radiosurgery for cerebral arteriovenous malformations. J Neurosurg 1992;77:1–8.

12 Pollock BE, Flickinger JC, Lunsford LD, Bissonette D, Kondziolka DS: Hemorrhage risk after stereotactic radiosurgery of arteriovenous malformations. 2nd Congr Int Stereotact Radiosurg Soc, Boston, June 1995, p 28.

13 Guo WY, Karlsson B, Ericson K, Lindqvist M: Even the smallest remnant of an AVM constitutes a risk of further bleeding. Acta Neurochir 1993;121:212–215.

14 Anderson CM, Edelman RR, Turski PA: Magnetic resonance angiography of vascular malformations; in Anderson CM (ed): Clinical Magnetic Resonance Angiography. New York, Raven Press, 1993, pp 247–285.

15 Yousem DM, Balakrishnan J, Debrun GM, Bryan RN: Hyperintense thrombus on GRASS MR images: Potential pitfall in flow evaluation. Am J Neuroradiol 1990;11:51–58.

16 Guo WY: Radiological aspects of Gamma Knife radiosurgery for arteriovenous malformations and other non-tumoural disorders of the brain. Acta Radiol 1993;34(suppl):388.

Proc 7th Int Meeting Leksell Gamma Knife® Society,
Island of Lana'i, Hawaii, November 1995
Stereotact Funct Neurosurg 1996;66(suppl 1):85–92

Stereotactic and Functional Neurosurgery

An Evaluation of the Accuracy of Magnetic-Resonance-Guided Gamma Knife Surgery

W.Y. Guo[a], *W.C. Chu*[d], *M.C. Wu*[d], *W.Y. Chung*[b], *W.P. Gwan*[e], *Y.L. Lee*[e], *H.C. Pan*[b], *C.Y. Chang*[a]

[a] Department of Radiology,
[b] Neurological Institute, and
[c] Cancer Center, Veterans General Hospital-Taipei;
[d] Institute of Biomedical Engineering, and
[e] Department of Medical Technique, National Yang Ming University, Taipei, Taiwan

Key Words

Stereotactic Magnetic Resonance · Gamma Knife Radiosurgery · Dosimeter Gel

Abstract

An evaluation of the systematic accuracy of magnetic resonance (MR)-guided Gamma Knife surgery was performed. In two experiments, a cylinder phantom filled with dosimeter gel containing ferrous sulfate was fixed to a stereotactic frame. The gel phantom was irradiated with the Gamma Knife with a single shot using 4-mm collimators. The target point was set at the frame center of the stereotactic system giving coordinate values of X = 100, Y = 100, Z = 100. The maximum target dose was 15 Gy. MR imaging was undertaken immediately after the irradiation, using a superconductive 1.5-T MR scanner. Spin echo T_1-weighted images, with transaxial, coronal, and sagittal views, were obtained. On the images, points with the highest signals were defined as the target point which received the maximum dose. Within the dose range of the experiment, this definition is based on a linear relationship between the dose to the gel and the T_1 relaxation shortening after irradiation. The distances between the frame center and the target point defined on the MR images in the experiments were 0.12 mm (0.2375 pixels) and 0.43 mm (0.8515 pixels), respectively. Both are within the mechanical accuracy of the Gamma Knife. The imaging study confirms the accuracy of the Gamma Knife surgery used in the institution.

KARGER

E-Mail karger@karger.ch
Fax + 41 61 306 12 34
http://www.karger.ch

1011–6125/96/0665–0085$10.00/0

W.Y. Guo, MD, PhD
Department of Radiology
Veterans General Hospital-Taipei
Shih-pai, 11217 Taipei (Taiwan)

Introduction

In radiosurgery, a bladeless surgery, radiation to the surrounding tissues must be minimized. Thus, avoiding potential radiation-induced biological or physiological changes to the surrounding tissues is an essential factor in dose planning and dose prescription. This is in contrast to conventional radiotherapy, where a large volume (usually several hundred cubic centimeters) is irradiated with fractionated doses. In radiosurgery, a restricted target of a few cubic centimeters is radiated effectively during a single session, imposing the necessity for an accurate and precise targeting system. Though some other radiation machines may provide similar treatment effects, the Leksell Gamma Knife has set the standard with regard to safety, efficacy, and reliability [1–5].

During bladeless procedures, surgeons cannot visualize the target lesions directly. Stereotactic imaging precedes the procedure and is an essential component of the treatment. Magnetic resonance (MR) imaging is one of the most widely used diagnostic imaging methods and is ideally suited for this purpose [6]. However, to ensure treatment quality, the accuracy of the system has to be regularly checked for errors in the data and its transfer between the MR scanner and the Gamma Knife. In this study, a ferrous sulfate dosimeter gel was used to evaluate information about the radiation target. The rationale is that the T_1 relaxation rate of the gel varies linearly with the absorbed radiation dose [7–10]. The difference in T_1 relaxation created by the radiation provides signal contrast on MR images to enable location of the target.

Materials and Methods

Radiation

A cylindrical phantom (width 5.6 cm, height 15.2 cm) filled with ferrous sulfate dosimeter gel and subsequently fixed to a Leksell stereotactic frame system was used for this study. The radiation procedures followed the usual routine for Gamma Knife surgery. A single radiation shot was delivered using the 4-mm collimators. The target point for the radiation was set to be (X, Y, Z) = (100, 100 100). The radiation parameters are listed in table 1.

MR Imaging

Immediately after the radiation, stereotactic MR imaging was performed on a 1.5-T MR scanner (Signa) using the imaging parameters listed in table 2. Two experiments were undertaken using the same irradiation and imaging parameters.

During imaging, the center of the magnetic system of the MR scanner in the Z direction was aligned with the Leksell MR indicator box at Z = 100. Seven transaxial images were obtained, with the middle one (the fourth) passing through the frame center, using T_1-weighted spin echo pulse sequences. Coronal and sagittal views were obtained in the same way. The slice thickness and spacing were 3.0 and 0 mm, respectively.

Table 1. Parameters for the phantom Gamma Knife surgery

Parameter	Value
Gamma angle	90
Grid size	1.0 mm
Collimator size	4 mm
Weighted	1
Shots for superposition	1
Dose matrix center	100, 100, 100
Reference point for absolute dose	100, 100, 100
Desired dose at reference point	15 Gy
Focus position	dose matrix center

Table 2. Parameters for the MR imaging

Parameter	Value
MR scanner	GE Signa 1.5 T
Coil type	head coil
Pulse sequence	spin echo
Patient entry	head first
Image mode	2 Dim
Echo time	20 ms
Repetition time	500 ms
Number of echoes	1
Acquisition matrix	512×512
Scan thickness	3 mm
Field of view	26×26 cm^2

Location of the target point on the MR images was based on the reaction of the gel to ionizing radiation [7–10]. The components of the gel consist of a mixture of agarose, NaCl, H_2SO_4, $(NH_4)2Fe(SO_4)_2 \cdot 6H_2O$ and water. After irradiation, the ferrous (Fe^{2+}) ion transforms into a ferric (Fe^{3+}) ion with a concentration proportional to the irradiation dose it has received [11]. This change causes a T_1 shortening, which manifests as a signal enhancement on the MR images. A plot of this relationship is shown in figure 1.

To reduce calculation error, the center of mass (COM) method is adopted in all calculations, which gives results to a fraction of a pixel [12].

Determination of Stereotactic Frame Center on MR Images

The three-dimensional (3D) physical location of the frame center, X = 100, Y = 100, and Z = 100, is obtained by integrating the fiducial markers visualized on the MR images with the built-in cursor report system of the MR scanner. First, the (X, Y) coordinates of the

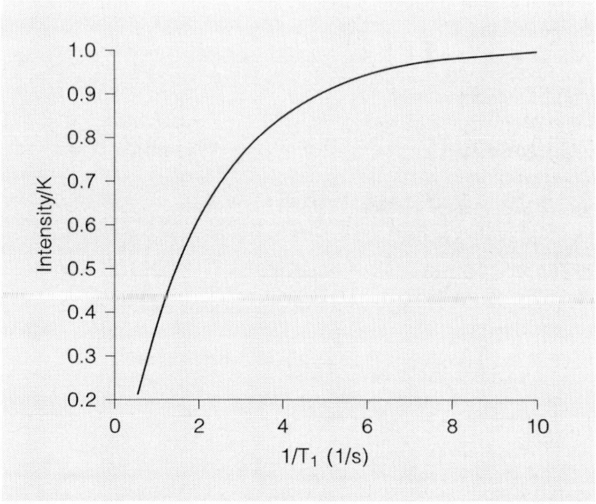

1

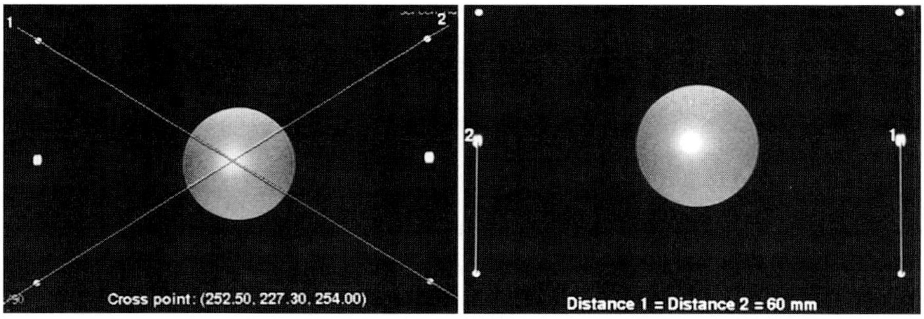

2

Fig. 1. A plot of intensity vs. $1/T_1$, where image intensity increases as $1/T_1$ increases. In the plot, repetition time/echo time (TE) = 500/20 ms. T_2 is assumed to be large compared to TE, so its decay is ignored. After irradiation, locations where high radiation dose absorption occurred will have a high image intensity.

Fig. 2. The line intersection (frame center projecting on the selected image) from the fiducial markers of the transaxial MR image is at (252.50, 227.30, 254.00), where the Z coordinate is calculated according to the procedure described in the text.

Fig. 3. The three different views – transaxial, coronal, and sagittal (from top to bottom) – of the irradiated phantom of the first experiment. Coordinates of the target point of irradiation are (252.40, 227.50, *), (253.00, *, 253.60), and (*, 227.30, 254.30), for transaxial, coronal and sagittal views, respectively, where * means the corresponding coordinate cannot be determined from that view. The mean value of the three gives the target point COM coordinates which are (252.70, 227.40, 253.95).

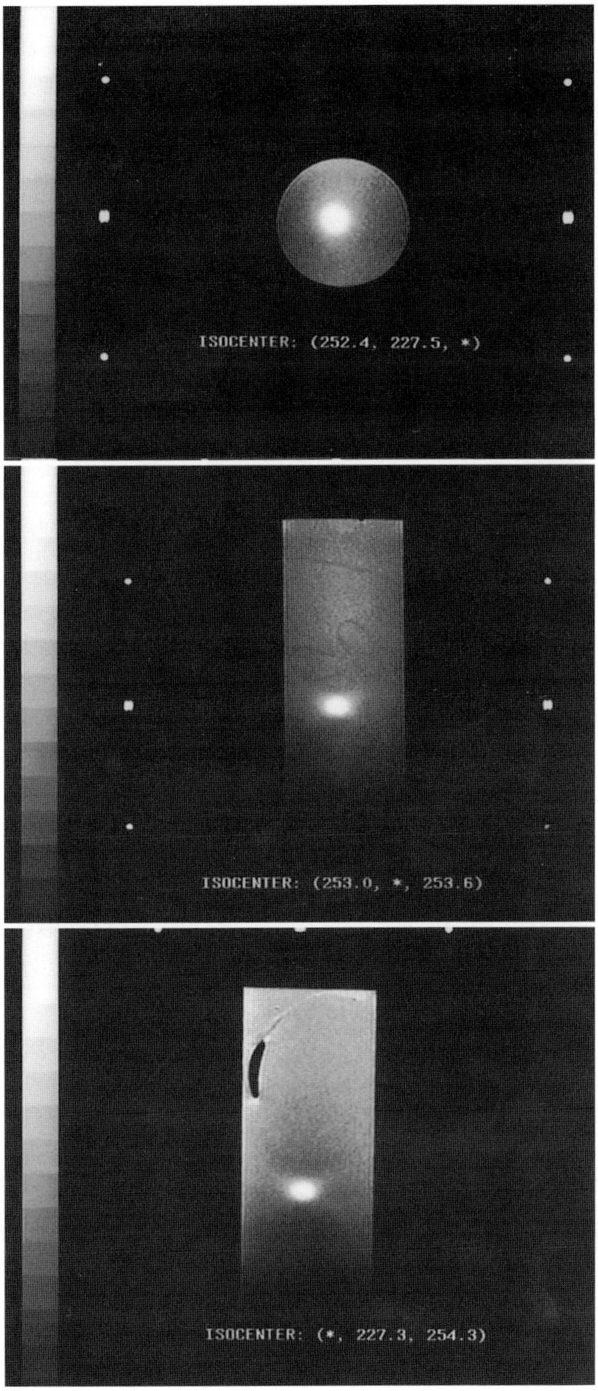
ISOCENTER: (252.4, 227.5, *)
ISOCENTER: (253.0, *, 253.6)
ISOCENTER: (*, 227.3, 254.3)

3

frame center are acquired from the intersections of the fiducial markers in the transaxial image (fig. 2). However, this method cannot be used for the direct determination of the (X, Z) and (Y, Z) coordinates of the frame center on the coronal and sagittal images, due to susceptibility artifacts derived from the indicator box and the metal basal ring of the stereotactic devices which can distort the MR images in nonaxial planes. Instead, in the current study, we selected a transaxial image that contains the highest target intensity for determination of Z coordinates. The image is usually the middle one; in the current study the fourth image. The Z coordinate of the selected plane is measured to be 100. On MR images, the plane usually has 's (superior) = 0' according to the MR coordinate system. This means that the plane passes through the isocenter of the magnetic system in the Z direction. These values are then transformed into pixel units via the cursor report system of the MR scanner. The frame center is, thereby, retrievable and can be displayed both on coronal and sagittal views with higher reliability than with a direct measurement. This coordinate determination method has been routinely used in our institution for Gamma Knife surgery.

Determination of the Irradiation Target Point on MR Images

Three different views – transaxial, coronal, and sagittal – of the irradiated phantom are shown in figure 3. The point which has the highest signal is the target point or, in other words, the radiation isocenter. By using the COM method, two coordinates are obtained pixelwise on each view. Mean coordinate values give the coordinates of the target point.

Results

In the first experiment, the coordinates of the frame center on MR images were (252.50, 227.30, 254.03), while the coordinates of the target point were (252.70, 227.40, 253.95). The difference between these two points was (0.2, 0.1, –0.08), which corresponds to 0.2375 pixels or 0.12 mm. In the second experiment, the point coordinates were (251.40, 227.50, 256.00) and (251.40, 227.45, 255.15), respectively. The absolute distance between the points was 0.8515 pixels or 0.43 mm (table 3). Both values are within the mechanical accuracy (0.5 mm) of the Gamma Knife [5].

Discussion

In these experiments we found that the deviations between the target point and the stereotactic frame center were small for the X and Y coordinates, while in the Z direction, a relatively larger deviation occurred, believed to be due to the 3.0 mm image thickness in the stereotactic MR imaging. The thickness causes partial volume effects, which summate all the signals within this thickness. As a result, in the worst situation, a maximum shift of one-half of a slice thickness may occur, as seen in figure 4. To keep this deviation to a minimum, careful control of the posi-

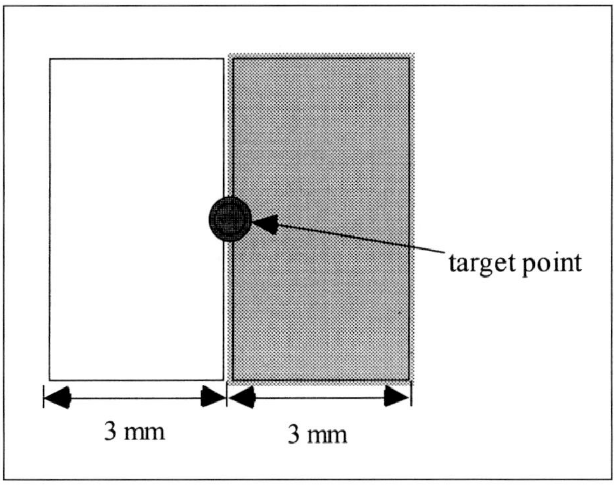

Fig. 4. Due to partial volume effects, a maximum shift of half a slice thickness may occur between the actual coordinate of the target point and the coordinate obtained from the image slice number on which it is assumed to be located.

Table 3. Coordinates of the target point (TP), frame center (FC) and their distances

	Experiment	
	1	2
Coordinates of FC on MR, X, Y, Z	252.50, 227.30, 254.03	251.40, 227.50, 256.00
Coordinates of TP on MR, X, Y, Z	252.70, 227.40, 254.95	251.40, 227.45, 255.15
Difference between FC and TP, pixels	0.2375	0.8515
Difference between FC and TP, mm	0.12	0.43

tioning of the scanned subject is recommended. A better alignment of the center of the Leksell MR indicator box with the center of the magnetic system of the MR scanner in the Z direction can reduce errors derived from partial volume effects. Another possibility would be the application of 3D MR imaging techniques. In 3D techniques, a thinner slice thickness is used, which can reduce the deviation derived from partial volume effects.

In conclusion, this dosimeter gel study has shown that (1) the accuracy of the MR-guided Gamma Knife surgery in our institution is equivalent to the mechanical accuracy of the Gamma Knife itself, (2) stereotactic MR imaging is suitable for both diagnosis and stereotactic purposes, and (3) regular system checks are necessary to ensure that everything is working properly and that a high quality of clinical treatment is provided.

Acknowledgment

This study was supported in part by research grant number NSC 85-2331-B-075-105 and Veterans General Hospital-Taipei research grant number 333, 1996.

References

1 Larsson B, Leksell L, Rexed B, Saurander P: The high energy proton beam as a neurological tool. Nature 1958;182:1222–1223.
2 Leksell L: The stereotactic method and radiosurgery of the brain. Acta Chir Scand 1951;102:316–319.
3 Leksell L: Stereotactic radiosurgery. J Neurosurg Psychiatry 1983;46:797–803.
4 Leksell DG: Stereotactic radiosurgery: Present status and future trends. Neurol Res 1987;9:60–68.
5 Leksell Gamma Unit User's Manual.
6 Guo WY: Radiological aspects of Gamma Knife radiosurgery for arteriovenous malformations and other non-tumoural disorders of the brain. Acta Radiol 1993;34(suppl):388.
7 Gore JC, Kang YS, Schulz RJ: Measurement of radiation dose distributions by nuclear magnetic resonance (NMR) imaging. Phys Med Biol 1984;29:1189–1197.
8 Olsson LE, Petersson S, Ahlgren L: Ferrous sulphate gels for determination of absorbed dose distributions using MRI technique: Basic studies. Phys Med Biol 1989;9:113–117.
9 Olsson LE, Fransson A, Ericsson A, Mattsson S: MR imaging of absorbed dose distributions for radiotherapy using ferrous sulphate gels. Phys Med Biol 1990;35:1623–1631.
10 Sperber GO, Ericsson AHA: A fast method for T_1 fitting. Magn Reson Med 1989;9:113–117.
11 Olsson LE, Appleby A, Sommer J: A new dosimeter based on ferrous sulphate solution and agarose gel. Appl Radiat Isot 1991;42:1081–1086.
12 Wu MC: The study and improvement about the measurement procedure of absorbed dose using ferrous sulphate gels. Master's thesis, Yang Ming University, 1995.

Proc 7th Int Meeting Leksell Gamma Knife® Society,
Island of Lana'i, Hawaii, November 1995
Stereotact Funct Neurosurg 1996;66(suppl 1):93–102

Stereotactic and Functional Neurosurgery

Effect of Gamma Knife Radiosurgery on Acoustic Neurinomas

Assessment by ^{99m}Tc-DTPA-Human Serum Albumin- and ^{201}TlCl-Single Photon Emission Computed Tomography

Y. Seo, S. Fukuoka, J. Nakagawara, M. Takanashi, S. Takahashi, K. Suematsu, J. Nakamura

Department of Neurosurgery, Nakamura Memorial Hospital,
Hokkaido Brain Research Foundation, Sapporo, Japan

Key Words

Brain neoplasms · Acoustic neurinoma · Radiosurgery · Single photon emission computed tomography

Abstract

Single photon emission computed tomography (SPECT) was performed on 16 patients with acoustic neurinoma before and 1 and 2 years after Gamma Knife surgery. ^{201}TlCl-SPECT was used to determine tumor viability. Early and delayed images of ^{99m}Tc-DTPA-human serum albumin (^{99m}Tc-HSA-D)-SPECT were used to assess tumor vascularity and permeability, respectively. There was a statistically significant decrease in the ^{99m}Tc-HSA-D index of the early image at 1 year ($p = 0.013$) and at 2 years ($p = 0.018$) after Gamma Knife surgery. On the other hand, the ^{201}Tl index and the ^{99m}Tc-HSA-D index of the delayed image were not significantly different from their pretreatment values. These observations demonstrate that a reduction in tumor vascularity without a decrease in tumor viability may be one of the effects of Gamma Knife surgery on acoustic neurinomas.

Introduction

Recent reports have shown that radiosurgery appears to be an effective treatment for acoustic neurinomas [1–3], with reported rates of tumor control in large series ranging from 88 to 97% [2, 3]. However, except for assessment by com-

KARGER

E-Mail karger@karger.ch
Fax + 41 61 306 12 34
http://www.karger.ch

1011–0125/96/0665–0093$10.00/0

Yoshinobu Seo, MD
Department of Neurosurgery
Nakamura Memorial Hospital
West-14 South-1, Chuo-ku
Sapporo 060 (Japan)

puted tomography (CT) or magnetic resonance imaging (MRI), there is little information on the posttreatment evaluation of the effects of Gamma Knife surgery on acoustic neurinomas. In this report we present the results of such an evaluation using single photon emission computed tomography (SPECT). Since thallium-201 chloride (^{201}TlCl)-SPECT is useful to identify viable tumor tissue [4–11], we employed this procedure to estimate the viability of the acoustic neurinomas. We used technetium-99m-DTPA-human serum albumin (^{99m}Tc-HSA-D), a blood pool scanning agent [12], to assess tumor vascularity in the early images and tumor permeability in the delayed images [13]. The volume of the acoustic neurinomas was determined by gadolinium-enhanced MRI (Gd-MRI). As far as we are aware, no such investigation has been performed previously.

Materials and Methods

Patient Population

The present study was carried out on 16 patients who underwent Gamma Knife surgery at our institution. Twelve were females and four were males (table 1). The mean age of the patients was 50.2 years (range: 26–76 years). Fifteen patients had a unilateral tumor. One had a neurofibromatosis 2 (NF2) neurinoma.

Radiation Dosimetry

The acoustic neurinomas of all patients were treated with multiple isocenters. The number of isocenters ranged from 5 to 12 (mean: 9.2). The dose to the periphery of the tumors ranged from 9 to 15 Gy (mean: 13.1 Gy), and to the center from 20 to 34 Gy (mean: 28.8 Gy).

^{99m}Tc-HSA-D-SPECT

^{99m}Tc-HSA-D-SPECT scanning was performed on the 16 acoustic neurinomas before treatment with Gamma Knife surgery. Follow-up scanning was carried out on 14 patients 1 year after radiosurgery, and on seven patients, 2 years after treatment.

^{201}TlCl-SPECT

A total of 11 acoustic neurinomas were studied by ^{201}TlCl-SPECT scanning before Gamma Knife surgery and 1 year after treatment. Of these, only three were studied 2 years after Gamma Knife surgery.

Imaging Protocol

Both ^{201}TlCl- and ^{99m}Tc-HSA-D-SPECT imaging were performed on the same day (dual isotope SPECT). After an intravenous injection of ^{201}TlCl (111 mBq), the patients underwent imaging with a triple gamma camera (Toshiba GCA-9300A/HG). Data acquisition began 30 min after tracer administration and continued for 20 min, collecting 90 projections with a 360° rotation of the high-resolution fan-beam collimators, and using an energy window of 71 ± 14 keV. Following completion of ^{201}TlCl-SPECT imaging, 740 mBq

Table 1. Clinical summary of 16 patients with acoustic neurinomas

Case	Age/sex	Tumor volume cm^3	Irradiation dose max/min, Gy	Number of isocenters	Tumor outcome	Follow-up period[a]
1	56/M	2.3	33/15	5	decreased	4y, 6m
2	76/F	10.7	22.5/9	11	decreased	4y, 4m
3	49/F	7.1	20/9	7	decreased	4y, 4m
4	30/F	1.7	30/12	10	unchanged	4y, 2m
5	58/F	1.2	30/15	6	decreased	4y, 1m
6	48/F	4.2	30/12	10	decreased	3y, 6m
7	57/F	5.4	30/12	10	increased	3y, 6m
8	40/M	2.4	28/14	6	decreased	3y, 5m
9	45/F	1.6	30/15	12	increased	3y, 4m
10	47/F	3.0	30/15	10	decreased	3y, 3m
11	62/F	5.2	25/12.5	10	unchanged	3y, 3m
12	26/F	1.1	30/15	9	unchanged	2y, 10m
13	50/M	8 5	28/14	11	decreased	2y, 8m
14	49/M	7.3	34/13.6	10	decreased	2y, 7m
15	43/F	4.0	28/14	11	decreased	2y, 6m
16	67/F	7.6	32.5/13	9	unchanged	2y, 4m

[a] y = Years; m = month(s).

of ^{99m}Tc-HSA-D was injected intravenously 1 h after the injection of ^{201}TlCl. Data acquisition began 10 min later and continued for 15 min using an energy window of 140 ± 28 KeV (early image). Another data acquisition period began 5 h after the injection of the tracer and continued for 20 min using the same energy window (delayed image). The ^{99m}Tc-HSA-D projections were processed in a similar way to the ^{201}TlCl-SPECT imaging. The transverse tomograms were displayed on a 128 × 128 matrix with a slice thickness of 2.4 mm. The spatial resolution of the method was 9 mm (fill width at half maximum).

Data Analysis

The indices of ^{201}Tl uptake (^{201}Tl index) and ^{99m}Tc-HSA-D uptake (^{99m}Tc-HSA-D index) were defined as the ratio of the average counts per pixel in the tumor to those in the normal contralateral cerebellum. The region of interest (ROI) was drawn around the region of maximum ^{201}Tl or ^{99m}Tc-HSA-D uptake, with a threshold of 70%. The ROI of the normal contralateral cerebellum was drawn with a diameter of more than 2 cm.

All results are expressed as means ± SE. Wilcoxon ranked-sign tests were used to compare the relative ^{201}Tl and ^{99m}Tc-HSA-D indices. A p value of less than 0.05 was considered to be statistically significant.

Results

Tumor Volume

Gd-MRI was used to determine tumor size. The volume of the treated tumors varied between 1.1 and 10.7 cm^3 (mean: 4.6 cm^3, table 1). A decrease in tumor volume was seen 1 year after Gamma Knife surgery in seven (43.8%) of the 16 patients. The volume was unchanged in two (12.5%) and increased in the remaining seven (43.8%). In comparison, 2 years after radiosurgery, the tumor volume was decreased in seven (43.8%), unchanged in six (37.5%) and increased in three (18.8%) patients.

At the last follow-up (range: 28–54 months after Gamma Knife surgery), MRI revealed that tumor volume had decreased in ten (62.5%) patients, was unchanged in four (25.0%) and had increased in two (12.5%) (table 1). The overall data indicated that the tumor volume was controlled in 56.3% of the patients 1 year after Gamma Knife surgery, in 81.3% 2 years after treatment, and in 87.5% at the last follow-up.

SPECT Analysis

^{201}TlCl-SPECT. The assessment of tumor viability determined by ^{201}TlCl-SPECT disclosed that no change in viability had taken place 1 year after radiosurgery. The mean ^{201}Tl indices in 11 patients before Gamma Knife Surgery and 1 year after treatment did not differ (2.03 ± 0.11 and 1.99 ± 0.16, respectively (table 2). As only three patients underwent ^{201}TlCl-SPECT 2 years after radiosurgery, the results obtained were not subjected to statistical analysis.

^{99m}Tc-HSA-D-SPECT (Early Images). Determination of the vascularity of the acoustic neurinomas by the early ^{99m}Tc-HSA-D-SPECT images disclosed a statistically significant reduction at 1 and 2 years after Gamma Knife surgery. As shown in table 2, the mean ^{99m}Tc-HSA-D early indices of the 14 patients obtained before and 1 year after treatment were 1.68 ± 0.08 and 1.50 ± 0.06 ($p = 0.013$), respectively, and those for the eight patients before and 2 years after Gamma Knife surgery, 1.62 ± 0.15 and 1.26 ± 0.13 ($p = 0.018$), respectively.

^{99m}Tc-HSA-D-SPECT (Delayed Images). Assessment of tumor permeability by the delayed ^{99m}Tc-HSA-D-SPECT images revealed the absence of significant changes 1 year after stereotactic radiosurgery. The mean values of the ^{99m}Tc-HSA-D delayed indices of the 14 patients before and 1 year after Gamma Knife surgery were 2.62 ± 0.26 and 2.45 ± 0.18, respectively, while those for the group of eight patients studied before and 2 years after radiosurgery were 2.28 ± 0.36 and 2.29 ± 0.37, respectively (table 2).

Table 2. ^{201}Tl and ^{99m}Tc-HSA-D indices before and after Gamma Knife surgery (GKS)

Index	n	Pre-GKS	Post-GKS	
			1 year	2 years
^{201}Tl	11	2.03±0.11	1.99±0.16	
^{99m}Tc-HSA-D (early image)	14	1.68±0.08	1.50±0.06*	
	8	1.62±0.15	(0.15)	1.26±0.13*
^{99m}Tc-HSA-D (delayed image)	14	2.62±0.26	2.45±0.18	
	8	2.28±0.36	(0.36)	2.29±0.37

Values are expressed as the mean ± SE. * $p < 0.05$ vs. pre-GKS value.

Illustrative Cases

Case 1 (fig. 1)

The patient was a 48-year-old woman with Recklinghausen's disease who had a left acoustic neurofibroma removed by surgery. Subsequent Gd-MRI revealed a right cerebellopontine tumor that was considered to be an acoustic neurofibroma. She had left deafness and mild facial paresis, but normal hearing acuity and no facial paresis on the right side. The patient underwent Gamma Knife surgery for the right acoustic neurofibroma. The dose at the margin was 12 Gy, and at the center, 30 Gy. The volume of the tumor was 4.2 cm^3.

The tumor had increased in size and there was ring-like contrast enhancement by Gd-MRI 8 months after radiosurgery. The tumor began to shrink thereafter. The uptake of ^{201}TlCl was not changed 1 year after Gamma Knife surgery, and was decreased 2 years after treatment. On the other hand, the uptake of ^{99m}Tc-HSA-D in the early images was significantly decreased 1 and 2 years after the treatment, but the uptake in the delayed images did not change.

Case 2 (fig. 2)

This patient was a 25-year-old woman with a left acoustic neurinoma who had suffered from a left-sided hearing disturbance since the age of 15. The patient underwent two partial surgical resections and received a ventriculoperitoneal shunt 1 month after the second operation. The patient was treated by Gamma Knife surgery 1 month after the shunt. The maximum diameter of the tumor was 3.0 cm and the tumor volume was 20.4 cm^3. The tumor received 9 Gy at its margin and 22.5 Gy at its center. The size of the tumor increased gradually, and the patient had progressive cerebellar dysfunction. She subsequently underwent a third surgical extirpation 18 months after radiosurgery. The histological examination of the specimen revealed proliferation of the internal membrane of the tumor vessels together with vessel obstruction.

a b c

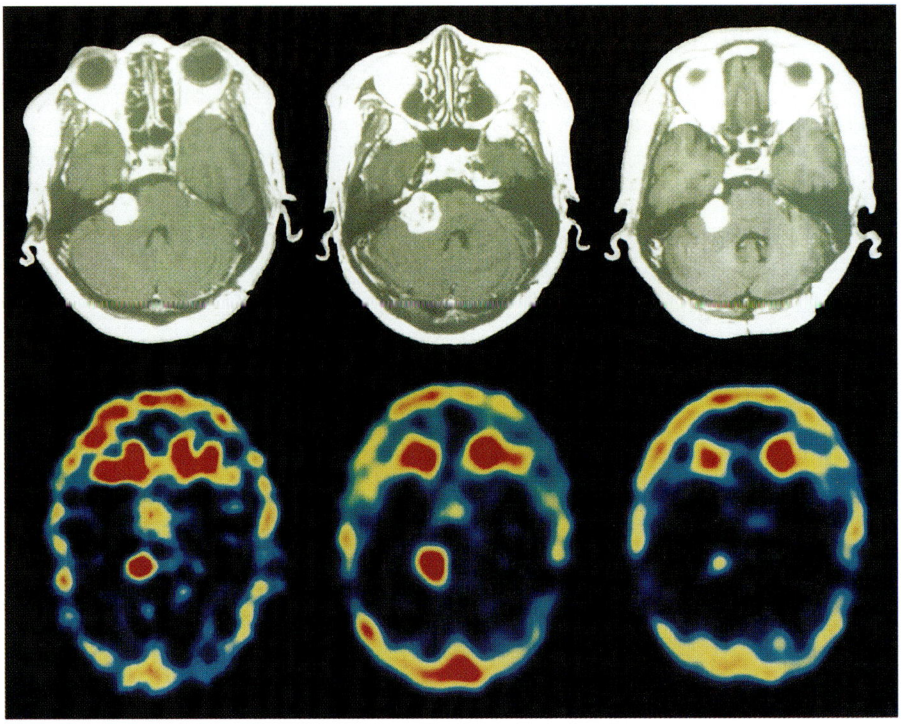

1

d e f

Fig. 1. Case 1. **a** Pretreatment Gd-MRI revealed an acoustic neurofibroma at the right cerebellopontine angle, the maximum diameter of which was 2.1 cm, and a tumor volume of 4.2 cm^3. **b** The tumor was enlarged and ring-like when contrast-enhanced by Gd-MRI 8 months after Gamma Knife surgery. **c** The following Gd-MRI revealed a reduction in tumor volume 2 years after treatment. **d** Pretreatment ^{201}TlCl-SPECT disclosed an abnormal uptake at the right cerebellopontine angle (^{201}Tl index = 3.0). **e** ^{201}Tl uptake in the tumor was not changed 1 year after treatment (^{201}Tl index = 2.9). **f** ^{201}Tl uptake in the tumor was decreased 2 years after treatment (^{201}Tl index = 2.1). **g** Pretreatment ^{99m}Tc-HSA-D--SPECT in the early image disclosed an abnormal uptake at the right cerebellopontine angle (^{99m}Tc-HSA-D early index = 1.8). **h** ^{99m}Tc-HSA-D early uptake in the tumor was not changed 1 year after treatment (^{99m}Tc-HSA-D early index = 1.7). **i** ^{99m}Tc-HSA-D early uptake in the tumor was decreased 2 years after treatment (^{99m}Tc-HSA-D early index = 1.3). **j** Pretreatment ^{99m}Tc-HSA-D-SPECT in the delayed image disclosed abnormal uptake at the right cerebellopontine angle (^{99m}Tc-HSA-D delayed index = 2.5). **k** ^{99m}Tc-HSA-D delayed uptake in the tumor was increased 1 year after treatment (^{99m}Tc-HSA-D delayed index = 2.5). **l** ^{99m}Tc-HSA-D delayed uptake in the tumor was slightly decreased 2 years after treatment (^{99m}Tc-HSA-D delayed index = 2.2).

Fig. 2. Case 2. Photomicrograph of the tumor specimen of an acoustic neurinoma 18 months after Gamma Knife surgery showing proliferation of the internal membrane of the tumor vessels and obstruction of the tumor vessels. HE. × 65.

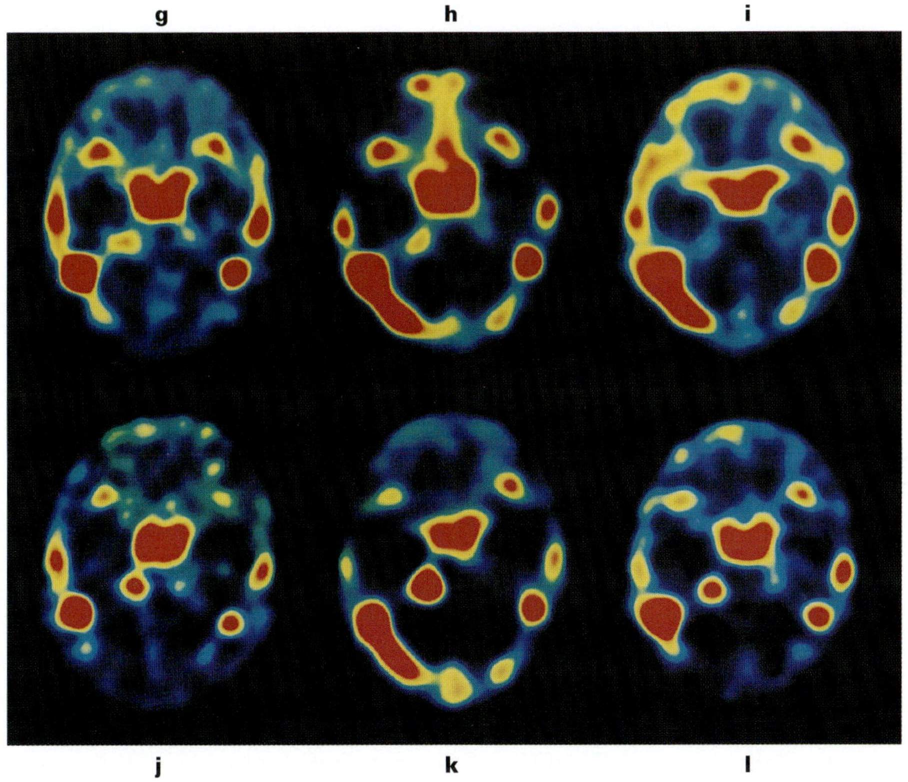

1

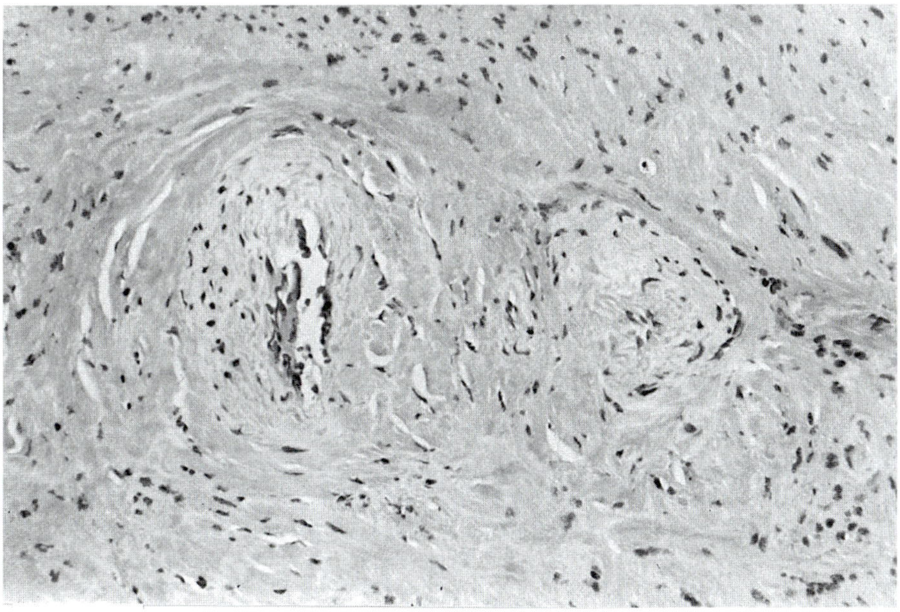

2

Discussion

Studies recently published indicate that many patients with acoustic neurinomas have received radiosurgery [1–3]. The aims of treatment have been control of tumor growth, maintenance of normal facial nerve activity, preservation of hearing and avoidance of complications [2]. Tumors which have decreased in size or remained unchanged have been considered to be controlled. The reported control rates of acoustic neurinomas range from 88 to 98%, with a minimum follow-up of 12 months [1–3, 14]. There are several studies in which CT and/or MRI were used after stereotactic radiosurgery [15–17]. However, there is no report on patient follow-up by other imaging methods, and there is little information regarding the vascularity, permeability and viability of acoustic neurinomas treated by Gamma Knife surgery.

Monovalent thallium has a greater affinity for the Na^+,K^+-ATPase pump than potassium [18], and its transport into cells and tissues is energy dependent. The uptake of ^{201}Tl within the brain is associated with tumor activity [6, 8] and several formulae for estimating ^{201}Tl uptake in a given brain tumor have been presented [4, 8, 9]. The formula introduced by Black et al. [4] relates the uptake in the tumor to that in the normal contralateral brain area (tumor/cerebral ratio). Because the ratios obtained by this simple computation have a high correlation with tumor malignancy and viability, we have adapted them (expressed as the respective index) to assess the effects of Gamma Knife surgery on acoustic neurinomas. As the present data show, there was no difference between the ^{201}Tl index before and 1 year after radiosurgery, indicating that tumor viability had not decreased. However, it is not known whether the ^{201}Tl index is indeed an absolute indicator of tumor viability, since a nonspecific reaction of the tumor tissue after Gamma Knife surgery could affect thallium uptake into the tumor. Hence, it is possible that different methods for caculating the ^{201}Tl index, or longer follow-up periods, might yield different results.

Cerebral blood volume (vascularity) can be assessed by ^{99m}Tc-HSA-D-SPECT, because the tracer has a high labeling yield and high blood retention in vivo [19, 20]. As albumin is exuded by degrees in experimental brain tumors [21], it is possible to estimate the capillary permeability of tumors using this substance. Thus, ^{99m}Tc-HSA-D-SPECT is used to determine the vascularity of tumors in the early images, and their permeability in the delayed images [13]. Our results indicate that a decrease in the ^{99m}Tc-HSA-D early index following radiosurgery was demonstrable before tumor shrinkage could be detected by Gd-MRI and before a decrease in tumor viability could be documented by ^{201}Tl-SPECT. As shown for case 2 (fig. 2), it is likely that proliferation of the internal membrane of the tumor vessels observed after Gamma Knife surgery may cause the reduction in tumor vascularity.

In conclusion, the data presented here document the usefulness of ^{201}Tl-SPECT for assessing the effects of stereotactic radiosurgery on acoustic neurinomas. With this method it is possible to obtain valuable information before changes in tumor size can be detected by Gd-MRI. When a reduction in ^{99m}Tc-HSA-D uptake is observed, it is possible that the tumor size may decrease after a longer posttreatment follow-up.

Acknowledgments

The authors would like to thank Yoshihiko Sakaue, RT, Hitoshi Yamagishi, RT, Mr. Masafumi Nakamura, Miss Akiko Kawamura, Mr. MarkAngelo Insalaco and Dr. Fritz Herz for their contributions in the preparation of the manuscript.

References

1 Steiner L, Lindquist C, Steiner M: Radiosurgery; in Symon L, Calliauw L, Cohadon F, Antunes JL, Loew F, Nornes H, Pásztor E, Pickard JD, Strong AJ, Yaşargil MG (eds): Advances and Technical Standards in Neurosurgery. Berlin, Springer, 1992, vol 19, pp 19–102.

2 Norén G, Greitz D, Hirsch A, Lax I: Gamma Knife surgery in acoustic tumours. Acta Neurochir 1993;58(suppl):104–107.

3 Lunsford LD, Kondziolka D, Flickinger JC: Radiosurgery as an alternative to microsurgery of acoustic tumors. Clin Neurosurg 1992;38:619–634.

4 Black KL, Hawkins RA, Kim KT, Becker DP, Lerner C, Marciano D: Use of thallium-201 SPECT to quantitate malignancy grade of gliomas. J Neurosurg 1989;71:342–346.

5 Carvalho PA, Schwartz RB, Alexander E III, Garada BM, Zimmerman RE, Loeffler JS, Holman BL: Detection of recurrent gliomas with quantitative thallium-201/technetium-99m HMPAO single-photon emission computed tomography. J Neurosurg 1992;77:565–570.

6 Kaplan WD, Takvorian T, Morris JH, Rumbaugh CL, Connolly BT, Atkins HL: Thallium-201 brain tumor imaging: A comparative study with pathologic correlation. J Nucl Med 1987;28:47–52.

7 Kim KT, Black KL, Marciano D, Mazziotta JC, Guze BH, Grafton S, Hawkins RA, Becker DP: Thallium-201 SPECT imaging of brain tumors: Methods and results. J Nucl Med 1990;31:965–969.

8 Mountz JM, Stafford-Schuck K, McKeever PE, Taren J, Beierwaltes WH: Thallium-201 tumor/cardiac ratio estimation of residual astrocytoma. J Neurosurg 1988;68:705–709.

9 Schwartz RB, Carvalho PA, Alexander E III, Loeffler JS, Forkerth R, Holman BL: Radiation necrosis vs high-grade recurrent glioma: Differentiation by using dual-isotope SPECT with ^{201}Tl and ^{99m}Tc-HMPAO. Am J Neuroradiol 1991;12:1187–1192.

10 Tonami N, Hisada K: Clinical experience of tumor imaging with 201-Tl-chloride. Clin Nucl Med 1977;2:75–81.

11 Vertosick FT Jr, Selker RG, Grossman SJ, Joyce JM: Correlation of thallium-201 single photon emission computed tomography and survival after treatment failure in patients with glioblastoma multiforme. Neurosurgery 1994;34:396–401.

12 Shirakami Y, Matsumoto Y, Yamauchi Y, Kurami M, Ueda N, Hazue M: Development of Tc-99m-DTPA-HSA as a new blood pool scanning agent. Jpn J Nucl Med 1987;24:475–478.

13 Nakagawara J, Fukuoka S, Takahashi S, Takahashi M, Satoh K, Suematsu K, Nakamura J: Assessment of vascularity and permeability in brain tumor using SPECT and ^{99m}Tc-DTPA-human serum albumin in relation to ^{201}Tl SPECT. Jpn J Nucl Med 1994;31:117–124.

14 Flickinger JC, Lunsford LD, Coffey RJ, Linskey ME, Bissonette DJ, Maitz AH, Kondziolka D: Radiosurgery of acoustic neurinomas. Cancer 1991;67:345–353.

15 Linskey ME, Lunsford LD, Flickinger JC: Neuroimaging of acoustic nerve sheath tumors after stereotaxic radiosurgery. Am J Neuroradiol 1991;12:1165–1175.

16 To SYC, Lufkin RB, Rand R, Robinson JD, Hanafee W: Volume growth rate of acoustic neurinomas on MRI post-stereotactic radiosurgery. Comput Med Imaging Graph 1990;14:53–59.

17 Oyama H, Kobayashi T, Kida Y, Tanaka T, Mori Y, Iwakoshi T, Niwa M, Kai O, Hirose M: Early changes in volume and non-enhanced volume of acoustic neurinoma after stereotactic gamma-radiosurgery. Neurol Med Chir (Tokyo) 1994;34:607–611.

18 Britten JS, Blank M: Thallium activation of the (Na^+-K^+)-activated ATPase of rabbit kidney. Biochim Biophys Acta 1968;159:160–166.

19 Ishii K, Nakazawa K, Tadokoro K, Ikeda T, Takamatsu T, Watanabe I, Yoda K, Matsubayashi T, Sakai F, Suzuki S: Local cerebral circulation dynamic study in patients with cerebral diseases: using ^{99m}Tc-HSA-D mainly compared with ^{99m}Tc-HSA. Jpn J Nucl Med 1989;26:35–44.

20 Nishizawa S, Tamaki N, Yonekura Y, Fujita T, Konishi J, Abe M, Fukuyama H, Miyoshi T, Harada K, Namura Y, Yamauchi H, Ishikawa M, Yamagata S, Nagata I, Kikuchi H: Clinical evaluation of ^{99m}Tc-DTPA-HSA in patients with cerebrovascular diseases: Assessment of perfusion reserve with SPECT. Jpn J Nucl Med 1988;25:1189–1200.

21 Tamura A, Matsutani M, Nakagomi T, Nagashima T, Tsujita Y, Sano K, Orii H: Changes of capillary permeability in experimental brain tumor. Brain Nerve 1988;40:149–156.

Proc 7th Int Meeting Leksell Gamma Knife® Society,
Island of Lana'i, Hawaii, November 1995
Stereotact Funct Neurosurg 1996;66(suppl 1):103–111

Stereotactic and Functional Neurosurgery

Acoustic Neurinomas with Macrocysts Treated with Gamma Knife Radiosurgery

G. Pendl[a], *J.C. Ganz*[a], *K. Kitz*[b], *S. Eustacchio*[a]

Departments of Neurosurgery,
[a] University of Graz, and
[b] University of Vienna, Austria

Key Words

Acoustic neurinoma · Cyst formation · Radiosurgery

Abstract

Six cases of acoustic neurinomas with macrocystic components are presented. In three cases the cystic portion was within the tumor, while in the other three, the cyst was peritumoral, in the form of a cul-de-sac within the arachnoid, in other words it was not a true tumor cyst. The six tumors are from a series of 74 acoustic neurinomas treated by radiosurgery with a minimum follow-up of 18 months. In all cases, enlargement of the associated cyst was observed as early as 4 months after radiosurgery. Clinical signs and symptoms such as facial weakness, trigeminal symptoms, vertigo and dizziness and coordination disorders developed between 4 and 8 months. In three cases (two intramural cysts and one combined peri- and intramural cyst), subacute microsurgery was performed to treat the progression of neurological symptoms. One case had spontaneous rupture of an intramural cyst, one case of a peritumoral cyst, after progression showed a slow spontaneous size decrease after 2 years, and one case is still under observation. In the reported series, the dose at the tumor margin ranged between 11 and 17 Gy (mean 13.8 ± 2.5 [SD] Gy) and the maximal dose between 24 and 40 Gy (mean 30.6 ± 6.2 Gy). In view of the findings in this study, one should perhaps be cautious in advising radiosurgery for this subgroup of acoustic tumors.

KARGER

E-Mail karger@karger.ch
Fax + 41 61 306 12 34
http://www.karger.ch

1011–6125/96/0665–0103$10.00/0

o. Univ. Prof. Dr. Gerhard Pendl
Universitätsklinik für Neurochirurgie
Auenbruggerplatz 29
A–8036 Graz (Austria)

Introduction

Acoustic neurinomas are in general solid, sharply delineated tumors. They appear in computerized tomography (CT) or magnetic resonance imaging (MRI) after administration of contrast medium as a homogeneous mass, often with slightly patchy areas due to regions of degenerative change within the tumor, sometimes as multiple cystic changes. Macrocysts, that is, cystic formations of at least one-third of the whole tumor volume, are not rare. They may be intramural or peritumoral, and the incidence may be as high as 28%. While macrocysts in acoustic neurinomas normally have no tendency to enlarge into a threatening form, the situation appears to be different after radiosurgery. The presence of a cyst between the tumor and the brain stem might represent added anatomical protection for the neuraxis. However, it would seem that this is of little value in practice for intramural cysts, since the cyst 'capsule' next to the brain stem is so thin. Our experience suggests that these macrocysts in acoustic neurinomas may enlarge rapidly after radiosurgery giving rise to acute clinical signs and symptoms due to their mass effect. Six cases are presented, of which three needed open microsurgical intervention for decompression.

Case Reports

Case 1

G.M., a 63-year-old female suffered from a recurrent acoustic neurinoma on the right side, with a peritumoral cyst sandwiched between the tumor and the brain stem. She received 16 Gy to the 50% isodose line with a maximal dose of 32 Gy. Eight months later, she developed slight deterioration in her permanent facial weakness. Fourteen months after Gamma Knife radiosurgery, MRI revealed a reduced tumor size but pronounced enlargement of the peritumoral cyst. She also suffered an increased number of attacks of dizziness. Thirty-four months later, following an unrelated accident with brain concussion, she experienced an amelioration of the dizziness, and MRI revealed a marked reduction in the size of the cyst (fig. 1).

Case 2

G.J., a 57-year-old female with an intramural macrocystic acoustic neurinoma on the right suffered from tinnitus, diminished hearing and slight trigeminal symptoms. Gamma Knife radiosurgery was performed with 11 Gy to the 45% isodose line and a maximum dose of 24 Gy (fig. 2). After 7 months, a marked increase in the trigeminal symptoms and deterioration of hearing loss were observed. MRI revealed enlargement of the cyst. One year after Gamma Knife treatment, she felt a sensation 'behind her right ear' followed by amelioration of trigeminal symptoms. MRI 2 weeks later no longer showed the cystic tumor compartment, and the solid tumor mass had shrunk markedly on MRI 24 months after Gamma Knife radiosurgery (fig. 3).

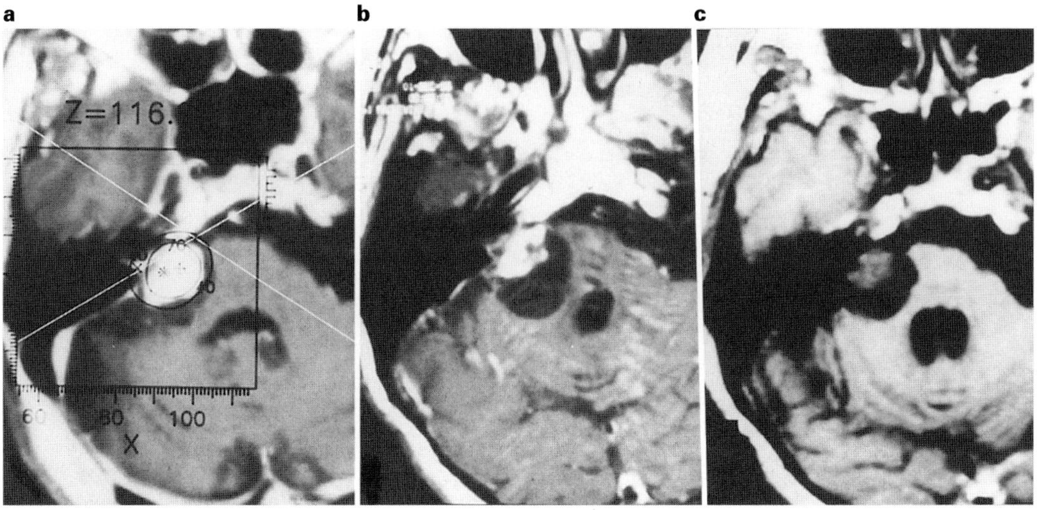

Fig. 1. Case 1. Acoustic neurinoma with a peritumoral cyst. **a** At Gamma Knife radiosurgery. **b** MR control 14 months after Gamma Knife radiosurgery and 6 months after deterioration of clinical signs and symptoms revealed a pronounced enlargement of the cyst but a decrease in the solid tumor volume. **c** Thirty-four months later (and 4 years after Gamma Knife radiosurgery), a spontaneous reduction of the cyst was seen with a further decrease in tumor volume.

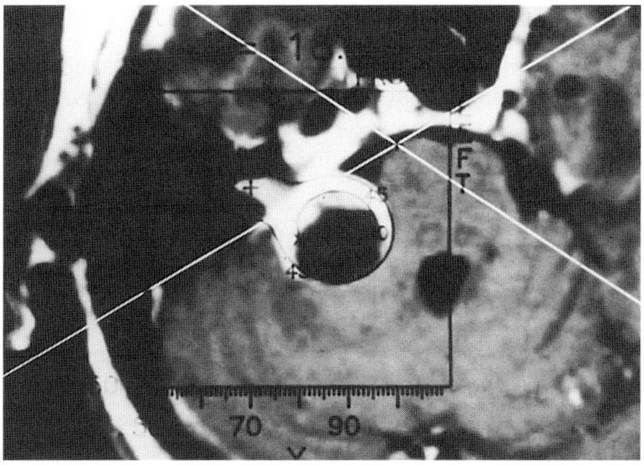

Fig. 2. Case 2. Dose plan for an acoustic neurinoma with a large intramural cystic component with the 45% isodose line covering the tumor margin.

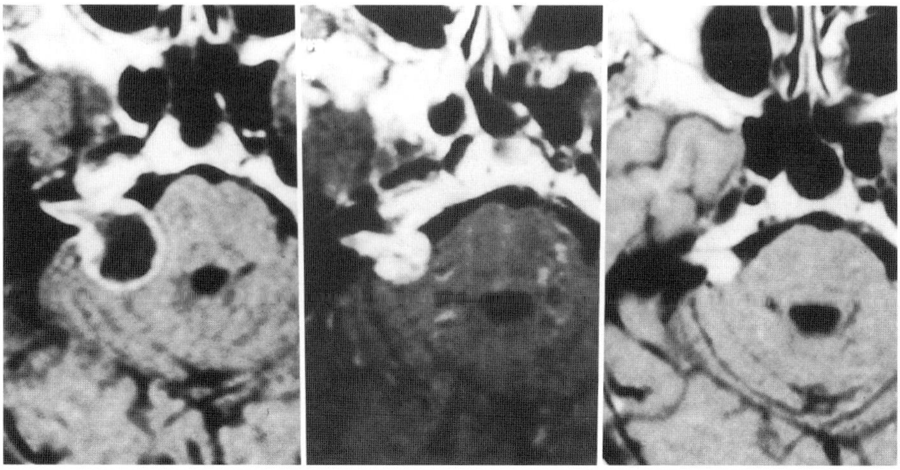

Fig. 3. Case 2. **a** Enlargement of an intramural cyst 7 months after Gamma Knife radiosurgery. **b** Sponanteous disappearance of the cystic component 1 year after Gamma Knife radiosurgery. **c** Additional tumor reduction 2 years after Gamma Knife radiosurgery.

Case 3

K.H., a 68-year-old-male suffered from gradual hearing loss on the right along with tinnitus, dizziness and episodes of vertigo for 6 years prior to Gamma Knife radiosurgery. CT revealed a cerebellopontine angle tumor 1 cm in diameter on the right with a 0.5-cm intramural cyst. He received 12 Gy to the 50% isodose line with a maximal dose of 24 Gy. Six months later, he developed increasing signs of vertigo, trigeminal symptoms, dysarthria, coordination disturbances in both legs and the left arm, as well as swallowing problems. CT showed an enlargement of a peritumoral cyst. Acute open surgery revealed a large, thin-walled arachnoid cyst as well as intramural tumor cyst formation. Postoperatively the clinical condition did not improve.

Case 4

Ten years prior to the Gamma Knife radiosurgery undertaken by us, I.A., a 61-year-old male, had received Gamma Knife radiosurgical treatment in another institution with only 2 Gy to the tumor margin. At first there was no tumor growth, but when the tumor began to enlarge again, there was an intramural cyst of at least 4 cm in diameter. In a second radiosurgical treatment, the solid portion of the tumor received 12 Gy to the 30% isodose line with a maximum dose of 40 Gy. One month later, he developed ataxia, dysarthria and coordination problems, increasing fatigue and drowsiness. CT and acute surgery 2 months after radiosurgery revealed a huge intramural cyst 6 cm in diameter. Only the cyst wall was removed, to try to preserve the facial nerve, the tumor having had sufficient radiosurgical treatment to be left in place. However, after surgery he developed a total paralysis of facial nerve function. The diagnosis of a schwannoma was confirmed with no particular evidence of radiation damage in the portions removed at surgery. The patient required a tarsorrhaphy.

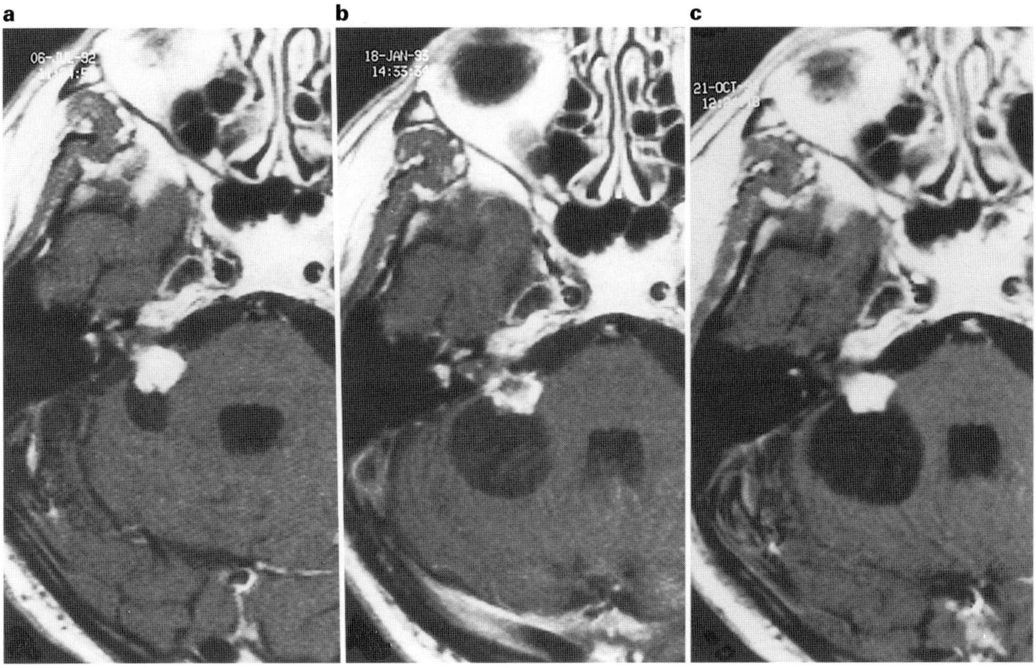

Fig. 4. Case 5. **a** MRI at the time of Gamma Knife radiosurgery of a recurrent acoustic neurinoma with a peritumoral cyst 27 years after open surgery. **b** Seven months later with transitory symptoms, MRI revealed a prominent enlargement of the peritumoral cyst. **c** Slight progression after 27 months.

Case 5

Z.K., a 66-year-old male patient had open surgery for an acoustic neurinoma on the right, 27 years before Gamma Knife radiosurgery. The recurrent tumor had been diagnosed 11 years previously. Radiosurgery was indicated because the tumor had begun to enlarge gradually. This 1-cm-diameter acoustic neurinoma was treated with an edge dose of 15 Gy to the 50% isodose line and a maximal dose of 30 Gy. Seven months later he developed pulsating headache in the right occipital region with dizziness. MRI revealed enlargement of a peritumoral cyst that had presented at the time of Gamma Knife treatment. Further control 27 months after Gamma Knife treatment showed further enlargement but no progress of clinical signs or symptoms. The patient is not willing to have an evacuation of the cyst and is kept under close observation (fig. 4).

Case 6

S.E., a 57-year-old female patient suffered from tinnitus for 15 years and hearing loss on the right 2 months before Gamma Knife radiosurgery. The acoustic neurinoma proved to be 2 cm in diamter with an intramural macrocyst. The tumor received 17 Gy to the 50% isodose line on the tumor margin with a total dose of 34 Gy. Five months after Gamma Knife radiosurgery, she developed facial weakness with nausea and ataxia. MRI revealed

a b c d

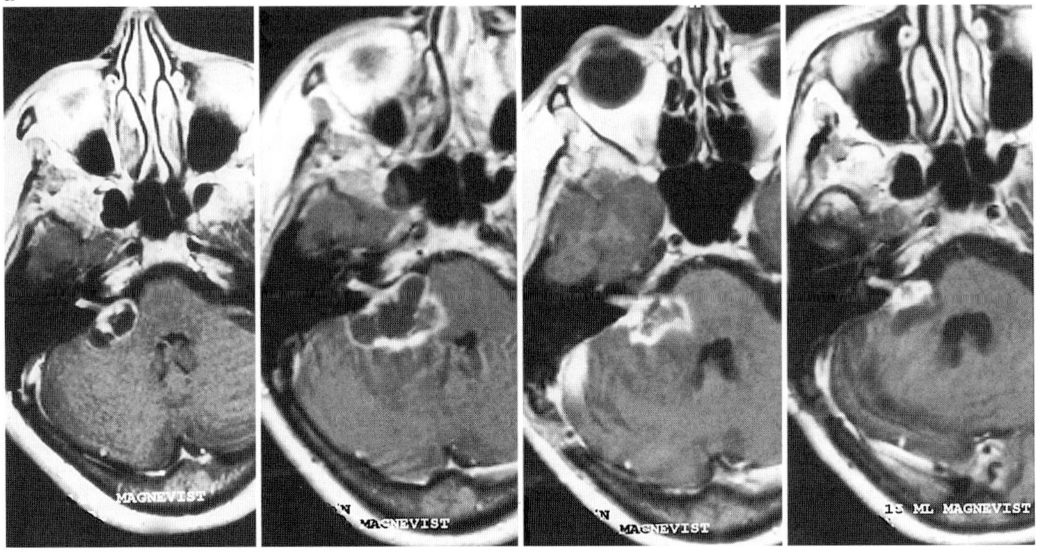

Fig. 5. Case 6. **a** MRI at the time of Gamma Knife radiosurgery. **b** 5 months after Gamma Knife radiosurgery with sudden clinical signs and symptoms with enlargement of the mostly cystic tumor. **c** 3 months after open surgery. **d** 17 months after Gamma Knife radiosurgery (12 months after open surgery) with marked reduction in tumor size.

marked enlargement of the cystic component of the tumor. Open surgery was performed with only partial resection of the cyst wall and mainly evacuation of the cyst. Histology revealed marked necrobiosis and fibrinoid vascular necrosis as radiation-induced changes. The tumor tissue itself was classified as Antoni type. MRI 3 months after surgery (8 months after radiosurgery) showed marked reduction of the still partially cystic acoustic neurinoma. Seventeen months after radiosurgery and 12 months after open surgery, only a small tumor nodule less than 1 cm in diameter remained (fig. 5).

Discussion

Cystic changes in acoustic neurinomas are expected in Antoni type B tissue. This variant, with its loose cell texture and tumor cell polymorphism is thought to be a degenerative phase of the compact and interwoven bundles of long bipolar spindle cells of Antoni type A neurinomas [1]. Although cystic acoustic neurinomas are quite often observed in neurosurgical routine, there is little discussed, especially concerning their neuropathology, in the literature. Russel and Rubinstein [2] mention only 'that the tumors may be partly or mainly cystic: this change

Table 1. Incidence of cystic acoustic neurinomas

Author	All tumors	Intramural cysts	Not specified	Peritumoral cysts
Kendall and Symon (1977) [5]	31		3 (10%)	
Robbins and Marshall (1978) [6]	29		8 (27.6%)	
Tali et al. (1993) [7]	80	9 (11.3%)		6 (7.5%)
Yokoh et al. (1993) [8]	55		14 (25.5%)	
Charabi et al. (1994) [9]	571	8 (1.4%)		15 (2.6%)
Own material	148	8 (5.4%)		1 (0.7%)

is particularly prone to occur in the spinal examples'. Zülch [3] describes regressive cystic changes in spinal neurinomas, but cites a single case from the literature. Even so, he describes the extramural cysts as frequently caudal to the tumor. In 1986, he described cystic degenerative changes of neurinomas as rare in the cerebellopontine tumors [4]. Peritumoral microcysts with acoustic neurinomas are the result of pseudocapsule formation by the arachnoid folds of the cerebellopontine angle, so that a cul-de-sac will fill with cerebrospinal fluid.

The frequency of cystic components to acoustic neurinomas varies between 4 and 27.6% (table 1) [5–9]. The average growth rate of acoustic neurinomas is 0.2 cm/year [10–14]. Ogawa et al. [15] found a mean volume doubling time of nonoperated acoustic neurinoma of 31.8 months Kameyama et al. [10] found in residual acoustic neurinoma after subtotal removal a significantly slower growth rate than in residual tumors with cyst formation. Degenerative or regressive changes in the tumor constitute a negative factor for regrowth [16, 17]. Cystic changes can cause sudden and rapid increases in tumor size [18, 19].

Cystic changes in the tumor are thought to be related to necrosis [7]. A large cyst formation may be produced by coalescence of microcysts. These secondary changes within acoustic neurinomas might be the result of thrombosis with ischemic necrosis and hemorrhages of teleangiectatic lesions in the cyst wall with ensuing liquefaction [20–22]. Radiosurgery itself, in the absence of preexisting cyst components, produced neither intramural nor peritumoral macrocysts in this material.

Peritumoral cysts are formed by arachnoid and the signal intensity is slightly higher than that of cerebrospinal fluid, in both T_1- and T_2-weighted images. These cysts seem to be formed by elevation and deformation of the leptomeninges by the enlarging tumors, causing adhesions between the leptomeninges surrounding the tumor and the posterior fossa structures. This process creates a cul-de-sac by pseudoduplication of the arachnoid and is usually some distance from the dura, sand-

Table 2. Postradiosurgery macrocyst enlargement

Case	Sex	Age years	Type of cyst	Gamma Knife surgery	Edge dose isodose Gy	Maximum dose Gy	Time from treatment to cyst months	Signs and intervention
(1) G.M.	F	63	peritumoral	Nov. 1992	16 Gy (50%)	32 Gy	8	spontaneous decrease
(2) G.J.	F	57	intramural	Feb. 1993	11 Gy (45%)	24 Gy	7	spontaneous rupture
(3) K.H.	M	68	intramural	Jun. 1989	12 Gy (30%)	24 Gy	6	open surgery
(4) I.A.	M	62	intramural	Apr. 1990	12 Gy (30%)	40 Gy	1	open surgery
(5) Z.K.	M	66	peritumoral	May 1992	15 Gy (50%)	30 Gy	7	observation
(6) S.E.	F	57	intramural	Jul. 1992	17 Gy (50%)	34 Gy	5	open surgery

wiched between the tumor and brain structures. Furthermore, leakage of hemorrhagic debris from the tumor to the surrounding leptomeninges might cause adhesions and formation of secondary arachnoid cysts [7]. The mechanism which promotes enlargement of preexisting intramural or peritumoral cysts after radiosurgery is poorly understood. One theory is that transudation of vessels in the tumor wall might occur. In addition, enforced coagulation necrosis of the tumor tissue might enhance osmotic tendencies [23].

Two patients, one with a peritumoral macrocyst (case 1) and another with an intramural macrocyst (case 2) experienced a spontaneous rupture of the gradually enlarging cyst after Gamma Knife radiosurgery. With peritumoral cysts the cause of spontaneous rupture might be a short period of raised intracapsular pressure with disruption of weaker areas of the leptomeningeal folds. In intramural cysts, disintegration of the cyst wall by radiation-induced necrosis might occur. Augmented transudation might precipitate rupture due to increased intracystic pressure.

Two cases (cases 3 and 6) with intramural cysts needed open surgical decompression within 6 and 5 months, respectively. However, in one case with peritumoral cyst enlargement, acute surgery was needed within 1 month after radiosurgery. Only one case with a large peritumoral cyst has not been reduced in volume. So far no rupture has occurred (case 5). The clinical onset of signs and symptoms caused by enlarging of the preexisting macrocysts was, in five cases, between 5 and 8 months, but in 1 case (case 4) as early as 1 month (table 2).

The dose given to the acoustic neurinoma seems not to be of any relevance, within the limits of dose used in this series.

References

1 Lundardi P, Missori P, Mastronardi L, Fortuna A: Cystic acoustic schwannomas. Act Neurochir 1991;110:120–123.

2 Russel DS, Rubinstein LJ: Pathology of Tumors of the Nervous System. London, Arnold, 1989.

3 Zülch KJ: Biologie und Pathologie der Hirngeschwülste; in Olivecrona H, Tönnis W (eds): Handbuch der Neurochirurgie. Berlin, Springer, vol 3, 1956.

4 Zülch KJ: Brain Tumors: Their Biology and Pathology. Berlin, Springer, 1986.

5 Kendall B, Symon L: Investigations of patients presenting with cerebellopontine angle syndromes. Neuroradiology 1977;13:65–84.

6 Robbins B, Marshall WH: Computed tomography of acoustic neurinoma. Radiology 1978;128: 367–370.

7 Tali ET, Yuh WTC, Nguyen HD, Feng G, Koci TM, Jinkins JR, Robinson RA, Hasso AN: Cystic acoustic schwannomas: MR characteristics. AJNR Am J Neuroradiol 1993;14:1241–1247.

8 Yokoh A, Kobayashi S, Tanaka Y, Gibo H, Sugita K: Preservation of cochlear nerve function in acoustic neurinoma surgery. Acta Neurochir 1993;123:8–13.

9 Charabi S, Tos M, Borgesen SE, Thomsen J: Cystic acoustic neuromas: Results of translabyrinthine surgery. Arch Otolaryngol Head Neck Surg 1994;120:1333–1338.

10 Kameyama S, Tanaka R, Honda Y, Hasegawa A, Yamazaki H, Kawaguchi T: The long-term growth rate of residual acoustic neurinomas. Acta Neurochir 1994;129:127–130.

11 Nedzelski JM, Canter RJ, Kassel EE, Rowed DW, Tator CH: Is no treatment good treatment in the management of acoustic neuromas in the elderly? Laryngoscope 1986;96:825–829.

12 Silverstein H, McDaniel A, Norrell H, Wazen J: Conservative management of acoustic neuroma in the elderly patient. Laryngoscope 1985;95:766–770.

13 Wazen J, Silverstein H, Norrell H, Besse B: Preoperative growth rates in acoustic neuromas documented with CT scanning. Otolaryngol Head Neck Surg 1985;93:151–155.

14 Valvassori GE, Shannon M: Natural history of acoustic neuromas. Skull Base Surg 1991;1:165–167.

15 Ogawa K, Kanzaki J, Ogawa S, Yamamoto M, Ikeda S, Shiobara R: The growth rate of acoustic neuromas. Acta Otolaryngol suppl (Stockh) 1991;487:157–163.

16 Amadasun JEO: The growth of acoustic neurinomas. Arch Otorhinolaryngol 1977;217:99–102.

17 Luetje CM, Whittaker CK, Davidson KC, Vergara GG: Spontaneous acoustic tumor involution: A case report. Otolaryngol Head Neck Surg 1988;98:95–97.

18 Nager GT: Acoustic neurinomas: Pathology and differential diagnosis. Arch Otolaryngol 1969;89: 252–279.

19 Drapkin AJ, Rose WS: Multicystic acoustic neuroma: Case report and differential diagnosis. Acta Radiol 1989;30:7–9.

20 Charabi S, Klinken L, Mantoni M, Tos M, Thomsen J: Histology and neuroimaging in cystic acoustic neuromas. Acta Otolaryngol (Stockh) 1993;113:519–523.

21 Prakash GS: Multicystic acoustic neuroma. Acta Radiol 1990;31:112.

22 Murakami S, Sotsu M, Hasegawa Y, Sanada S: Acoustic neurinoma associated with a totally thrombosed large cyst: A case report. Jikeikai Med J 1992;39:275–282.

23 Thompson BG, Coffey RJ, Flickinger JC, Lunsford LD: Stereotactic radiosurgery of small intracranial tumors: Neuropathological correlation in three patients. Surg Neurol 1990;33:96–104.

Proc 7th Int Meeting Leksell Gamma Knife® Society,
Island of Lana'i, Hawaii, November 1995
Stereotact Funct Neurosurg 1996;66(suppl 1):112–120

Stereotactic and Functional Neurosurgery

Gamma Knife Radiosurgery in Skull Base Meningiomas

Preliminary Experience with 50 Cases

A. Nicolato, P. Ferraresi, R. Foroni, A. Pasqualin, E. Piovan, F. Severi, B. Masotto, M. Gerosa

Department of Neurosurgery, University Hospital, Verona, Italy

Key Words

Stereotactic radiosurgery · Gamma Knife · Meningioma · Skull Base

Abstract

Gamma Knife radiosurgery was performed on 50 patients (10 males and 40 females) with skull base meningiomas (SBMs) between February 1993 and September 1995. The patients ranged in age from 25 to 78 years (mean age 56 years). The location of the tumors was anterior fossa (n = 4), sphenoorbital (n = 2), sellar region (n = 5), cavernous sinus (n = 26), petroclival (n = 12), and occipital foramen (n = 1). The tumor volume ranged from 0.6 to 20 cm^3 (mean 8.6 cm^3). The mean values for dose planning were edge isodose (EI) 46.7%, edge dose (ED) 18.0 Gy, maximum dose 39.8 Gy, average dose (AD) 25.4 Gy, and average number of isocentres 5.7. The patients were analyzed for five parameters: tumor volume (<7.5 vs. ≥7.5 cm^3); EI (<50 vs. ≥50%); ED (<18 vs. ≥18 Gy); AD (<25 vs. ≥25 Gy), and primary versus residual or recurrent tumors. The overall frequency of tumor growth control (TGC) was 98%, with 1- and 2-year TGC rates of 97% and 100%, respectively. The most favorable neurological results were obtained with a tumor volume <7.5 cm^3 ($p < 0.05$), EI ≥50% (NS), ED ≥18 Gy (NS) and with primary SBMs ($p < 0.01$). A favorable TGC was demonstrated at follow-up imaging examinations when the tumor volume was ≥7.5 cm^3 (100% TGC rate), EI <50% (100%), ED ≥18 Gy (100%), AD >25 Gy (100%), in both primary SBMs (100%) and residual or recurrent SBMs (96.5%). To date, only 3 (6%) of the 50 patients have presented signs of neurological worsening related to the Gamma Knife radiosurgery. While no early complications were noted, neuroradiological follow-up did show delayed transient imaging complications (3 edema and 1 radionecrosis; 8% of all patients). In conclusion, our preliminary results seem to confirm that Gamma Knife radiosurgery is an effective and safe adjuvant or a feasible alternative primary treatment in controlling or preventing SBM progression.

KARGER

E-Mail karger@karger.ch
Fax + 41 61 306 12 34
http://www.karger.ch

1011–6125/96/0065–0112$10.00/0

Antonio Nicolato, MD
Department of Neurosurgery
University Hospital
Piazzale Stefani 1
I–37126 Verona (Italy)

Introduction

Skull base meningiomas (SBMs) represent approximately 35–50% of all intracranial meningiomas [1]. Despite recent advances in microsurgical techniques, anesthetic management, and postoperative intensive care, surgical access to such tumors is still very difficult, and related mortality and morbidity rates remain high [1–7]. A consequence of the high risk of the surgical approach and removal of such tumors (Simpson's grade 1 or 2) [8] is that total resection is seldom performed [9–11]. This results in a high percentage of subtotal removal and tumor recurrence or regrowth [3, 5, 12–17].

The role of conventional external-beam fractionated radiation therapy (RT) in the treatment of meningiomas remains controversial. In different studies, tumor growth control (TGC) after RT varies from 50 to 90% [9, 16, 18, 19]. Other authors report that fractionated RT does not appear to show any benefit in either preventing recurrence or controlling regrowth [6, 14, 20–22]. On the other hand, Gamma Knife radiosurgery has been proposed by some authors as an adjuvant treatment of residual SBMs or an effective alternative to microsurgical removal of primary tumors in pursuing preservation of neurological function and prevention of further tumor growth [5, 22–24]. Moreover, meningiomas are considered to be an ideal tumor type for radiosurgery due to their demarcation from normal brain, accurate localization by computed tomography (CT) and magnetic resonance (MR) scanning, and slow growth. These characteristics could allow adequate time for cytotoxic and obliterative vascular effects to develop following radiation [1].

This study presents the preliminary results from a series of 50 patients treated with Gamma Knife radiosurgery for SBMs. Particular reference is made to (1) tumor volume (<7.5 vs. ≥ 7.5 cm^3), (2) edge isodose (EI; <50 vs. $\geq 50\%$), (3) edge dose (ED; <18 vs. ≥ 18Gy), (4) average dose (AD; <25 vs. >25 Gy), and (5) primary versus residual or recurrent tumors.

Clinical Material and Methods

Between February 1993 and September 1995, stereotactic radiosurgey using the 201-source cobalt-60 Gamma Knife was performed on 97 patients with endocranial meningiomas (n = 116) at the University Hospital in Verona. In 51 patients (10 males and 41 females), 53 SBMs were treated. a 49-year-old man with meningiomatosis, harboring three cranial base tumors, was excluded from treatment. The 50 remaining cases ranged in age from 25 to 78 years (mean 56). The meningioma locations were categorized as follows: anterior fossa, 4 cases (8%), sphenoorbital, 2 cases (4%), sellar region, 5 cases (10%), cavernous sinus, 26 cases (52%), petroclival, 12 cases (24%), and occipital foramen, 1 case (2%). The Karnofsky performance status (KPS) score and Order's grading classification [25] were used for pre- and postradiosurgical treatment clinical and neurological evaluations, respectively.

Gamma Knife radiosurgery was performed on the basis of the following criteria: (1) the tumor volume should be less than 20.0 cm^3; (2) the associated neurological risk for primary or additional microsurgery was too high; (3) the patient was of advanced age; (4) the medical condition precluded general anesthesia; (5) the patient refused open surgery. There were 28 residual or recurrent (56%) and 22 primary (44%) SBMs. All demonstrated the characteristic clinical and imaging findings of meningiomas with documented tumor recurrence on repeated neuroradiological examination before radiosurgery. Tumors were localized using thin-slice contrast-enhanced CT or MRI. Sophisticated in-house computerized three-dimensional reconstruction planning was used for tumor volume evaluation and dose planning optimization.

The mean tumor volume was 8.6 cm^3 (range 0.6–20.0 cm^3). Dose planning parameters were as follows: mean EI was 46.7% (range 30–80%); mean ED was 18 Gy (range 10–28 Gy); mean maximum dose was 39.8 Gy (range 24–66.7 Gy); mean AD was 25.4 Gy (range 14.8–45.2 Gy); the mean number of radiation shots was 5.7 (range 1–12). The treatment dose level at the tumor margin was selected after evaluations of the size, location, and the projected radiobiological risk to adjacent critical structures (for example, brain stem, cranial nerves, hypophysis).

All patients were discharged within 24 h after radiosurgical treatment. Follow-up imaging studies and neurological examinations were scheduled at 4 months after Gamma Knife radiosurgery, then at 6-month intervals for the first 2 years and annually thereafter. None of the patients underwent conventional external-beam fractionated RT either before or after the radiosurgery. Statistical significance was evaluated using the χ^2 test.

Results

Although the follow-up period (4–31 months, mean 14 months) is still too brief to be conclusive, some interesting preliminary conclusions may be drawn from the findings. At the end of the study (September 1995), all 50 patients are alive. Follow-up neurological examination was normal, improved, or stable in 43 (86%), with only 6% (3/50) experiencing any radiosurgery-related worsening. This was mostly mild, and with no influence on the overall clinical outcome. In fact, the mean post-treatment KPS score (90%, range 60–100%) had improved slightly when compared with the preradiosurgery score (mean 84.4%, range 70–100%). With respect to Order's neurological status classification, the posttreatment grade I/II rates of patients (82%/14%) did not demonstrate any significant change compared with the preradiosurgery values (80%/20%). Clinical worsening from grade II to grade III occurred in only 2 patients (4%). In one case, a 47-year-old man, the cause of clinical deterioration was unrelated to Gamma Knife treatment of the SBM recurrence, but rather to the slow progression of his postoperative cerebrovascular disease. The other case was a 63-year-old woman who had the only radiosurgery nonresponding tumors of the current series. From the neuroradiological point of view, the last follow-up imaging examination showed an overall TGC rate of 98% (table 1) with 1- and 2-year progression-free rates of 97 and 100%, respectively.

Table 1. Tumor growth control

	Tumor control	Percent tumor control
Total (n = 50)	49/50	98.0
At 12 months (n = 30)	29/30	97.0
At 24 months (n = 3)	3/3	100.0

Table 2. Imaging results related to tumor volume, EI, ED, AD, and primary versus residual/recurrent SBMs

Group	Shrank/ disappeared	Unchanged	Progression	Central CE loss	p
Tumor volume					
<7.5 cm (n = 26)	13 (50)	12 (46)	1 (4)	3 (11.5)	
≥7.5 cm (n = 24)	14 (58)	10 (42)	0 (0)	3 (12.5)	NS
EI					
<50% (n = 29)	15 (52)	14 (48)	0 (0)	4 (14)	
≥50% (n = 21)	12 (57)	8 (38)	1 (5)	2 (9.5)	NS
ED					
<18 Gy (n = 21)	9 (43)	11 (52.5)	1 (4.5)	2 (9.5)	
≥18 Gy (n = 29)	18 (62)	11 (38)	0 (0)	4 (14)	NS
AD					
<25 Gy (n = 26)	14 (54)	11 (42.5)	1 (3.5)	3 (11.5)	
≥25 Gy (n = 24)	13 (54)	11 (46)	0 (0)	3 (12.5)	NS
Primary	12 (54.5)	10 (45.5)	0 (0)	3 (14)	
Residual/recurrent	15 (53.5)	12 (43)	1 (3.5)	3 (11)	NS

Values in parentheses are percentages. CE = Central enhancement; NS = not significant.

Central contrast enhancement loss was documented in 6 cases (12%; table 2). No evidence of early imaging complications was observed. However, there were delayed transient imaging complications in 4 patients (8%): edema in 3 patients, and in 1 case, more profound radiation-induced changes which had resolved at the most recent MRI examination.

Patients harboring SBMs smaller than 7.5 cm^3 had the best neurological result, with radiosurgery-associated worsening in only 1/26 patients (4%). On the

Table 3. Neurological deficits related to tumor volume, EI, ED, AD, and primary versus residual/recurrent SBMs

Group	None	Improved	Unchanged	Worsening	RS-related worsening	p
Tumor volume						
<7.5 cm (n = 26)	9 (35)	5 (19)	11 (42)	1 (4)	1 (4)	
⩾7.5 cm (n = 24)	2 (8.5)	7 (29)	9 (37.5)	6 (25)	2 (8.5)	<0.05
EI						
<50% (n = 29)	5 (17)	8 (27.5)	10 (34.5)	6 (21)	2 (7)	
⩾50% (n = 21)	6 (28.5)	4 (19)	10 (48)	1 (4.5)	1 (4.5)	NS
ED						
<18 Gy (n = 21)	2 (9.5)	7 (33.5)	8 (38)	4 (19)	1 (21)	
⩾18 Gy (n = 29)	9 (31)	5 (17)	12 (41.5)	3 (10.5)	2 (7)	NS
AD						
<25 Gy (n = 26)	4 (15)	9 (35)	9 (35)	4 (15)	1 (4)	
⩾25 Gy (n = 24)	7 (29)	3 (12.5)	11 (46)	3 (12.5)	2 (8)	NS
Primary	10 (45.5)	5 (23)	4 (18)	3 (13.5)	1 (4.5)	
Residual/recurrent	1 (3.5)	7 (25)	16 (57)	4 (14.5)	2 (7)	<0.01

Values in parentheses are percentages. RS = Radiosurgery; NS = not significant.

other hand, there was radiosurgical-related worsening in 8.5% of patients with tumor volumes over 7.5 cm^3 (table 3). These differences were significant ($p < 0.05$). Nonetheless, it was also demonstrated that TGC was achieved in 100% of patients with large SBMs.

Analysis of dose planning parameters (tables 2, 3) showed that better radiosurgery-related neurological results were obtained when the EI was ≥50%, the ED was ≥18 Gy, and the AD was <25 Gy. Higher TGC rates were observed in cases treated with EI <50%, with ED ≥18 Gy, and with AD ≥25 Gy. However, these differences showed no statistical significance. On the other hand, patients with primary SBMs had a more favorable neurological result after Gamma Knife treatment than did those with residual/recurrent tumors (table 3, $p < 0.01$).

With the 1-year progression-free rates related to the different parameters (table 4), 100% TGC was demonstrated in patients with tumor volumes ≥7.5 cm^3, with primary SMBs and using an EI <50%, ED ≥18 Gy, and AD ≥25 Gy. The worst TGC rate (86%) in this series occurred when the ED was less than 18 Gy. Our preliminary data demonstrated that with the low risk of neurological worsen-

Table 4. 1-Year progression-free survival according to various parameter end points

Tumor volume		Primary	Residual/ recurrent	EI		ED		AD	
<7.5 cm^3	≥7.5 cm^3			<50%	≥50%	<18 Gy	≥18 GY	<25 Gy	≥25 Gy
15 (94)	14 (100)	14 (100)	15 (94)	15 (100)	14 (93)	6 (86)	23 (100)	11 (92)	18 (100)

Values in parentheses are percentages.

ing, excellent TGC results can be obtained in both primary and residual or recurrent SBMs. Good results were also obtained in larger tumors (volume ≥7.5 cm^3) using an EI <50%, an ED ≥18 Gy, and an AD ≥25 Gy.

Discussion

The management of SBMs remains a formidable challenge. Despite recent improvements in microsurgical techniques, anesthetic management, and postoperative intensive care, surgical-related risks are still high. Recent series have reported surgical mortality rates of 5–9% [3, 4, 15, 26] and permanent morbidity rates of 24–43% [2, 3, 10, 26–29]. Moreover, there is an additional risk of permanent neurological deficit after microsurgery in 24–63% of cases [3, 23]. Because of these risks, SBM surgery is often incomplete, with subtotal removal rates varying between 24 and 74% [3, 6, 11, 15, 16, 29, 30], and thus moderate to high recurrence rates (12–41%) are reported [3, 6, 14, 15, 26], with 5- and 10-year probability of progression rates of 25–46% and 35–64%, respectively [3, 14, 16].

In an attempt to improve TGC, associated conventional external-beam fractionated RT after surgery has been suggested. Many studies have reported a beneficial effect of RT in controlling the progression of intracranial benign residual meningiomas, with 5-year progression-free survival rates of 77–88% [17, 18, 30, 31]. In an 84-patient series with subtotal removal of meningiomas, where most cases were SBMs, Barbaro et al. [30] described a 40% TGC rate in the nonirradiated patients, compared to a 68% TGC rate in patients with RT. Taylor et al. [17] reported a 10-year TGC rate of 82% for subtotal removal associated with RT, and 18% for subtotal excision alone. The UCSF group [9] reported a series of 117 patients with benign meningiomas treated surgically with subtotal removal and RT. The 5-year progression-free survival rates in 44 parasellar and 14 anterior fossa meningiomas were 88 and 79%, respectively. The relative risk of progression was 4.5-fold greater than that of all other sites combined.

Other authors maintain that RT does not decrease the recurrence or regrowth rates of intracranial meningiomas [6, 20, 21]. In particular, Mahmood et al. [14] reported nearly the same regrowth rates with (33%) or without (39%) irradiation following subtotal removal and they concluded that RT did not significantly improve the TGC rate.

Even if RT is usually associated with zero [17] or with very low morbidity rates (<4.9%) [9], there is a 38% risk of radiation complications with fractionated irradiation for benign tumors in adults [32]. Glaholm et al. [18] reported that 4 of 186 patients (2%) achieved late persistent neurological impairment following RT for intracranial meningiomas. Three of these patients were treated for parasellar tumors.

The role of RT in controlling the progression of meningiomas remains controversial, due to the variability of the reported success rates and the associated occasional risk of developing major neurological complications. In the recent literature, there are preliminary results for Gamma Knife treatment for these lesions. To data, Gamma-Knife-related mortality rates have not been documented, neither in our series nor in published studies [5, 23, 24]. We noted a permanent morbidity associated with radiosurgical treatment in 3 (6%) of our 50 patients. These complications consisted of a mild added cranial nerve deficit or slight worsening of a preexisting cranial nerve deficit. These findings are similar to those reported by Duma et al. [23] (9%) and by Pendl et al. [24] (7.5%). These rates are lower than those described in other surgical series (24–63%).

Even though the SBM follow-up periods of the radiosurgical studies are shorter than surgical or RT series, the progression-free survival rates following Gamma Knife radiosurgery are typically very favorable, exceeding 95% in this series and in the literature [23, 24]. Only Ganz et al. [5] reported a 1-year TGC rate of 80% in a series of 20 patients, harboring primarily SBMs. In that material, there was tumor progression in 4 cases where the ED was less than 10 Gy. Our experience confirms these results, as we also noticed a lower 1-year progression-free survival rate (86%) when we administered lower EDs (<18 Gy). On the other hand, the 1-year TGC rate was excellent (100%) for margin doses equal to or in excess of 18 Gy.

One additional promising finding was that the results were extremely rewarding in large SBMs (tumor volume ≥7.5 cm^3) treated with higher doses (ED ≥18 Gy and AD ≥25 Gy). We observed extremely promising TGC rates with slight risk of short-to middle-term neurological complications.

In conclusion, although longer follow-up studies are needed, our preliminary results suggest that Gamma Knife radiosurgery is a useful adjuvant form of therapy for selected patients with residual or recurrent SBMs and an effective and safe alternative primary treatment in older patients for whom microsurgery represents an unacceptable risk.

Randomized investigations on radiosurgical treatment optimization are needed to improve these results further, while reducing the risk for delayed sequelae.

Acknowledgment

The authors wish to thank Mrs. Victoria Marie De Micheli for her excellent help in reviewing the manuscript.

References

1 Wright DC, Sekhar LN: Cranial base meningiomas; in Salcam M (ed): Current Techniques in Neurosurgery. Philadelphia, Current Medicine, 1993, pp 2.1–2.13.
2 Black P McL: Meningiomas. Neurosurgery 1993;32:643–657.
3 DeMonte F, Smith HK, Al-Mefty O: Outcome of aggressive removal of cavernous sinus meningiomas. J Neurosurg 1994;81:245–251.
4 Dolenc VV, Kregar T, Ferluga M, Fettich M, Mozrina A: Treatment of tumors invading the cavernous sinus; in Dolenc VV (ed): The Cavernous Sinus: Multidisciplinary Approach to Vascular and Tumorous Lesions. Vienna, Springer, 1987, pp 377–391.
5 Ganz JC, Backlund EO, Thorsen FA: The results of Gamma Knife surgery of meningiomas related to size of tumor and dose. Stereotact Funct Neurosurg 1993;61(suppl 1):23–29.
6 Marks SM, Whitewell HL, Lye RH: Recurrence of meningiomas after operation. Surg Neurol 1986; 25:436–440.
7 Ojeman RG: Skull base surgery: A perspective. J Neurosurg 1992;76:569–570.
8 Simpson D: The recurrence of intracranial meningiomas after surgical treatment. J Neurol Neurosurg Psychiatry 1957;20:22–39.
9 Goldsmith BJ, Wara WM, Wilson CB, Larson DA: Postoperative irradiation for subtotally resected meningiomas: A retrospective analysis of 140 patients treated from 1967 to 1990. J Neurosurg 1994;80:195–201.
10 Maroon JC, Kennerdell JJ, Vidovich DV, Abla A, Sternau L: Recurrent spheno-orbital meningiomas. J Neurosurg 1994;80:202–208.
11 Newmann SA: Meningiomas: A qest for the optimum therapy. J Neurosurg 1994;80:191-194.
12 Philippon J: Meningiomi; in Cohadon F (ed): Tumori del sistema nervoso e dei suoi involucri. Rome, Antonio Delfino, Medicina-scienze, 1994, pp 455–473.
13 Lunsford LD: Contemporary management of meningiomas: Radiation therapy as an adjuvant and radiosurgery as an alternative to surgical removal? J Neurosurg 1994;80:187–190.
14 Mahmood A, Qureshi NH, Malik GM: Intracranial meningiomas: Analysis of recurrence after surgical treatment. Acta Neurochir 1994;126:53–58.
15 Mayberg MR, Symon L: Meningiomas of the clivus and apical petrous bone: Report of 35 cases. J Neurosurg 1986;65:160–167.
16 Mirimanoff RO, Dosoretz DE, Linggood RM: Meningioma: Analysis of recurrence and progression following neurosurgical resection. J Neurosurg 1985;62:18–24.
17 Taylor BW Jr, Marcus RB Jr, Friedman WA, Ballinger WE, Million RR: The meningioma controversy: Postoperative radiation therapy. Int J Radiat Oncol Biol Phys 1988;15:299–304.
18 Glaholm J, Bloom HJG, Crow JH: The role of radiotherapy in the managment of intracranial meningiomas: The Royal Marsden Hospital experience with 186 patients. Int J Radiat Oncol Biol Phys 1990;18:755–761.
19 Solan MJ, Kramer S: The role of radiation therapy in the management of intracranial meningiomas. Int J Radiat Oncol Biol Phys 1985;11:675–677.

20 Adegbite AB, Khan MI, Paine KWE: The recurrence of intracranial meningiomas after surgical treatment. J Neurosurg 1983;58:51–56.
21 Chan RC, Thompson GB: Morbidity, mortality and quality of life following surgery for intracranial meningiomas: A retrospective study in 257 cases. J Neurosurg 1984;60:52–60.
22 Kondziolka D, Lunsford LD, Coffey RJ, Flickinger JC: Stereotactic radiosurgery of meningiomas. J Neurosurg 1991;74:522–559.
23 Duma CM, Lunsford LD, Kondziolka D, Harsh GR IV, Flickinger JC: Stereotactic radiosurgery of cavernous sinus meningiomas as addition or alternative to microsurgery. Neurosurgery 1993;32: 699–705.
24 Pendl G, Shröttner O, Friehs GM, Legat J, Leber K, Mokry M, Papaefthymiou G, Langman G: Radiosurgery with the first Austrian cobalt-60 gamma unit: A one year experience. Acta Neurochir 1994;127:170–178.
25 Order SE, Hellman S, Von Essen CF, Kligerman MM: Improvement in quality of survival following whole-brain irradiation for brain metastasis. Radiology 1968;91:149–153.
26 Andrews BT, Wilson CB: Suprasellar meningiomas: The effect of tumor location on postoperative visual outcome. J Neurosurg 1988;69:523–528.
27 Al-Mefty O, Smith RR: Surgery of tumors invading the cavernous sinus. Surg Neurol 1988;30: 370–381.
28 Sekhar LN, Moller AR: Operative management of tumors involving the cavernous sinus. J Neurosurg 1986;64:879–889.
29 Sekhar LN, Sen CN, Jho HD, Vanecka IP: Surgical treatment of intracavernous neoplasm: A four-year experience. Neurosurgery 1989;24:18–30.
30 Barbaro NM, Gutin PM, Wilson CB, Sheline GE, Boldrez EB, Ward WM: Radiation therapy in the treatment of partially resected meningiomas. Neurosurgery 1987;20:525–528.
31 Miralbell R, Linggood RM, de la Monte S: The role of radiotherapy in treatment of subtotally resected benign meningiomas. J Neurooncol 1982;13:157–164.
32 Al-Mefty O, Kersh JE, Routh A, Smith RR: The long-term side effects of radiation therapy for benign brain tumors in adults. J Neurosurg 1990;73:502–512.

Proc 7th Int Meeting Leksell Gamma Knife® Society,
Island of Lana'i, Hawaii, November 1995
Stereotact Funct Neurosurg 1996;66(suppl 1):121–128

Stereotactic and Functional Neurosurgery

Gamma Knife Treatment of 100 Consecutive Meningiomas

W.R. Hudgins, J.L. Barker, D.E. Schwartz, T.D. Nichols

Departments of Neurosurgery and Radiation Oncology, Presbyterian Hospital of Dallas, Tex., USA

Key Words

Meningioma · Gamma Knife · Radiosurgery · Outcome studies

Abstract

Clinical and imaging results of Gamma Knife treatment of 100 consecutive patients with intracranial meningiomas are reported. Only 1 patient refused follow-up imaging and her symptoms remain improved after 1 year. Mean values for the patient and treatment parameters were age 61 years, duration of symptoms 3.6 years, time since diagnosis 3 years, average tumor diameter 2.4 cm, surface radiation dose 15 Gy and number of isocenters 5. Clinical outcomes revealed that 6 were improved, 75 were unchanged and 17 had deteriorated. Of the latter, 8 were operated, 4 were treated medically and 5 died. Imaging follow-up showed no growth in 87 patients. The size of tumors treated ranged from 0.66 to 6.8 cm average diameter. In the 77 patients with tumors with an average diameter of 3 cm or less, only 2 (3%) showed further growth, and none died of tumor-related causes.

Introduction

The preferred treatment for a meningioma is total surgical resection. However, this is not always sensible or possible. Some of these tumors are seen to be surgically difficult on preoperative imaging studies. Others cannot be completely resected at craniotomy, and some recur after an apparent total removal. Other

KARGER

E-Mail karger@karger.ch
Fax + 41 61 306 12 34
http://www.karger.ch

1011–6125/96/0665–0121$10.00/0

W. Robert Hudgins, MD
8230 Walnut Hill Lane
Suite 620
Dallas, TX 75231 (USA)

patients may have medical contraindications to general anesthesia and surgery. Radiation is not usually considered for these benign tumors. However, Wara et al. [1] reported in 1975 that of 58 patients followed after subtotal resection of meningiomas, 75% recurred, while the recurrence rate was only 30% among 34 similar patients who had also received postoperative radiotherapy.

When our hospital installed a Gamma Knife, we expected the majority of referrals to be patients with arteriovenous malformations (AVMs) or acoustic neuromas, according to the previous experience in other centers. However, after 5 years, we have treated more meningiomas (28% of all patients) than any other diagnostic category. Outcomes in the first 100 consecutively treated patients are reported here.

Materials and Methods

We treated patients only after review and acceptance by a group of physicians including a neurosurgeon, a neuroradiologist and a radiation oncologist. Our clinical guidelines contained a size limitation of 3 cm in average diameter, but we made exceptions in special circumstances for patients without other good options. Most patients were elderly, with an average age of 61 years (range 32–88 years). The duration of symptoms ranged from zero (asymptomatic patients) to 25 years, averaging 3.6 years. The interval from diagnosis to treatment varied from a few weeks up to 20 years (mean 3 years).

Figure 1 shows the location of all the tumors treated. All but 9 patients had recurrent/residual tumor after previous surgery. Eighteen patients had previous partial resection, 34 had subtotal resection, 30 had 'complete' resection, and 9 had undergone multiple (2–6) previous operations. Two patients (in addition to the 9 mentioned above) were treated without histological confirmation, the diagnosis being based on images alone. They were subsequently found to have a different diagnosis: one had an intracavernous aneurysm and the other a metastasis along the sphenoid wing. We excluded both of these patients from this group of 100.

We estimated tumor size by measuring the maximum diameter in the three orthogonal (X, Y, Z) planes used in treatment planning and targeting. The smallest tumor treated measured 0.8 × 0.6 × 0.6 cm, the largest 6 × 6.5 × 8 cm. The mean was 2.45 × 2.47 × 2.35 cm. Treatment required from 1 to 12 isocenters of radiation, averaging 5 'shots' in these often irregularly shaped tumors. The maximum central radiation dose ranged from 13 to 67 Gy, averaging 33 Gy. The surface dose ranged from 8 to 25 Gy, averaging 15 Gy. The lowest surface isodose shell was 20%, the highest 80%, with an average of 46%.

Clinical follow-up was by office visit, letter or telephone interview, and all patients were recommended to have magnetic resonance imaging (MRI) with and without contrast enhancement at 6 months, 1 year, and then annually for 5 years. We obtained contrast-enhanced computed tomography if MRI was contraindicated. At each follow-up, we reviewed all serial imaging studies with a neuroradiologist and completed a standard form, which recorded tumor size, any evidence of radiation-induced edema or radionecrosis, and clinical outcome data.

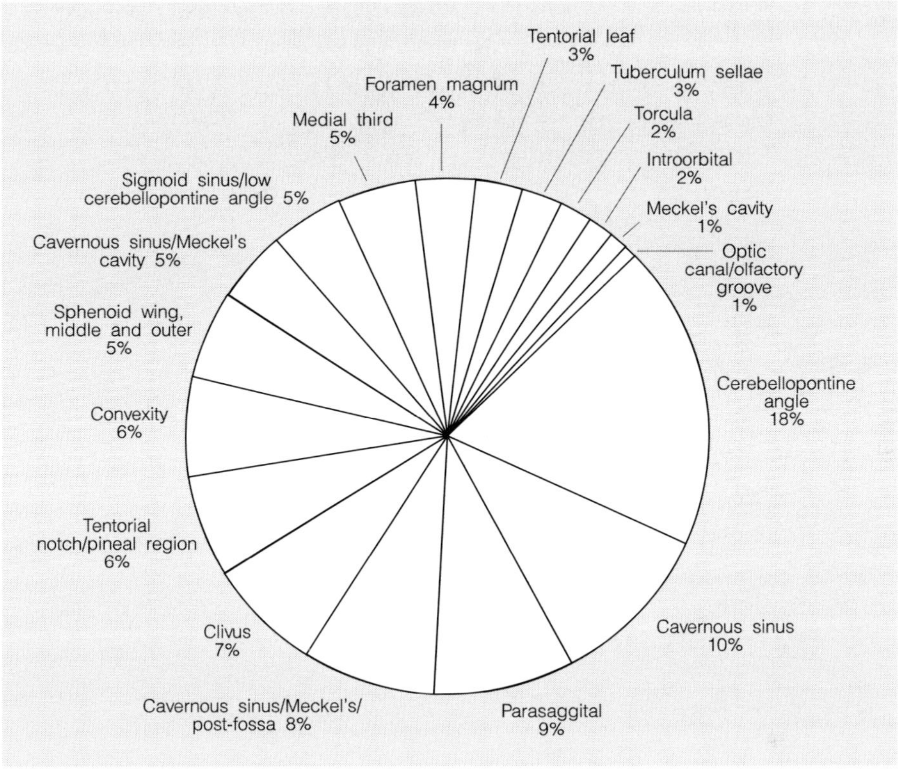

Fig. 1. Pie graph showing the locations of the first 100 consecutive meningiomas treated by Gamma Knife radiosurgery.

Results

Figure 2 compares the number of follow-up imaging studies obtained related to the number requested. For each interval, some patients had less than or more than the expected number. Those who had fewer were doing well and frequently refused requests for follow-up scans, while those with more than the usual number of scans had new or unusual symptoms requiring more frequent follow-up. Only 1 patient has not had a follow-up scan. She feels well, is caring for her husband who has cancer, and lives in a remote area from which she cannot come in for a study.

Table 1 summarizes the clinical outcomes. Four of the patients who remain worse than before treatment are being treated medically and followed. Two of them were permanently worse. One had brain stem radionecrosis after a second

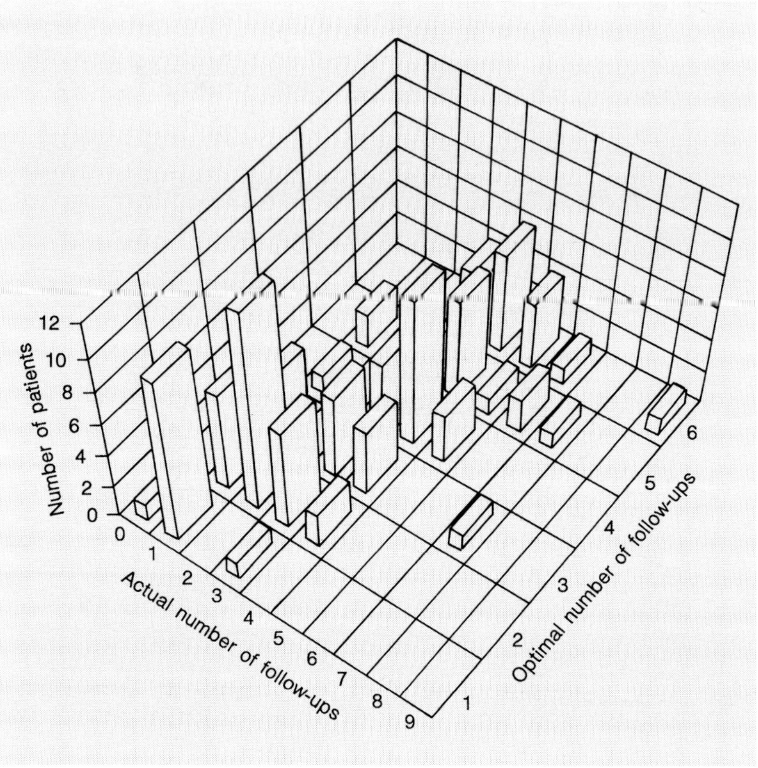

Fig. 2. Comparison of the number of follow-up imaging studies obtained to the number requested. Only 1 patient, treated less than 1 year ago, has had no imaging follow-up.

treatment in the posterior fossa and died later from recurrent bilateral posterior fossa tumors. The other lost useful vision in one eye, due either to radionecrosis or a slight transient increase in size of a parasellar meningioma. Ten patients were temporarily worse, from either cerebral edema or cranial neuropathy. Eight patients had increased symptoms from tumor growth and were submitted to surgery. So far, 6 patients have died, 1 from cardiovascular disease and 5 from continued growth of their meningioma. Of these 5 patients, 1 is mentioned above, 2 died postoperatively after further attempts at resection, and 2 died of malignant menigioma, 1 of which metastasized to the lung. New meningiomas were found in 6 patients on follow-up, 3 of which were treated with the Gamma Knife after subsequent follow-up showed growth. In the subset of 77 patients with tumors less than 3.1 cm in average diameter, no tumor-related deaths or permanent complications occurred and no growth was seen in 75 (96%) of them.

Table 1. Clinical outcomes of 100 patients

	All patients	<30 mm	>30 mm
Improved	8	7	1 (4)
Unchanged	74	64	10 (43)
Worse			
Followed	4	3	1 (4)
Retreated	0	0	0
Operated	8	2	6 (26)
Died			
Tumor	5	0	5 (22)
Other	1	1	0
Total	100	77	23
Complications			
Wrong diagnosis	2	2	
From radiation			
Transient	10	7	3 (13)
Permanent	2	0	2 (9)
New tumors found	6	6	0

Values in parentheses are percentages.

Figure 3 illustrates the imaging results. One patient had no imaging follow-up, 9 tumors grew after treatment, 44 showed no growth, and in 47 tumors showed a size reduction. However, if tumors with an average diameter over 3 cm are excluded, growth was controlled in 75 of 77 patients (97%). In 4 of the 23 patients with tumors greater than 3 cm average diameter, treatment stopped tumor growth, but the patients required subsequent surgery to relieve persistent mass effects or radiation-induced edema.

Figure 4 shows the surface dose of radiation prescribed to each tumor plotted against the average diameter ($\sqrt[3]{(X^2 + Y^2 + Z^2)}$) of each tumor. The straight line represents an extrapolation of the 1% risk of necrosis from the data of Kjellberg [2] on proton beam therapy of AVMs. Our conservative 'first do no harm' approach is apparent from the appearance of most data points below this line. Figure 5 shows the 9 tumors that increased in size, equally distributed above and below the 1% risk line. However, it is interesting and possibly significant that all but one of them had an average diameter greater than 3 cm. Figure 6 illustrates the dose/volume relationships of all patients with adverse affects. The 9-mm tumor was an intracavernous meningioma, and this patient had a transient third and fifth cranial nerve neuropathy. The 2 patients with permanent sequelae were the only patients with adverse effects whose tumors were over 3 cm in diameter.

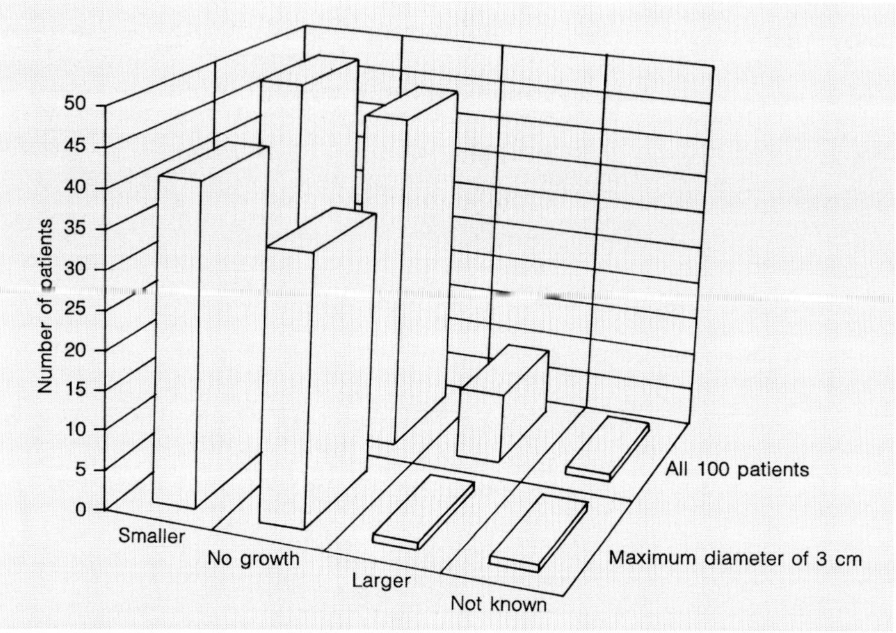

3

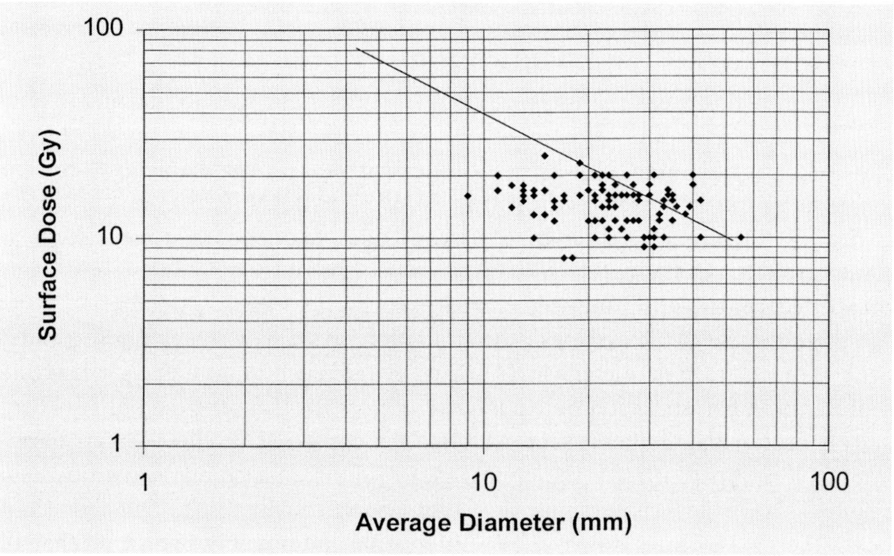

4

Fig. 3. Follow-up findings in 100 patients with meningiomas treated with the Gamma Knife.

Fig. 4. Scatter-plot on a log/log scale of the surface dose of Gamma Knife radiation versus the average diameter of all meningiomas treated. The straight line represents approximately a 1% risk of radionecrosis in single-dose radiosurgery (see text).

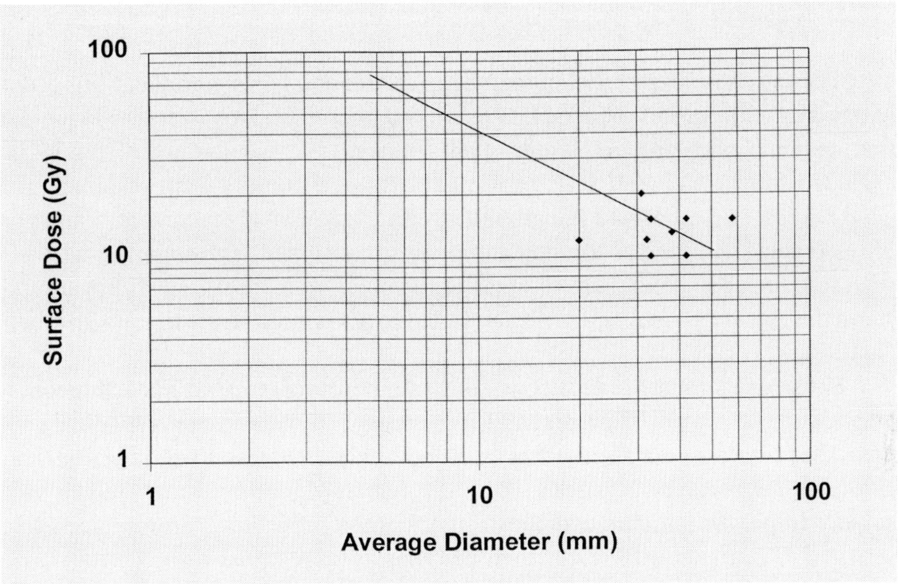

5

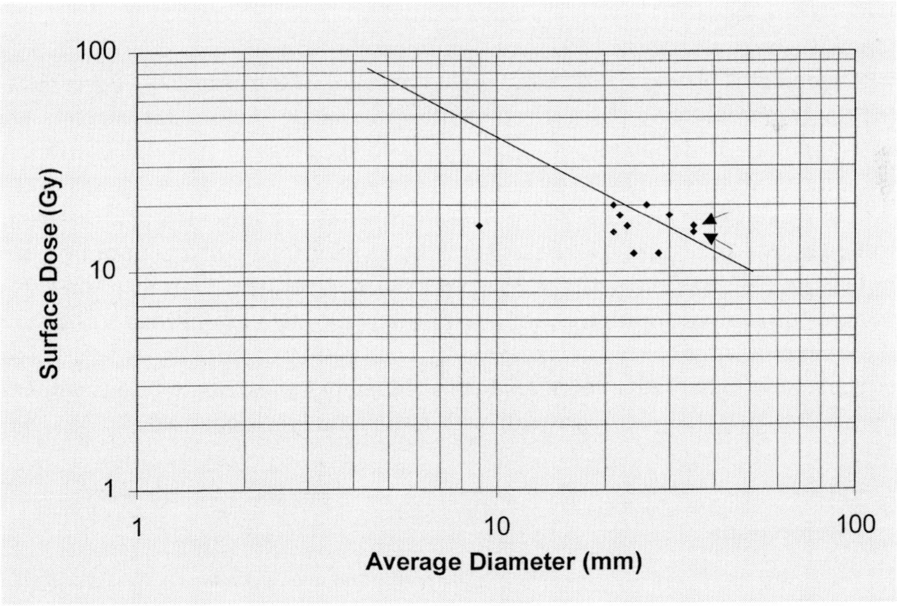

6

Fig. 5. The same scatter-plot as in figure 4, showing only those meningiomas that increased in size after Gamma Knife radiosurgery.

Fig. 6. Scatter-plot showing the dose/volume relationship of all meningiomas in patients having an adverse clinical effect (excluding asymptomatic edema) after Gamma Knife radiosurgery. The arrows point out the 2 patients with permanent complications.

Discussion

These results suggest that outcomes are better and fewer complications occur in patients with tumors 3 cm or less in average diameter. However, it is not clear that patients with tumors larger than 3 cm in average diameter should be excluded from treatment. Half of the patients with tumors 3 cm or larger had good clinical outcomes and the growth of either aggressively recurrent tumors or unresectable skull base or torcular tumors was controlled. Treatment of patients with tumors larger than 3 cm in average diameter seems justified if they understand the increased risks and lower success rate of Gamma Knife therapy for their condition.

Skull base surgical teams, consisting of a neurosurgeon, an ENT surgeon, a plastic surgeon, and even an oral surgeon, are now in place in many medical centers. They can carry out approaches to difficult meningiomas involving long, dangerous and expensive operations. However, one may question whether skull base surgery improves patients enough to justify these procedures. In one operative series of 41 patients with clivus meningiomas, total removal without recurrence was obtained in about 70%, but complications included a mortality rate of 2%, major neurological deficits in 7% and a cranial nerve palsy requiring tracheotomy (cranial nerves IX, X) in 12%. Leakage of cerebrospinal fluid occurred in 9%, with meningitis in 5% [3]. Ojemann [4] has questioned the propriety of ever causing lower cranial nerve palsies in patients with benign tumors. He suggests the best approach is debulking of easily removed intracranial portions of tumor, avoiding morbidity, followed by radiation therapy.

In conclusion, Gamma Knife treatment of intracranial meningiomas controlled growth in about 90% of this small series of 100 patients, with tumor size reduction in 45% of the patients. We observed no treatment mortality and a 2% permanent complication rate. Long-term follow-up data are needed to be sure these tumors will not resume growing in later years. Considering its safety and effectiveness, Gamma Knife radiosurgery of meningiomas should be a treatment option considered for many patients with intracranial meningiomas.

References

1 Wara WM, Sheline GE, Newman H, Townsend JJ, Boldrey EB: Radiation therapy of meningiomas. Am J Roentgenol Radiat Ther Nucl Med 1975;123:453–458.

2 Kjellberg RN: Isoeffective dose parameters for brain necrosis in relation to proton radiosurgical dosimetry; in Szikla G (ed): Stereotactic Cerebral Irradiation. Amsterdam, Elsevier-North Holland, 1979, pp 157–166.

3 Sekhar LN, Janetta PJ, Burkhart LE, Janosky JE: Meningiomas involving the clivus: A six-year experience with 41 patients. Neurosurgery 1990;27:764–781.

4 Ojemann RG: Skull-base surgery: A perspective. J Neurosurg 1992;76:560–570.

Proc 7th Int Meeting Leksell Gamma Knife® Society,
Island of Lana'i, Hawaii, November 1995
Stereotact Funct Neurosurg 1996;66(suppl 1):129–133

Stereotactic and Functional Neurosurgery

Radiation-Induced Edema after Gamma Knife Treatment for Meningiomas

J.C. Ganz, O. Schröttner, G. Pendl

Department of Neurosurgery, Karl Franzens University School of Medicine, Graz, Austria

Key Words
Meningioma · Gamma Knife · Radiosurgery · Edema

Abstract

A retrospective study was performed to analyze some parameters in a consecutive series of 35 Gamma Knife treatments in 34 patients with benign meningiomas. The minimum dose to the tumors was never less than 12 Gy. The follow-up period was from 1 to 3 years. A semiquantitative method of tumor volume assessment was used to measure the tumor response to treatment. The presence and clinical significance of postradiation edema were noted. Even in this short follow-up period, 11 of the 35 tumors were reduced in volume. No tumors increased in size. Edema developed preferentially in nonbasal tumors, especially those around the midline and sagittal sinus. In all but one case where radiation-induced edema was observed was the margin tumor dose 18 Gy or more. It is suggested that doses of 18 Gy or more should probably be avoided in the Gamma Knife treatment of meningiomas and that the greatest care should be taken in selecting non-skull base tumors for this form of treatment.

Introduction

The use of Gamma Knife surgery for the treatment of intracranial meningiomas is a relatively recent development. In 1991, some authors were advocating extreme care as the results seemed to be disappointing [1]. Others were reporting

KARGER

E-Mail karger@karger.ch
Fax + 41 61 306 12 34
http://www.karger.ch

1011–6125/96/0665–0129$10.00/0

Jeremy C. Ganz, MA, PhD, FRCS
Department of Neurosurgery
School of Medicine
Karl Franzens University
A–8036 Graz (Austria)

early results which looked most promising [2, 3]. Later reports confirmed the initial cautious optimism [4–6]. The correct dose has yet to be determined, as have other dose planning parameters. One study suggests that a margin dose of 12 Gy is adequate while less than 12 Gy may be unsatisfactory [5]. The earlier reports mentioned a risk of postradiation edema without a more detailed analysis of its degree and consequences. Moreover, no analysis was done which clarified the factors producing edema.

The purpose of the present study was to analyze clinical material to acquire information about the relationships between dose, dose plan and therapeutic success, and between radiosurgery dose planning parameters and the incidence of complications.

Materials and Methods

Thirty-nine patients with menigiomas received 41 Leksell Gamma Knife treatments between May 1, 1992 and April 30, 1994. The minimum follow-up for this material was 1 year and the maximum, 3 years. One patient had no follow-up studies, and 1 patient was treated twice but had inadequate follow-up studies. Three patients had malignant meningiomas. The remaining 35 treatments in 34 patients form the basis of this retrospective study.

The KULA dose planning system was used for all patients. Patients were assessed after treatment with either computed tomography or magnetic resonance imaging (MRI). The size of the tumor was measured semiquantitatively. The maximum diameter was measured on the images in the three stereotactic directions X, Y and Z. These diameters were then summated and the sum divided by three to give a mean diameter [7]. In all cases, the measurements were compared between the dose planning images and those taken from the most recent follow-up images. Only changes in excess of 10% were registered as such.

The age and sex of the patients were recorded, as were the location of the tumor, its size and the margin and center dose. Clinical changes were registered as were alterations in the size of the tumor and changes occurring in the surrounding brain.

Differences between groups were measured using the χ^2 test. Results were considered significant at $p < 0.005$.

Results

Background Data

There were 35 treatments in 34 patients. In 1 patient, 2 treatments were directed at different targets. In no case was the same target treated twice. The mean age of the patients was 55.5 years (range 30–76 years). The male:female sex ratio was 3.9:1.

Tumor locations were grouped into basal and nonbasal (table 1). Most of the basal tumors were adjacent to the cavernous sinus. All but 1 of the nonbasal tumors were related to the midline.

Table 1. Tumor location

Location	Number
Basal	
Parasellar	8
Sphenoid wing	5
Frontal	2
Orbit	4
Sphenoid wing tent	2
Base temporal	1
Tentorium	1
Clivus	3
Sella-suprasellar	1
Nonbasal	
Falx	5
Parasagittal	1
Parietal convexity	1

The margin dose varied between 12 and 25 Gy (mean 15 Gy). The maximum dose varied between 21 and 57 Gy (mean 33.9 Gy). The edge isodose varied between 25% and 80% (mean 46.7%). In 20 of 35 treatments, the 50% isodose or higher was used.

Tumor Changes after Radiation

Eleven tumors decreased in size, some quite dramatically, while 24 remained unchanged for the duration of the follow-up period. None increased in volume. There was no relation between the change in tumor size and the initial size of the tumor, the location of the tumor, the dose of the tumor margin, the age of the patient or the development of cerebral edema.

Development of Postradiation Edema

Edema was found in 7 of the 34 patients. The timing of its development was difficult to quantify due to variation in follow-up routines. There was no clear-cut evidence of clinical disturbance in 6 of the 7 patients, and the edema resolved in every case.

There was no relationship between the development of edema and the central or margin dose. There was also no relationship between tumor size and the development of edema. However, there was a significant relationship between the margin dose and the development of edema: all but 1 of the patients who developed edema had a margin dose of 18 Gy or more. The remaining patient received

15 Gy in the 25% marginal isodose. There was also a significant relationship between location and the development of edema. Of 28 basal tumors, 2 developed edema, while 5 of 7 nonbasal tumors developed edema.

Discussion

This is a limited retrospective study on a small sample over a short period. However, it still indicates some areas of interest that might reward further study. The material was sequential. Only 3 patients were lost to follow-up. Quite a variety of dose planning strategies were used during the 2 years of the study. This reflects the uncertainty current at the time the patients were treated concerning the right dose and the correct way to perform dose planning.

This study confirms previous work [5] which indicated that a margin dose of 12 Gy was adequate to prevent further growth of most meningiomas treated with Gamma Knife radiosurgery. However, this study goes a stage further in that it examines the relationship between dose, dose planning parameters and the appearance of edema. It is likely that the incidence of edema is underestimated, since T_2 MRI studies were not done routinely in the follow-up of these patients. It is also important to emphasize that the edema with these tumors, at these doses, caused little clinical disturbance and that disturbance was temporary. Nonetheless, it would seem from the results described here that caution is required if doses in excess of 15 Gy are to be considered, and that doses of more than 18 Gy should perhaps be avoided.

Two other studies in this volume [8, 9] found a relationship between meningioma size and complications, which we did not. This is most probably due to the relatively low doses used in most cases and the relatively small size of the tumors.

The relationship between tumor location and the development of edema is more interesting. At the time of writing, no literature has been published on this subject, to the best of our knowledge. However, there is mention made of this phenomenon at another center in another study in the present volume [10]. This lends credence to the notion that it is a real phenomenon rather than a chance observation. If true, then at present there is no explanation. Many possible mechanisms could be adduced relating to the varying biology of meningiomas, such as sex hormone receptors, production of vasoactive peptides, and so on. However, most of these factors could apply to meningiomas anywhere. The one factor that is different for midline supratentorial meningiomas is their proximity to cerebral veins which drain a territory with few or no anastomoses. It is possible that it is involvement of these veins which underlies the edema observed in this study. However, at the time of writing this remains, necessarily, speculative.

Conclusions

(1) With Gamma Knife radiosurgery, it would seem to be wise to limit the margin dose to meningiomas to not more than 15 Gy and definitely not more than 18 Gy.

(2) Radiosurgery of non-basal meningiomas should be carried out with great care or perhaps should be avoided.

References

1 Steiner L, Lindquist C, Steiner M: Meningiomas and Gamma Knife radiosurgery; in Al-Mefty O (ed): Meningiomas. New York, Raven Press, 1991, pp 263–272.

2 Kondziolka D, Lunsford LD, Coffey RJ, Flickinger JC: Gamma Knife radiosurgery of meningiomas. Stereotact Funct Neurosurg 1991;57:11–21.

3 Kondziolka D, Lunsford LD, Coffey RJ, Flickinger JC: Stereotactic radiosurgery of meningiomas. J Neurosurg 1991;74:522–559.

4 Kondziolka D, Lunsford LD: Radiosurgery of meningiomas. Neurosurg Clin North Am 1992;3: 219–230.

5 Ganz JC, Backlund EO, Thorsen FA: The results of Gamma Knife surgery of meningiomas related to size of tumor and dose. Stereotact Funct Neurosurg 1993;61(suppl 1):23–29.

6 Duma CM, Lunsford LD, Kondziolka D, Harsh GR IV, Flickinger JC: Stereotactic radiosurgery of cavernous sinus meningiomas as an addition or alternative to microsurgery. Neurosurgery 1993;32: 699–705.

7 Norén G, Arndt J, Hindmarch T: Stereotactic radiosurgery in cases of acoustic neurinomas: Further experiences. Neurosurgery 1983;13:12–22.

8 Nicolato A, Ferraresi P, Foroni R, Pasqualin A, Piovan E, Severi F, Masotto B, Gerosa M: Gamma Knife radiosurgery in skull base meningiomas. Preliminary experience with 50 cases. Stereotact Funct Neurosurg 1996;66(suppl 1):112–120.

9 Hudgins WR, Barker JL, Schwartz DE, Nichols TD: Gamma Knife treatment of 100 consecutive meningiomas. Stereotact Funct Neurosurg 1996;66(suppl 1):121–128.

10 Nakamura S, Hiyama H, Arai K, Nakaya K, Sato H, Hayashi M, Kawamata T, Izawa M, Takakura K: Gamma Knife radiosurgery for menigiomas: Four cases of radiation-induced edema. Stereotact Funct Neurosurg 1996;66(suppl 1):142–145.

Proc 7th Int Meeting Leksell Gamma Knife® Society,
Island of Lana'i, Hawaii, November 1995
Stereotact Funct Neurosurg 1996;66(suppl 1):134–141

Stereotactic and Functional Neurosurgery

Gamma Knife Radiosurgery for Acoustic Schwannoma: Effects of Low Radiation Dose and Functional Prognosis

M. Hirato, H. Inoue, A. Zama, C. Ohye, T. Shibazaki, Y. Andou

Department of Neurosurgery, Gunma University School of Medicine,
Hidaka Hospital, Maebashi, Japan

Key Words

Gamma Knife radiosurgery · Schwannoma · Acoustic neurinoma · Hearing

Abstract

The effects of relatively low dose Gamma Knife irradiation on acoustic schwannoma were evaluated in 29 patients followed over 2 years after treatment. The mean dose delivered to the tumor periphery was 12.1 Gy. Lowering of the magnetic resonance signal intensity in the tumor center appeared in 69% and signs of tumor shrinkage appeared in 59% of cases. The cyst in the tumor enlarged in 3 cases, and 2 cases developed hydrocephalus. The percentage of pure-tone hearing preservation was 82% at 3 months, 73% at 6 months, 68% at 12 months, 64% at 18 months and 59% at 24 months in 22 out of 29 cases. Relatively low dose Gamma Knife radiosurgery was effective in suppressing tumor growth, with preservation of hearing.

Introduction

With the recent advances in early diagnosis and microsurgical techniques, total removal of acoustic schwannoma with preserved facial function can generally be achieved. However, comparison of the results of radiosurgery with those of microsurgery suggests that radiosurgery is the treatment of choice [1, 2]. The Gamma Knife is now used widely for the treatment of acoustic tumors [1–7], not

KARGER

E-Mail karger@karger.ch
Fax + 41 61 306 12 34
http://www.karger.ch

1011–6125/96/0665–0134$10.00/0

M. Hirato, MD
Department of Neurosurgery
Gunma University School of Medicine
3-39-15, Showa-machi
Maebashi, Gunma 371 (Japan)

only in elderly patients, but also in patients with medical problems, bilateral tumors, a tumor in the only functioning ear, a recurrent tumor, or in patients who refuse surgical removal. Recently, hearing preservation [8] has become a major target of the treatment of acoustic schwannoma by both Gamma Knife radiosurgery and microsurgery [7, 9–11].

Acoustic schwannoma has been treated by Gamma Knife radiosurgery with a relatively high radiation dose [3–6], but lower doses have been recommended [2, 12]. We report our experience in treating acoustic schwannoma with a relatively low radiation dose [13], and have followed patients for 2 years. We studied changes in the tumor appearance by magnetic resonance imaging (MRI) and the clinical course, especially changes in hearing acuity.

Materials and Methods

Twenty-nine patients, 12 males and 17 females, were studied. The mean age was 47.7 years (range 24–71). Two patients had bilateral tumors. Five were already deaf on the tumor side when treated. Tumor size was from 5 mm (intrameatal) to 31 mm. Dosimetry was carefully planned in both the axial and coronal planes. Special attention was paid to the porus and the internal auditory meatus, using computed tomography (CT) scans to correct the distortion of the MRI. The mean maximum dose was 25.2 Gy (range 17–34 Gy) and the mean dose to the tumor margin was 12.1 Gy (range 9.9–17 Gy). The mean follow-up time was 27.6 months (range 24–40 months).

The following variables were studied: (1) the time when signal change or shrinkage of the tumor was observed on MRI; (2) the original tumor size (approximate volume); (3) the central dose; (4) the margin dose, and (5) the time course of the changes in hearing. The changes in the different variables were then correlated with each other.

Results

MRI Study

Lowering of the MR signal intensity in the tumor center appeared in 20 of 29 cases (69%). The mean latency from treatment to the observation of this change was 5.7 months. In 13 of these cases, there was tumor shrinkage. In the whole series there were signs of tumor shrinkage in 17 of 29 cases (58.6%) with a latency from treatment to observation of 17.8 months. In 2 cases, the MR signal intensity and the tumor size remained unchanged. In 9 of the 29 cases (31%), the tumor size remained unchanged (fig. 1). A tumor cyst was observed in 3 patients after Gamma Knife surgery, although the solid component of these tumors had shrunk. Surgical removal of the tumor was carried out in 2 of these cases.

Tumors receiving less than 12 Gy to the margin took longer to shrink than those receiving 12 Gy or more. Moreover, in tumors receiving less than 12 Gy,

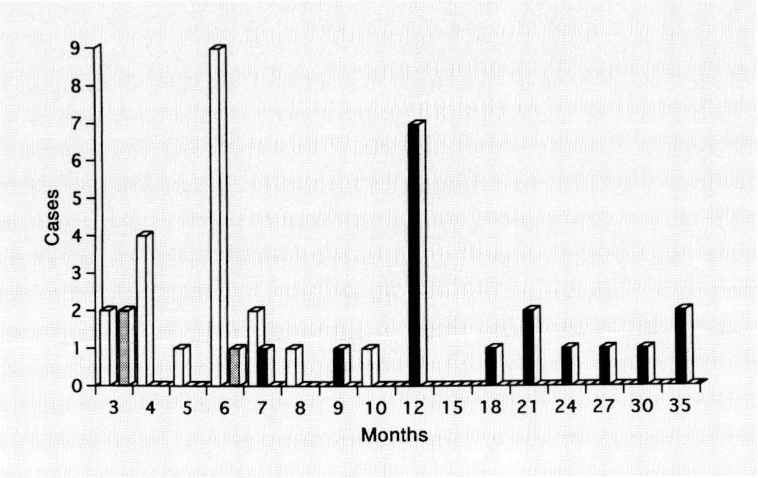

Fig. 1. Onset of MR signal intensity changes in the central area, and tumor shrinkage. Open bars represent patients with lowering of the MR signal intensity; filled bars represent patients with tumor shrinkage; hatched bars indicate patients with tumor enlargement.

there was a tendency for the tumor volume to remain unchanged despite the appearance of changes in MR signal intensity in the tumor center. Nonetheless, even with a margin dose as low as 10 Gy, a lowering of MR signal intensity and tumor shrinkage were observed (fig. 2).

Clinical Study

Follow-up examination revealed trigeminal neuropathy in 1 patient and facial weakness in 3 patients. These deficits were temporary. No patient developed lower cranial nerve deficit. Two patients had transient vertigo appearing just after treatment. Another 2 patients required implantation of a shunt following development of hydrocephalus.

Hearing acuity was studied in 22 of 29 patients after radiosurgery; 7 patients were excluded because 5 were already deaf at the time of treatment and the remaining 2 underwent subsequent surgery. Hearing acuity for pure tone was preserved in 18 (82%) at 3 months, 16 (73%) at 6 months, 15 (68%) at 12 months, 14 (64%) at 18 months and 13 (59%) at 24 months. Speech discrimination studies detected subtle changes of hearing. In cases with a pure tone loss of more than 50 dB, speech tone acuity fell markedly after treatment, resulting in useless hearing. This was also true for a small tumor (less than 10 mm diameter). In 2 cases with pure-tone hearing loss of less than 50 dB, useful hearing was preserved over

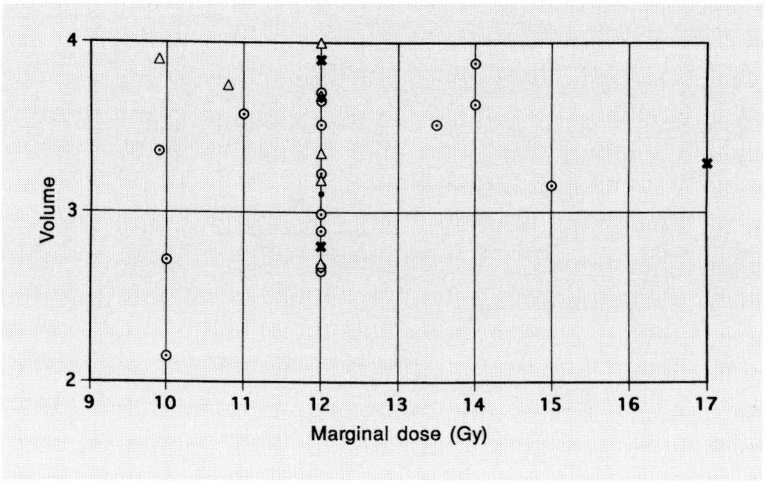

Fig. 2. Change of MR signal intensity, tumor shrinkage, original tumor size and margin dose. The circled dots show tumor shrinkage with and without MR signal intensity change; triangles show MR signal intensity change in the tumor center without tumor shrinkage; solid dots show no tumor shrinkage or MR signal intensity change; crosses show an enlarging cyst after treatment. Tumor volumes are shown as the logarithm of the volume in mm^3 in the vertical axis.

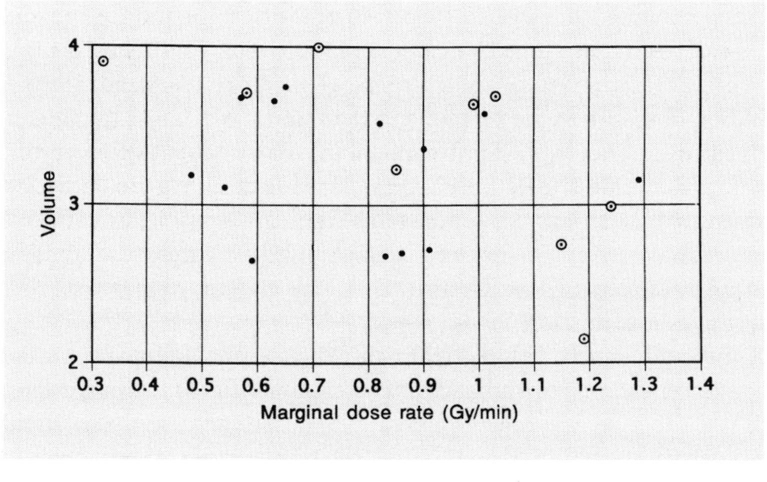

Fig. 3. Changes in auditory acuity, original tumor size and dose rate to the tumor margin. Circled dots show patients with a decrease in hearing after radiosurgery; solid dots indicate patients with preserved hearing. Tumor volumes are shown as the logarithm of the volume in mm^3 in the vertical axis.

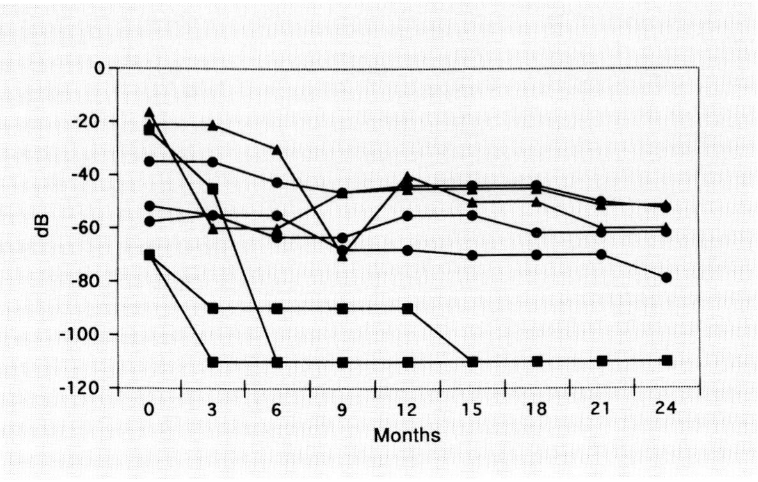

Fig. 4. Decrease of auditory acuity during follow-up. Circles show patients with a gradual decrease in auditory acuity. Squares show patients with a rapid decrease in auditory acuity. Triangles show patients with recovery of auditory function after an initial rapid decrease.

2 years. In 2 cases where pure-tone hearing loss was between 50 and 70 dB, the pure tone acuity remained unchanged, while speech discrimination decreased markedly. In 3 cases with pure-tone hearing loss of more than 70 dB, hearing was almost lost.

The radiation dose rate to the margin and the tumors was larger in patients who showed hearing deterioration after treatment (fig. 3). A patient with neurofibromatosis type 2 showed a late deterioration of hearing despite a low radiation dose rate. However, this patient did not have useful hearing prior to treatment. There was no definite correlation between the risk of hearing deterioration and either the margin or the center dose. Even 10 Gy to the margin could be associated with a deterioration in hearing.

Auditory function levels before treatment and during follow-up varied among 9 patients with hearing disturbance after treatment (fig. 4). In one patient, periodic auditory function was not observed. Three patients showed a rapid decrease in hearing acuity within 3 months and 3 showed a more gradual deterioration. One patient had a pure-tone loss of 35 dB and a speech discrimination score of 100% prior to treatment. After 2 years, the results were 52.5 dB and 50%, respectively. Interestingly, 2 patients showed a rapid deterioration in hearing followed by recovery over a few months. One patient had 16.3 dB pure-tone loss and a speech discrimination of 100% prior to treatment. After 3 and 6 months, the scores were 60 dB and 55%, respectively. At 9 months they were 46.3 dB and 100% and at 12 months 45 dB and 95%, respectively. At 21 and 24 months they were 51.3 dB and 85%, respectively. Half the patients retained tinnitus after radiosurgery with exacerbation in some.

Discussion

Our study suggests that Gamma Knife radiosurgery is effective in suppressing the growth of acoustic schwannomas with a relatively low radiation dose. Of course, the follow-up period is still short. Lowering of MR signal intensity occurred in 69% of patients, 5–6 months after treatment, and tumor shrinkage occurred in 58.6%, 17–18 months after treatment. In 31% of cases, the tumor size remained unchanged. Thus, arrest of tumor growth was achieved in nearly 90% of cases. Previous reports have observed a tumor control rate of 90% with higher doses of radiation [3–6]. Low radiation doses of 10–15 Gy achieved arrest of tumor growth in 81% of cases. Previous reports have also shown reduction of MR signal intensity in 70% of cases and signs of shrinkage appearing within the first 2 years after treatment in 30% of cases [2, 12]. The nature and timing of the MR signal changes were similar in this study and in the work of others with both high and low irradiation doses. The tumor shrinkage rate was higher than previously reported with low radiation dose but the latency interval from treatment to shrinkage was longer. It was interesting that tumor shrinkage was observed with margin doses in the range of 10–17 Gy and center doses in the range of 17–34 Gy. However, tumors receiving less than 12 Gy to the margin took longer to shrink, compared with those receiving 12 Gy or more. Moreover, the lower doses were associated with a greater tendency for the tumor to remain unchanged. Thus a minimum margin dose of 12 Gy would seem to be appropriate for obtaining tumor growth suppresion. This is rather lower than previously recommended doses.

A parallel histological study following radiosurgery demonstrated various changes, both destructive and proliferative, in the tumor blood vessel walls [13]. These vascular changes may be related to changes in MR signal intensity or tumor shrinkage following radiosurgery. However, further study is needed to clarify the mechanisms of tumor growth suppression and the minimum dose required to achieve it [14]. Enlargement of tumors after treatment was caused by cyst expansion in this series. The treatment of this enlargement remains difficult and surgery was performed in 2 of these cases. Hydrocephalus developed in another 2 patients requiring shunting. The mechanisms underlying cyst enlargement and hydrocephalus remain unkonwn. It is necessary to remember that such complications may develop after radiosurgery [12].

In this study, 68% of patients retained pretreatment levels of hearing at 1 year, and 59% retained such hearing at 2 years after treatment. Recent good surgical series recording the results for acoustic schwannoma show that the chance of retaining useful hearing is 52% if the tumor diameter is less than 2 cm. If the diameter is less than 1 cm, useful hearing preservation can be achieved in 83% of cases [11]. The classification of pretreatment auditory function and the definition of useful hearing remain matters of debate [7, 8, 10]. Nonetheless, the results of this series are acceptable and comparable with the results of good surgery. The follow-up time in this series is short. Previous studies have shown that deterioration in hearing begins from 1 week to 12 months after treatment [3]. However, comparison of hearing acuity at 1 year and 5 years showed little change [12]. Therefore we may expect that the hearing acuity recorded in this series will be maintained over a longer period. There was no significant correlation between hearing deterioration and either the margin or the center dose. The minimum dose producing a hearing disturbance was 10 Gy. Thus, risk factors related to dose [15] were not significant within the dose range used in this study.

Since all the patients in this series were treated over the last 2 years, the selection of collimators might be important. With larger collimators, dose planning is less precise, which is particularly important with smaller intrameatal tumors. Great attention to the dose plan is required in the treatment of acoustic schwannomas. Moreover, imaging factors can be important. In this series all dose planning was performed using both CT and MRI to enable precise stereotactic localization with CT and better anatomical definition with MRI. The paucity of cranial nerve neuropathies and their temporary course may be attributed at least in part to the precise imaging.

In conclusion, low-dose Gamma Knife radiosurgery effectively suppressed the growth of acoustic schwannomas, with an acceptable rate of hearing preservation and a low complication rate. Further improvements may be expected as dose planning becomes even more precise and as more information is available about the optimal dose to these tumors.

References

1 Pollock BE, Lunsford LD, Kondziolka D, Flickinger JC, Bissonette DJ, Kelsey SF, Jannetta PJ: Outcome analysis of acoustic neuroma management: A comparison of microsurgery and stereotactic radiosurgery. Neurosurgery 1995;36:215–229 .

2 Steiner I, Lindquist C, Steiner M: Radiosurgery; in Symon L, Calliauw L, Cohadon F, Lobo Antunes J, Loew F, Nornes H, Pasztor E, Pickard JD, Strong AJ, Yasargil MG (eds): Advances and Technical Standards in Neurosurgery. Vienna, Springer, 1992, vol 19, pp 19–102.

3 Linskey ME, Lunsford LD, Flickinger JC: Radiosurgery for acoustic neurinomas: Early experience. Neurosurgery 1990;26:736–745.

4 Linskey ME, Lunsford LD, Flickinger JC: Stereotactic radiosurgery for acoustic nerve sheath tumors; in Lunsford LD (ed): Stereotactic Radiosurgery Update. New York, Elsevier, 1992, pp 321–334.
5 Norén G, Arndt J, Hindmarsh T: Stereotactic radiosurgery in cases of acoustic neurinoma: Further experiences. Neurosurgery 1983;13:12–22.
6 Norén G, Arndt J, Hindmarsh T, Hirsch A: Stereotactic radiosurgical treatment of acoustic neurinomas; in Lunsford LD (ed): Modern Stereotactic Neurosurgery. Boston, Nijhoff, 1988, pp 481–489.
7 Ogunrinde OK, Lunsford LD, Flickinger JC, Kondziolka D: Stereotactic radiosurgery for acoustic nerve tumors in patients with useful preoperative hearing: Results at 2-year follow-up examination. J Neurosurg 1994;80:1011–1017.
8 Gardner G, Robertson JH: Hearing preservation in unilateral acoustic neuroma surgery. Ann Otol Rhinol Laryngol 1988;97:55–66.
9 Glasscock ME, Hays JW, Minor LB, Haynes DS, Carrasco VN: Preservation of hearing in surgery for acoustic neuromas. J Neurosurg 1993;78:864–870.
10 Kondziolka D, Lunsford LD: Preservation of hearing in acoustic neurinoma surgery. J Neurosurg 1993;78:154–156.
11 Post KD, Eisenberg MB, Catalano PJ: Hearing preservation in vestibular schwannoma surgery: What factors influence outcome? J Neurosurg 1995;83:191–196.
12 Norén G, Greitz D, Hirsch A, Lax I: Gamma Knife radiosurgery in acoustic neurinoma; in Steiner L, Lindquist C, Forster D, Backlund EO (eds): Radiosurgery: Baseline and Trends. New York, Raven Press, 1992, pp 141–148.
13 Hirato M, Inoue H, Nakamura M, Ohye C, Hirato J, Shibazaki T, Andou Y: Gamma Knife radiosurgery in acoustic neurinoma: Early effects and the preservation of hearing. Neurol Med Chir (Tokyo) 1995;35:737–741.
14 Ganz JC, Mathisen JR, Thorsen F, Backlund EO: Acoustic neurinoma: Early results related to radiobiological variables; in Lunsford LD (ed): Stereotactic Radiosurgery Update. New York, Elsevier, 1992, pp 359–363.
15 Urie MM, Fullerton B, Tatsuzaki H, Birnbaum S, Suit HD, Convery K, Skates S, Goitein M: A dose response analysis of injury to cranial nerves and/or nuclei following proton beam radiation therapy. Int J Radiat Oncol Biol Phys 1992;23:27–39.

Proc 7th Int Meeting Leksell Gamma Knife® Society,
Island of Lana'i, Hawaii, November 1995
Stereotact Funct Neurosurg 1996;66(suppl 1):142–145

Stereotactic and Functional Neurosurgery

Gamma Knife Radiosurgery for Meningiomas: Four Cases of Radiation-Induced Edema

S. Nakamura, H. Hiyama, K. Arai, K. Nakaya, H. Sato, M. Hayashi, T. Kawamata, M. Izawa, K. Takakura

Department of Neurosurgery, Tokyo Women's Medical College, Tokyo, Japan

Key Words

Meningioma · Gamma Knife radiosurgery · Radiation-induced edema · Edema · Complications

Abstract

We review 48 cases of meningioma treated with Gamma Knife radiosurgery. The mean marginal dose was 15 Gy and the mean follow-up was 12 months. Follow-up computed tomography and magnetic resonance imaging showed tumor shrinkage in 19 cases, central necrosis in 1 case, loss of contrast enhancement in 1 case, and no change in 27 cases. We noted 4 cases of radiation-induced edema in supratentorial meningiomas.

Introduction

We review 48 cases of meningioma treated with Gamma Knife radiosurgery. Among them we observed 4 cases of radiation-induced edema.

Material and Methods

From May 1993 to March 1995, 48 cases of meningioma were treated with Gamma Knife radiosurgery (table 1). The male:female ratio was 1:2 and their mean age was 55 years. Most of the tumors were less than 3 cm in diameter. The mean maximum dose was 34 Gy and the mean marginal dose was 15 Gy. The mean follow-up period was 12 months.

KARGER

E-Mail karger@karger.ch
Fax + 41 61 306 12 34
http://www.karger.ch

1011–6125/96/0665–0142$10.00/0

S. Nakamura, MD
Department of Neurosurgery
Tokyo Women's Medical College
8-1 Kawada-cho, Shinjuku
Tokyo (Japan)

Table 1. Clinical characteristics of 48 patients with meningiomas

Characteristic	Cases
Females:males	32:16
Location	
Skull base	32
Supratentorial	9
Falcotentrial	3
Ventricular	3
Others	1

Table 2. Follow-up results on CT/MRI demonstrating consistent increase in the response rate

Shrinkage	19 (40%)
Central necrosis	1
Loss of enhancement	1
No change	27 (56%)

Results

Follow-up computed tomography (CT)/magnetic resonance imaging (MRI) revealed a decrease in tumor size in 19 cases, central necrosis in 1 case, loss of contrast enhancement in 1 case, and no change in 27 cases (table 2). Radiation-induced edema was noted in 4 cases (table 3, fig. 1, 2), located supratentorially. One was at the falx and 2 were parasagittal; 2 were recurrences of preexisting edema. The patients' ages were 73, 67, 63 and 38 years and the dose to the tumor margin was 24, 18, 15 and 20 Gy, respectively. Their neurological status deteriorated, but subsequently resolved in 1 patient.

Discussion

Although the follow-up period was relatively short in these cases, 48 meningiomas treated with the Gamma Knife were reviewed. Supratentorial meningioma, preexisting edema and old age may be risk factors for the development of radiation-induced edema.

Table 3. Complication due to radiation-induced edema in 4 cases

Age	Sex	Location	Size ml	Maximum dose Gy	Marginal dose Gy	Symptom
67	F	falx	9	36	18	hemiparesis
73	F	convexity	4	30	24	frontal ataxia
38	F	parasagittal	15	50	20	hemiparesis
63	F	parasagittal	12	38	15	hemiparesis visual field disturbance

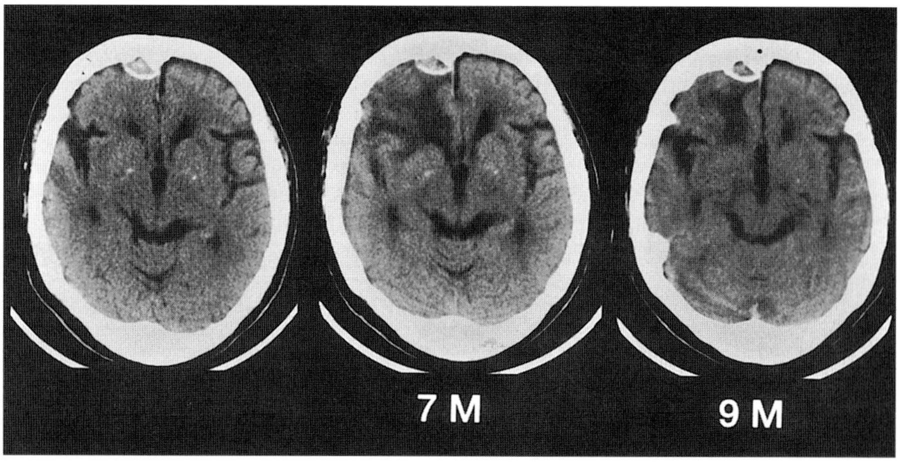

Fig. 1. Case 1. A convexity meningioma treated with Gamma Knife radiosurgery with a margin dose of 24 Gy. Four months after radiosurgery, the patient developed headache and ataxia. The follow-up CT demonstrated radiation-induced edema in the left frontal lobe 7 months later. The edema diminished and the symptoms resolved over the next 2 months.

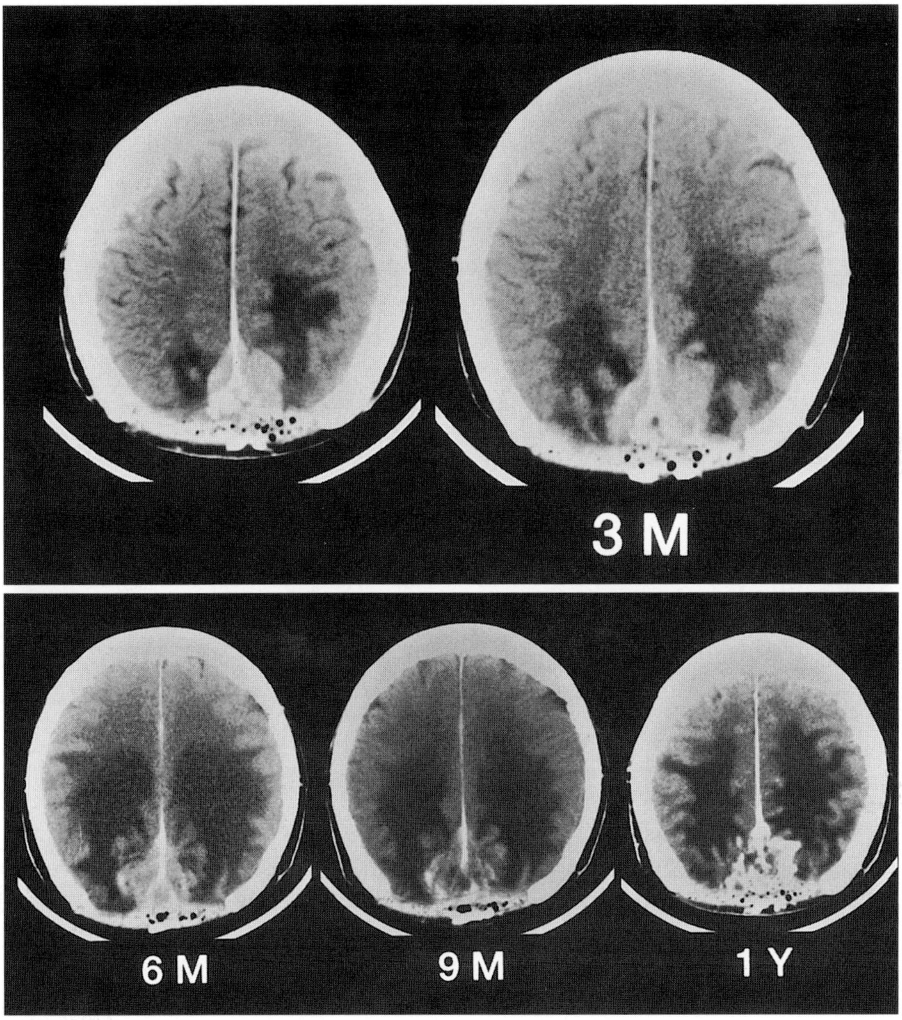

Fig. 2. Case 2. A parasagittal meningioma with preexisting edema treated with Gamma Knife radiosurgery, after an operation, with a margin dose of 15 Gy. The patient developed hemiparesis and a visual-field disturbance 2 months later. The follow-up CT demonstrated radiation-induced edema. Gradual tumor shrinkage was seen on subsequent CT examinations. However, the clinical deficits remain unchanged 1 year after treatment.

Proc 7th Int Meeting Leksell Gamma Knife® Society,
Island of Lana'i, Hawaii, November 1995
Stereotact Funct Neurosurg 1996;66(suppl 1):146–156

Stereotactic and Functional Neurosurgery

Dose Distribution and Shrinkage of Acoustic Neurinomas 2 Years after Gamma Knife Treatment

H. Nagano[a], *K. Tanohata*[a], *E. Kato*[a], *S. Nakayama*[b], *H. Fujino*[b], *S. Matsubara*[c]

Departments of [a] Radiology and [b] Neurosurgery, Yokohama Rosai Hospital, and [c] Department of Radiology, Yokohama City University, Yokohama, Japan

Key Words

Dose-volume histogram · Stereotactic radiosurgery · Acoustic neurinoma · Dose optimization · NIH-image

Abstract

To examine the relationship between dose distribution and tumor shrinkage of acoustic neurinomas, correlation coefficients between distribution probabilities of some dose areas and residual tumor ratios of 21 cases were studied at 2 years. Approximating a dose-volume histogram to beta-distribution, two essential dose areas for tumor control were extracted: a dose area from 14.2 to 24.7 Gy contributed to tumor shrinkage, whereas a dose area from 27.3 to 29.4 Gy was contraindicated. Given that there are at least two different dose areas with reverse characters, a formula with two opposing logistic components is proposed to predict tumor control. With this formula, Gamma Knife treatment of acoustic neurinomas may be optimized.

Introduction

Gamma Knife treatment for acoustic neurinoma is said to be as effective as microsurgery, without the risk of infection, bleeding or leakage of cerebrospinal fluid [1]. It is viewed as an important option for treating acoustic tumors in those patients who have no symptomatic brain stem or cerebellar compression from a large tumor [2]. Despite its acceptance as a safe and effective treatment for acous-

KARGER
E-Mail karger@karger.ch
Fax + 41 61 306 12 34
http://www.karger.ch

1011–6125/96/0665–0146$10.00/0

Hisato Nagano, MD
3211-1 Kozukue Cho, Kohouku-Ku
Yokohama, Kanagawa 222 (Japan)

Table 1. Patients' age, and treatment dose characteristics

	Minimum	Mean	Maximum	SD
Age, years	21.0	55.1	74.0	13.2
Tumor volume, cm^3	0.5	3.9	17.0	4.0
Peripheral isodose, %	45	52.4	70.0	6.6
Minimum dose, Gy	12.0	15.9	18.0	2.0
Mean dose, Gy	15.1	20.0	24.8	3.0
Maximum dose, Gy	24.0	30.5	37.8	4.3

tic tumors, however, it has been questioned whether there is a relationship between dose distribution characteristics and tumor shrinkage [3]. There is an increasing demand for objective evaluation of competing treatment plans and computer optimization of the dose distribution [4]. Because Gamma Knife treatment inevitably produces an inhomogeneous dose distribution, it may be necessary to integrate the effect of every dose area of a target to evaluate the total irradiation effect. Dose-volume histograms (DVHs) have been generally used to analyze stereotactic radiosurgery under these inhomogeneous dose conditions [5].

Previously, assuming a normally distributed DVH, it was revealed that a distribution probability of a dose area of 15.8–22.3 Gy produced tumor shrinkage, whereas 25.9–26.0 Gy did the reverse. Linear combination of the two correlated somewhat to the residual tumor ratio (see below) with a correlation coefficient of 0.61, but if the DVH did not fit a normal distribution, a dose area far from the mean value might not be analyzed precisely.

The aim of this study was to reveal a relationship between the DVH and tumor shrinkage using beta-distribution and to propose a formula predicting tumor shrinkage. Using this formula, the dose distribution may be optimized to achieve good tumor shrinkage.

Materials and Methods

Patients

The relationship between dose distribution and tumor shrinkage was analyzed in 21 of 31 patients treated from February 1992 to March 1993 in our institution and followed by magnetic resonance imaging (MRI) at 24 ± 6 months. The mean age of the patients was 55.1 years. Tumor volumes ranged from 0.5 to 17 cm^3 (mean 3.9 cm^3). The patients received 12–18 Gy to the tumor margin with a maximum dose of 24–37.8 Gy in a single fraction (table 1).

DVH and Beta-Distribution

The KULA system calculates a three-dimensional dose distribution and saves 31*31*31 matrix data as a temporal file named 'DOSE.DAT.' Although the matrix value is the central point of each voxel, the volume of which is a cube of the grid size, each voxel is small enough to neglect inhomogeneity of the dose distribution within it. The class width of the histogram was 1% of the maximum dose. The cumulative DVH of the target was approximated to a cumulative beta-distribution using the least-squares method.

The distribution probability of some dose areas may be related to tumor shrinkage. The distribution probability from dL to dU Gy is hereafter expressed as beta-distribution[dL–dU].

Residual Tumor Ratio (R)

R was defined as the tumor volume at 2 years divided by that at treatment. The volume was calculated by summing tumor areas on the MR images using the truncated-cone model. Each area was estimated with an NIH-image. The truncated-cone model could only be used when the tumor shadow was seen on at least three slices of the MRI films, since with fewer slices, the error in the calculated volume is large. Overestimation of the volume might be within 5 to 20% if the volume of the tumor was within the ordinal limits of the Gamma Knife treatment, so the error of the value R will be 15% or less (see Appendix).

R versus Distribution Probability

Each R was plotted against beta-distribution[dL–dU], and the correlation coefficient calculated. Lower and upper limits of the dose area were scanned from the periphery to the maximum dose. If the correlation coefficient between R and beta-distribution[d1–d2] is close to –1, the dose area from d1 to d2 Gy may be the most effective. If the coefficient between R and beta-distribution[d3–d4] is large, the area from d3 to d4 Gy may be ineffective, and may even cause enlargement when the value is positive. Two dose areas may be extracted using this method: one is effective, the other ineffective or even detrimental.

Predictive Formula Using Beta-Distribution

A linear combination of the above two probabilities, beta-distribution[d1–d2] and beta-distribution[d3–d4] produces the following predictive formula:

$$\text{CalcR} = a + b*\text{beta-distribution}[d1-d2] + c*\text{beta-distribution}[d3-d4] \qquad (1)$$

where a, b and c are constants, d1 and d2, the lower and upper limits of the effective dose area respectively, and d3 and d4, the lower and upper limits of the ineffective dose area, respectively.

The three constants, a, b and c, may be calculated by minimizing the summation of squares of the remainder CalcR – R, or by the least-squares method. If the correlation coefficient between R and CalcR is large enough (as is probable from the previous consideration using the normal distribution), the two dose regions which are extracted as above are essential to tumor control.

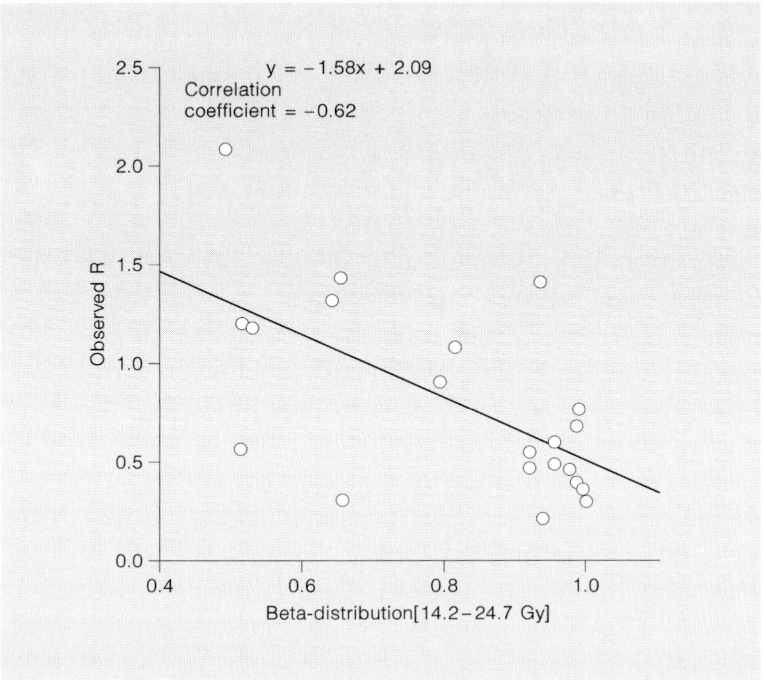

Fig. 1. R plotted against beta-distribution[14.2–24.7 Gy]. As the beta-distribution increased, R decreased.

Results

R vs. Distribution Probability

The DVH approximated well to the beta-distribution. The standard deviation of the error was within 1.1%. The probability of the distribution from 14.2 to 24.7 Gy, beta-distribution[14.2–24.7 Gy] correlated with R (correlation coefficient = –0.62). For cases with a high probability of being in this dose area, tumor size was well controlled in size, but for those with a low probability, the results varied (fig. 1). The correlation coefficient between beta-distribution[27.3–29.4 Gy] and R was 0.61. The value was positive, and it might be possible that this dose area was characterized by tumor swelling (fig. 2). The probability of this dose area correlated well (coefficient = –0.74) with the error (beta-distribution[14.2–24.7 Gy] – R) (fig. 3).

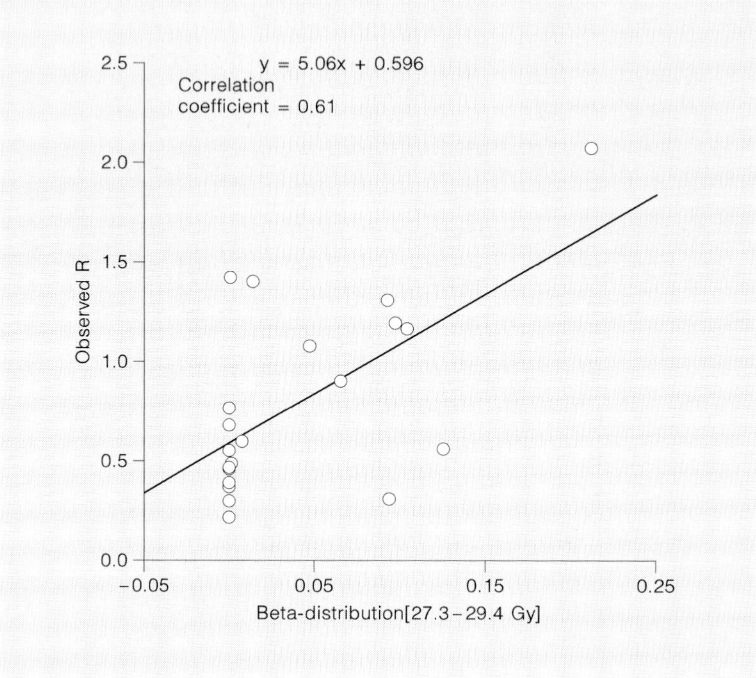

Fig. 2. R plotted against beta-distribution[27.3–29.7 Gy]. As the subvolume irradiated with this dose range increased, tumor size increased.

Predictive Formula Using Beta-Distribution

The upper and lower limits of the two dose areas were inserted in equation (1):

CalcR = a + b*beta-distribution[14.2–24.7 Gy] + c*beta-distribution[27.3–29.4 Gy] (2)

All constants in equation (2) were estimated by the least-squares method (see below), yielding a = 1.47, b = – 0.93 and c = 2.39. The correlation coefficient between R and CalcR was calculated as 0.65. Figure 4 plots R against CalcR.

Discussion

Predictive Formula Using Beta-Distribution

R and CalcR were well correlated. This means that the two extracted regions were crucial for tumor control. The areas were similar but wider than those estimated using the normal distribution, because that beta-distribution approximated the DVH more precisely than does a normal distribution.

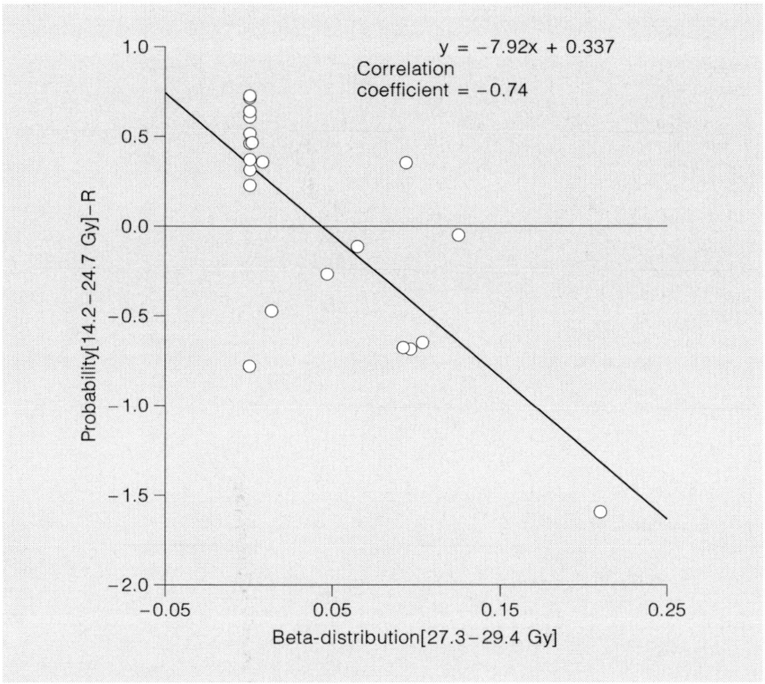

Fig. 3. The error in figure 1 (beta-distribution[14.2–24.7 Gy] – R) correlated well with beta-distribution[27.3–29.4 Gy]. A combination of these two dose distribution areas may correlate with R.

Expansion of Equation (1)

From the viewpoint of the DVH, beta-distribution[dL–dU] is identical to the normalized tumor volume within the range from dL to dU Gy. When v(d) is defined as the normalized partial volume of the tumor-irradiated d Gy class, summation of v(d) from the class containing dL Gy to the class containing dU Gy equals beta-distribution[dL–dU], if the class width is small enough. As the v(d) is normalized by the whole tumor volume, summation of v(d) from the peripheral to the maximum tumor dose classes equals 1. Then equation (1) can be modified as below.

$$\mathrm{CalcR}' = \mathrm{SUM}\{[a + r'(d)]*v(d)\} \tag{3}$$

$$\text{where: } r'(d) = \begin{cases} b \text{ [from d1 to d2 Gy classes]} \\ c \text{ [from d3 to d4 Gy classes]} \\ 0 \text{ [other dose classes]} \end{cases} \tag{4}$$

$$\mathrm{SUM}\,\{a*v(d)\} = a \tag{5}$$

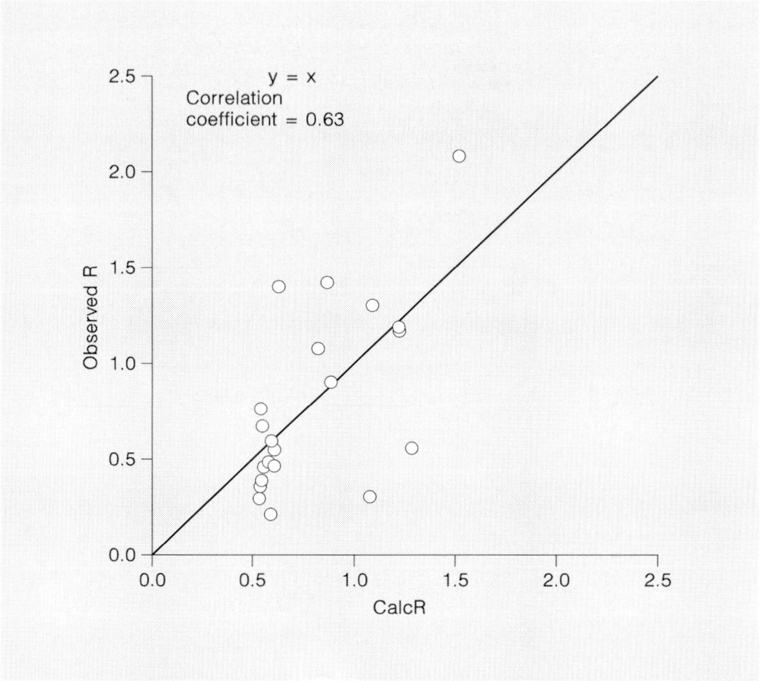

Fig. 4. The result of the predictive formula CalcR.

SUM means summation of values from peripheral to maximum dose classes. When a + r′(d) is replaced by r(d), equation (3) is simplified:

$$\text{CalcR}' = \text{SUM}\{r(d)*v(d)\} \qquad (6)$$

where

$$r(d) = a + r'(d) \qquad (7)$$

Because only two dose areas could be extracted by the method, r(d) took only three values. These two areas were essential, as mentioned above, but this also led to dispersed values of r(d). The next step is to expand equations (4) or (7) to be able to keep a succession along all the dose classes.

Predictive Formula on DVH Itself

A formula with two opposing logistic components was proposed on the supposition that there were at least two different dose areas with reverse characteristics. Each constant of the equation was defined by the least-squares method.

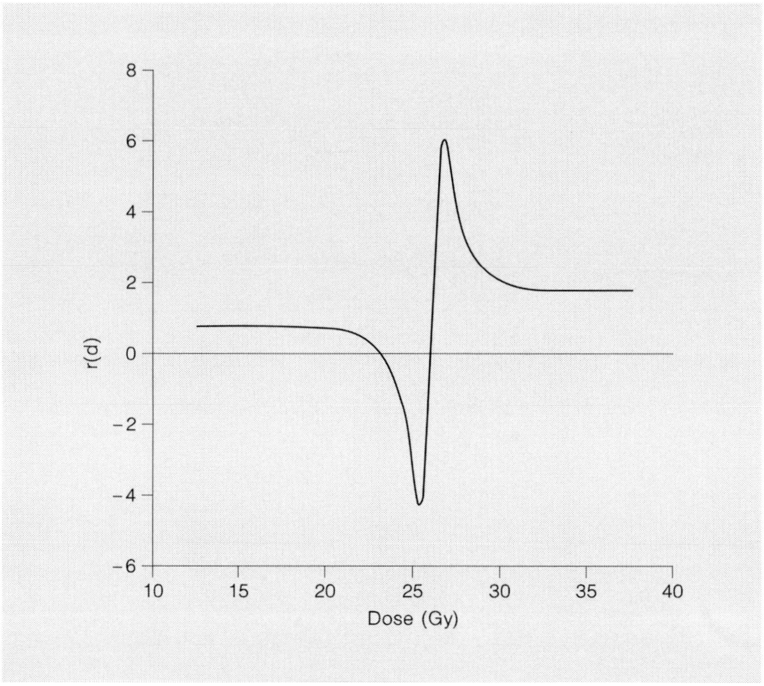

Fig 5. The expanded 'residual rate' of a unit volume irradiated by dose d, r(d), plotted against dose. There was a large fault at 25.9 Gy. The value of r(d) was large in the high-dose area.

$$r(d) = 0.8 - 11.3/\{1 + \exp[(25.9 - d)/1.1]\} + 12.3/\{1 + \exp[(25.9 - d)/0.02]\} \quad (8)$$

Figure 5 shows r(d) as a function of the dose. There is a large fault at 25.9 Gy, lying between a steep trough and peak. This is radiobiologically controversial, but, as shown in figure 6, CalcR′ correlated well with R (correlation coefficient = 0.76).

Radiobiological Considerations

From an analytical point of view, equation (6) states that the initial subvolume of the tumor irradiated with d Gy, v(d), will become r(d)*v(d), 2 years after treatment. r(d) may be called the residual rate of a unit volume at 2 years. However, the problem then arises that the value r(d) is negative just before the fault at 25.9 Gy. What does the negative residual volume rate mean? Does it work like a 'black hole?' Returning to the beginning, equation (6) derives from equations (1) and (2) with the expansion of r(d) to maintain a succession along the whole dose

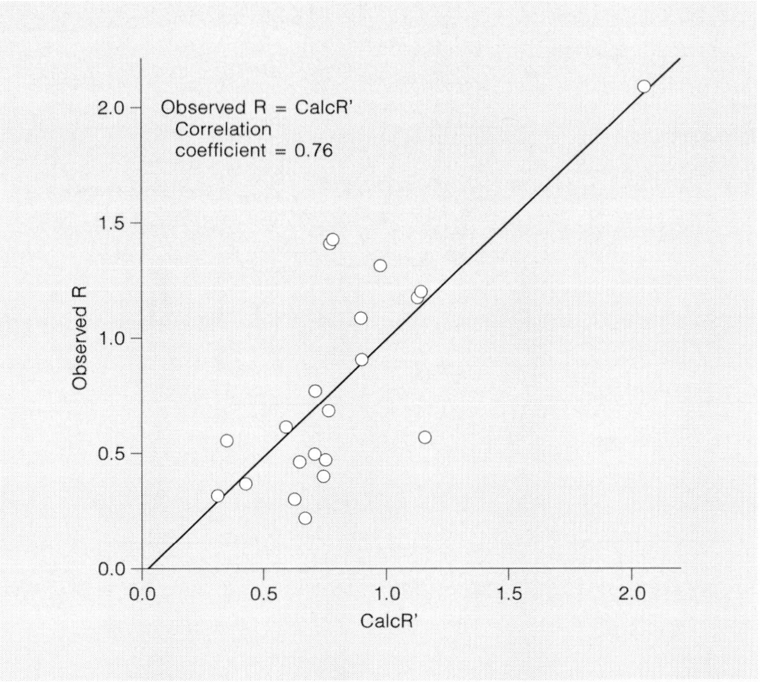

Fig. 6. The result of the expanded predictive formula CalcR′. R and CalcR′ correlated well.

area. And since equations (1) and (2), on statistical grounds, are only concerned with some dose areas, it would be unreasonable to assume radiobiological significance directly from equation (8).

As for the fault, the dose 25.9 Gy is very similar to the 50% central-necrosis-forming dose which we presented previously. We can propose no radiobiological basis for this phenomenon. However, it is believed that the tumor stroma may be destroyed above that dose. From a radiobiology perspective, killing of a functional subunit or clonogen should be dose dependent [4, 5]. More tumor cells should be killed as the irradiation dose increases. This is in contradiction to the subvolume increase seen above the fault. It is probable that this is not tumor growth, but mass swelling, which would then be a sequela of high-dose irradiation.

At least empirically, from a clinical perspective, it is possible to predict whether or not the mass will have shrunk at 2 years. Too high a dose may be contraindicated for tumor shrinkage. All previous optimization efforts aimed only at maximizing the irradiation dose without increasing normal-tissue damage should be reconsidered, at least for acoustic neurinomas.

Full Optimization

To fully optimize a treatment plan, a method is needed which can determine the probability of complications for normal tissues affected by the treatment [6]. The work reported here was concerned only in obtaining good mass shrinkage. Referring to the value of CalcR′, estimated from the predictive formula, a good result can be obtained with careful dose determination. The formula may reject a higher dose because r(d) becomes larger when the dose increases over 25.9 Gy. This may contribute to full optimization, because the probability of normal-tissue damage will probably also be reduced when the irradiation dose is kept low.

Using the beta-distribution, two critical dose areas for tumor control were obtained. Linear combination of the beta-distribution of these two areas provided a predictive formula, which was expanded to cover the whole dose area. The expanded formula agreed more precisely with the clinical observations. Full optimization of the treatment, including a determination of the complication probability, is the target of the next study.

Appendix

The truncated-cone model was used to estimate the tumor volume (V).

$$V = SUM\{[vi + sqr(vi*vi + 1) + vi + 1]/3\} \quad (9)$$

where

SUM{Ai}: summation of Ai from A0 to An;
sqr(A): square root of A;
n: number of slices;
ch: height of a tumor on coronal MRI;
st: thickness of a slice;
si: area of a shadow of the tumor on axial MRI;
$v0 = vn + 1 = 0$; $v1 = s1*[ch - st*(n - 2)]/2$;
$vn = sn*[ch - st*(n - 2)]/2$; $vi = si*st$ ($i = 2$ to $n - 1$);

When n is large enough, v1 and vn may be calculated as vi ($i = 2$ to $n - 1$).

Figure 7 represents the result of a hypothetical experiment. Spherical masses with radii ranging from 3 to 18 mm were sliced by an imaginary MRI. The slice thickness was set from 0.3 to 3 mm. Slice position, the position of the central slice relative to the center of the mass, ranged from 0 to st/2 from the center of mass in five steps. ch was radius*2. Except for the central slice, the area of the shadow was estimated on the surface of the slice near the center of the mass, in order to gather the total partial volume. The area of the central slice is

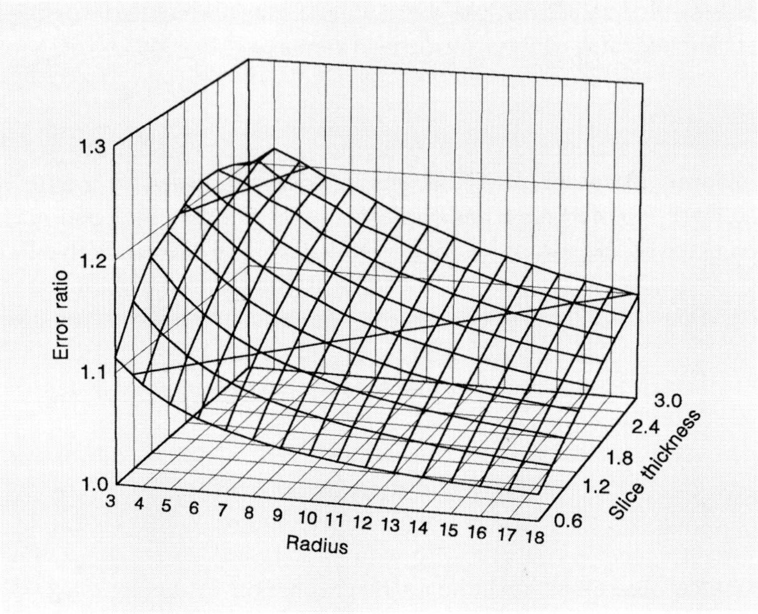

Fig. 7. The surface represents an error ratio of an overestimation of the volume calculated by the truncated-cone model to the true volume of the sphere, the radius of which ranged from 3 to 18 mm. The slice thickness was set from 0.3 to 3 mm.

calculated as 3.14*radius^2. The mass volume was calculated at all five steps of the slice position, and the mean value estimated. This mean value was then divided by the mathematically estimated mass volume (= 4/3*3.14*radius^3), to give the error ratio. The surface of figure 7 shows this error ratio.

References

1 Norén G, Greitz D, Hirsch A, Lax I: Gamma Knife surgery in acoustic tumours. Acta Neurochir 1993;58:104–107.

2 Lunsford LD, Kondziolka D, Flickinger JC: Radiosurgery as an alternative to microsurgery of acoustic tumors. Clin Neurosurg 1992;38:619–634.

3 Flickinger JC, Lunsford LD, Linskey ME, Duma CM: Gamma Knife radiosurgery for acoustic tumors: Multivariate analysis of four year results. Radiother Oncol 1993;27:91–98.

4 Andrzej N, Michael G: Modeling of normal tissue response to radiation: The critical volume model. Int J Radiat Oncol Biol Phys 1992;25:135–145.

5 Colombo F, Francescon P, Cora S, Testolin A: Evaluation of linear accelerator radiosurgical techniques using biophysical parameters (NTCP and TCP). Int J Radiat Oncol Biol Phys 1995;31: 617–628.

6 Lyman JT: Complication probability as assessed from dose-volume histograms. Radiat Res Suppl 1985;8:13–19.

Proc 7th Int Meeting Leksell Gamma Knife® Society,
Island of Lana'i, Hawaii, November 1995
Stereotact Funct Neurosurg 1996;66(suppl 1):157–163

Stereotactic and Functional Neurosurgery

Radiosurgery for Pineal Tumors: Is Biopsy Indicated?

C.B. Chasan[a], *S. Goetsch*[b], *K. Ott*[c]

[a] Radiation-Oncology Department, Sharp Chula Vista Medical Center, Chula Vista, Calif., and
[b] San Diego Gamma Knife Center, Scripps Memorial Hospital, La Jolla, Calif., USA

Key Words

Pineal · Neoplasm · Biopsy · Radiosurgery · Imaging

Abstract

Pineal region tumors can be difficult to biopsy, given the critical structures in the location of the pineal gland. Modern computerized imaging techniques like computed tomography and magnetic resonance imaging used in association with tumor markers and the age at presentation may enable treatment without biopsy using a rational treatment algorithm.

Introduction

Prior to the widespread use of microsurgery, operation for pineal region tumors was associated with a combined morbidity and mortality between 50 and 70% [1], due to the anatomic complexity of the pineal region. There are vital midbrain structures immediately adjacent to the pineal region as well as critical blood vessels, including the internal cerebral veins, the basal vein of Rosenthal, the vein of Galen, and the precentral cerebellar vein. Due to the high risk of surgery, conservative management was popular in the 1950s and 1960s. This included fractionated radiation therapy administered without the benefit of histological diagnosis [1, 3]. Therapeutic test doses of radiation became standard in the treatment of pineal region tumors. This empirical approach to radiation therapy resulted in unnecessary or ineffective brain irradiation in many patients with benign or radioresistant tumors [4]. The development of microsurgical techniques

KARGER

E-Mail karger@karger.ch
Fax + 41 61 306 12 34
http://www.karger.ch

1011–6125/96/0665–0157$10.00/0

Cynthia Bajada Chasan, MD
Sharp Chula Vista Medical Center
Radiation-Oncology Department
751 Medical Center Court
Chula Vista, CA 91911 (USA)

has enabled surgery of the region to be undertaken with fewer risks. Thus, a change in the management of pineal region tumors occurred with the test dose of radiation being replaced by microsurgical resection or biopsy [5, 6]. Even so, morbidity and mortality persisted despite the use of microsurgical techniques. However, advances in neurodiagnostic imaging techniques and stereotactic-guided surgery provide an acceptable and effective method of obtaining histological diagnosis of pineal region tumors [7, 8]. Recent literature on the diagnosis and management of pineal region tumors advocates biopsy to confirm the histological diagnosis prior to deciding appropriate treatment [9, 10].

In the last few years, many centers have begun to report on radiosurgery in the treatment of pineal region tumors [9, 10]. As a consequence of these pilot studies, the necessity for biopsy in every case has been questioned. This paper will outline the current imaging and diagnostic techniques that can be used to determine whether or not a biopsy is required prior to treating pineal region tumors with radiosurgery.

Histologic Possibilities in the Pineal Region

There are several nonneoplastic lesions that may arise in the pineal region, including arachnoid cysts, pineal cysts, and vascular lesions such as cavernous malformation, arteriovenous malformation (AVM), and aneurysm of the vein of Galen. Neoplastic lesions are also reasonably common in the pineal region. Lesions of pineal parenchymal origin include pineocytoma, pineoblastoma, or mixed pineocytoma/blastoma. Glial-origin tumors may also present in this region, including glioma, ganglioma, neurinoma, and ganglioglioma. Meningioma may also occur. Germ cell tumors may originate in the pineal region, either germinomas or nongerminomas. The latter may be either benign or malignant. Benign lesions include teratomas and dermoid tumors. The malignant lesions include choriocarcinoma, embryonal carcinoma, yolk sac tumor, and mixed nongerminoma germ cell tumors. There are thus a multitude of tumors that can arise in the pineal gland region. Consequently one can understand why the use of tumor markers and age distribution in addition to radiographic imaging could be imperative in achieving a diagnosis.

Imaging Characteristics of Pineal Region Tumors

Pineoblastomas, malignant teratomas, and malignant nongerminomatous germ cell tumors are usually more than 4 cm in diameter at presentation and are irregular in shape. Dermoid and mature teratomas may show a fat signal on mag-

Table 1. Imaging characteristics of pineal region tumors

Tumor	MRI characteristics
Pineoblastoma/malignant teratoma	>4 cm and irregular shape
Malignant nongerminoma germ cell tumors	
Dermoid/mature teratoma	fat signal
Choriocarcinoma	hemorrhage
Glioma/pineocytoma	originate from collicular plate or surrounding temporal lobe
Germinoma	(males with diabetes insipidus and Parinaud's syndrome)

Table 2. Tumor markers for pineal region tumors

Histology	AFP	β-HCG	PAP
Germinoma	–	+/–	+
Malignant teratoma	+/–	+/–	+/–
Endodermal sinus tumor	+	–	+/–
Pineocytoma/blastoma	–	–	–
Germ cell tumor	+/–	+/–	+/–
Choriocarcinoma	–	+	+/–
Embryonal cell tumor	+	+	+/–
Teratoma	–	–/+[a]	+/–

[a] Rare.

netic resonance imaging (MRI). Choriocarcinoma may present as a hemorrhagic lesion. Gliomas and pineocytomas originate from the collicular plate or the surrounding temporal lobe (table 1).

Tumor Markers

Tumor markers have often been used to aid the diagnosis of pineal region tumors. α-Fetoprotein (AFP), β-human chorionic gonadotropin (β-HCG), and placental alkaline phosphatase (PAP) have been found to be elevated in certain germ cell tumors, embryonal cell tumors, and choriocarcinoma (table 2). Pineal cytomas and pinealoblastomas do not excrete any specific tumor markers.

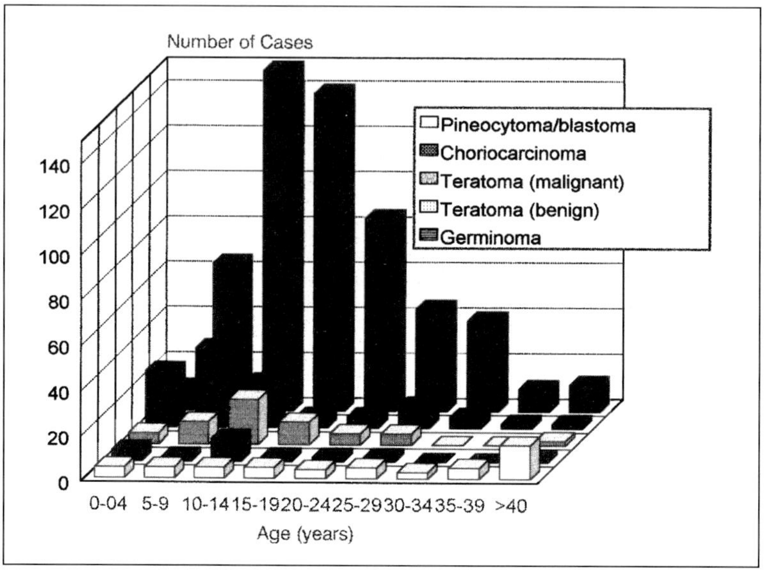

Fig. 1. Histology of pineal region tumors based on age.

Incidence of Pineal Region Tumors Based on Histology

The most common pineal region tumors are germinomas which comprise approximately 35% of all cases. Astrocytomas represent 15% of the tumors. Another 15% are pineoblastomas. These three lesions thus contribute approximately 65% of all lesions seen in the pineal region in people less than 40 years of age. The histology of pineal region tumors can be further subclassified in relation to the age of the patient at presentation, as shown by Oi [11] (fig. 1). The incidence of germinomas reaches a peak between the ages of 15 and 30 and falls rapidly thereafter. The tumor is rarely seen after the age of 40. Choriocarcinoma, benign and malignant teratomas all tend to be tumors of childhood. Pineocytomas tend to have a low incidence in childhood and increase in incidence after 40 years of age.

Treatment Algorithms for Pineal Region Tumors

A treatment algorithm can be suggested for pineal region tumors, based on the diagnostic data mentioned above, derived from MRI scans, tumor markers, and age at diagnosis (fig. 2). For patients under the age of 40, a rigorous histologi-

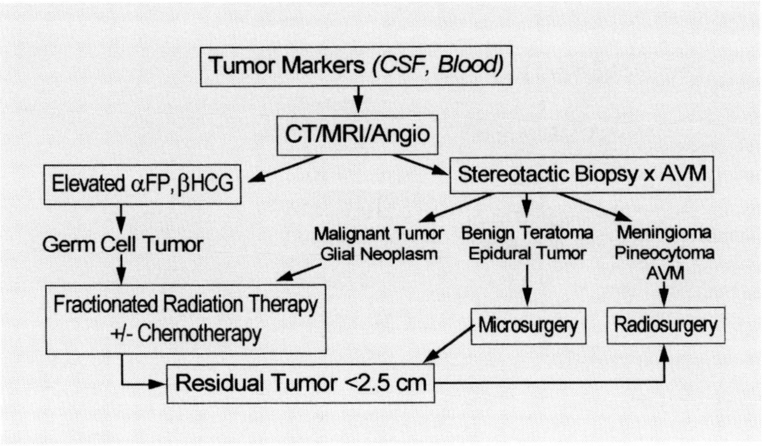

Fig. 2. Treatment algorithm for patients under 40 years old. CSF = Cerebrospinal fluid; Angio = angiography; αFP = α-fetoprotein.

cal diagnosis must be obtained because many of these patients will need comprehensive radiation therapy and chemotherapy. Two algorithms are proposed, one for patients of 40 years of age or less and the other for patients over 40 years of age.

Patients Under 40 Years Old

These patients should initially be evaluated with a CT and MRI scan. An angiogram should be used if the lesion is thought to be vascular. The patient must then undergo cerebrospinal fluid and blood studies for AFP, β-HCG, and PAP. A chest X-ray is performed to exclude a midline mass. Routine blood studies should also be obtained. Patients with markedly elevated β-HCG may proceed directly to chemotherapy and radiation therapy protocols [12]. After this workup, the patient would undergo a stereotactic biopsy of the lesion if an AVM and/or cavernous malformation have been excluded. If the tumor is found to be a benign teratoma or an epidermoid tumor, the patient should be referred for microsurgery. Residual disease of less than 2.5 cm should be treated with radiosurgery. If the patient is found to have a germ cell tumor, malignant tumor or glial neoplasm, he should proceed to fractionated radiation therapy plus or minus standard chemotherapeutic protocols. If the tumor is found to be a meningioma, pineocytoma or an AVM, the patient may proceed straight to radiosurgery, provided the lesion is not too large.

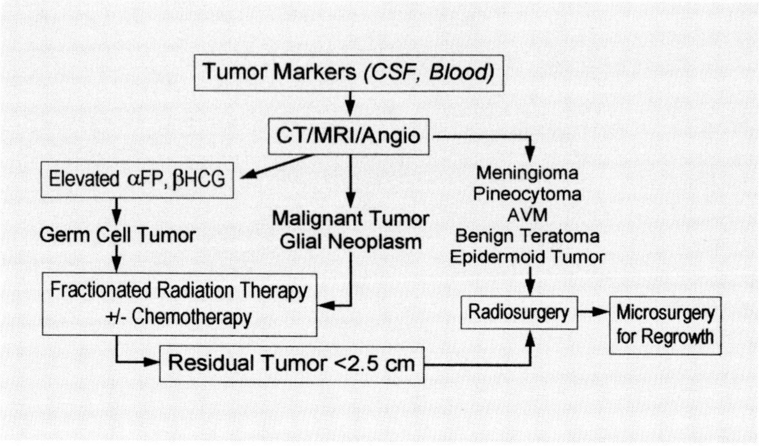

Fig. 3. Treatment algorithm for patients over 40 years old. CSF = Cerebrospinal fluid; Angio = angiography; αFP = α-fetoprotein.

Patients Over 40 Years Old

For these patients a CT and MRI scan are performed initially with an angiogram for lesions that are felt to be vascular. If the MRI shows a noncystic, fat-free, smooth circular lesion, less than 3 cm in diameter, the probable diagnoses are meningioma, pineocytoma, or low-grade glioma. Radiosurgery in such cases could be undertaken before biopsy. It is necessary to exclude from such treatment patients who need surgical decompression. If MRI characteristics and tumor marker studies are not indicative of a meningioma, pineocytoma, low-grade glioma, or AVM, the patient should have a stereotactic biopsy. Following the stereotactic biopsy, treatment recommendations can be given based on the algorithm (fig. 3).

Conclusions

There have been several recently reported cases of pineal region tumors being treated with radiosurgery. To date, all lesions have been subjected to biopsy or surgical resection for a histologic diagnosis prior to radiosurgery. However, given the anatomy of the pineal gland and the surrounding vascular structures, this procedure is not without risk. Using the information obtained in this report, the surgeon may elect to proceed with radiosurgery based on imaging results, tumor markers, and the age of the patient. This would certainly not be recommended in patients less than 40 years of age unless the β-HCG was markedly elevated. The reason for such caution is that many of these lesions may require comprehensive fractionated radiotherapy as well as chemotherapy. However, there are tumors that do give a classic appearance on MRI scan, do not secrete tumor markers, and are generally found in an elderly population, which would be appropriate for radiosurgery. Radiosurgery could then be considered without the additional risk of stereotactic biopsy.

Acknowledgment

Special thanks are given to Chris Urbaniak for her help in preparing this manuscript.

References

1 Rand RW, Lemmen LJ: Tumors of the posterior portion of the third ventricle. J Neurosurg 1953; 10:1–18.
2 Genkin RD, Simpson WJK, Keen CW: Pineal and suprasellar germinomas: Results of Radiation treatment. J Neurosurg 1978;48:99–107.
3 Pertuiset B, Visot A, Metzger J: Diagnosis of pineoblastomas by positive response to cobalt teletherapy. Acta Neurochir (Wien) 1976;34:451–452.
4 McDonnel DE: Pineal epidermoid cyst: Its surgical therapy. Surg Neurol 1977;7:387–391.
5 Chapman PH, Linggood RM: The management of pineal area tumors: A recent appraisal. Cancer 1980;46:1253–1257.
6 Neuwelt EA: An update on the surgical treatment of malignant pineal region tumors. Clin Neurosurg 1985;32:397–428.
7 Conway LW: Stereotaxic diagnosis and treatment of intracranial tumors including initial experience with cryosurgery for pinealomas. J Neurosurg 1973;38:453–460.
8 Moser RP, Backlund EO: Stereotactic techniques in the diagnosis and treatment of pineal region tumors; in Neuwelt ER (ed): Diagnosis and Treatment of Pineal Region Tumors. Baltimore, Williams & Wilkins, 1984, pp 234–253.
9 Dempsey PK, Lunsford LD: Stereotactic radiosurgery for pineal region tumors. Stereotact Radiosurg 1992;3:245–253.
10 Baumgartner JE, Edwards MSB: Pineal tumors. Pediatr Neurooncol 1992;4:853–862.
11 Oi S, Matsumoto S: Controversy pertaining to therapeutic modalities for tumors of the pineal region: A world wide survey of different patient populations. Child Nerv Syst 1992;8:332–336.
12 Edwards MSB, Hudgins RJ, Wilson CB, Levin VA, Wara WM: Pineal region tumors in children. J Neurosurg 1988;68:689.

Proc 7th Int Meeting Leksell Gamma Knife® Society,
Island of Lana'i, Hawaii, November 1995
Stereotact Funct Neurosurg 1996;66(suppl 1):164–173

Stereotactic and Functional Neurosurgery

Pineal Region Tumors: The Role of Stereotactic Radiosurgery

L. Manera[a,b], *J. Régis*[a], *O. Chinot*[a], *D. Porcheron*[a], *O. Levrier*[b], *P. Farnarier*[b], *J.C. Peragut*[a]

Departments of
[a] Neurosurgery, and
[b] Neuroradiology, La Timone Hospital, Marseilles, France

Key Words

Radiosurgery · Gamma Knife radiosurgery · Pineal region tumors · Germinomas · Pinealoblastoma

Abstract

Between July 1992 and August 1995, 11 patients with pineal region tumors (PRTs) were treated at our center. Ages ranged from 8 to 72 years (median 21). Diagnosis was confirmed by histological examination in 7 patients. The remaining cases had strong neuroradiological and marker evidence of the diagnosis, so that a stereotactic biopsy could be avoided. The pathological diagnoses were pinealocytoma (n = 1), tectal astrocytoma (n = 1), germinoma (n = 2), pinealoblastoma (n = 2), and meningioma (n = 3). The marginal dose to these tumors ranged from 12 to 18–20 Gy. Conventional external radiotherapy was never used in this series. With a median follow-up of 12.3 months (range 2–34), all tumors responded to treatment and disappeared or ceased growing. We observed no mortality or major morbidity. One patient (tectal astrocytoma) had a mild radiation-induced reaction, with headache and transient worsening of an abducent nerve palsy, which were controlled with steroids. In germinomas and pinealoblastomas, recovery of normal cerebrospinal fluid circulation was observed in less than 7 days, in parallel with major tumor shrinkage. In this study we confirm that radiosurgery can be an effective and safe alternative for the treatment of pinealocytomas and low-grade tectal gliomas. Moreover, we consider that the characteristics of the radiosurgery technique suggest the method should be evaluated for the treatment of malignant PRTs.

KARGER

E-Mail karger@karger.ch
Fax + 41 61 306 12 34
http://www.karger.ch

1011–6125/96/0665–0164$10.00/0

J. Régis, MD
Gamma Unit, Hôpital de La Timone
Bd Jean Moulin
F–13385 Marseille Cedex 5 (France)

Introduction

Pineal region tumors (PRTs) are uncommon and constitute approximately 1 and 8% of all intracranial tumors in adults and children, respectively. The diagnostic and therapeutic dilemmas posed by PRTs are due to their strategic location and to their pathological variability. Many different types of neoplasm may develop in the pineal region [1].

It has recently been reported that 36–50% of pineal tumors are either benign or radioresistant [2]. As a result of advances in microsurgical techniques, the mortality and morbidity rates associated with pineal region surgery have diminished significantly. However, the risk of cerebrospinal fluid (CSF) seeding after surgical procedures must be kept in mind [2]. Germinomas and pinealoblastomas are radiosensitive tumors which respond well to conventional radiotherapy. Nevertheless, the literature reflects differences of opinion concerning the place of irradiation and that of chemotherapy.

In the last decade, the optimal therapy for pineal tumors has been a combination of microsurgery, chemotherapy, and radiotherapy. The exact combination would be determined on a case-by-case basis, depending on the clinical problems and the tumor histology. More recently, the use of a 'radiosurgical boost' to standard radiotherapy has been described by Casentini and Colombo [3]. Moreover, radiosurgery alone without conventional radiotherapy was proposed for the treatment of low-grade tectal astrocytomas or pinealocytomas [4, 5].

However, the place of radiosurgery alone in the treatment of PRTs is not well defined. Thus, the discussion of results after Gamma Knife radiosurgery of PRTs could help to deepen our understanding of the use of radiosurgery for these tumors.

Clinical Material and Methods

Clinical Material

Of the 877 cases treated with the Leksell Gamma Knife in our department over a 38-month period since July 1992, 11 have had PRTs. Patients' ages ranged from 8 to 72 years. There were 5 males and 6 females. All patients had a Karnofsky performance score of more than 90. Clinical symptoms included headache, nausea, vomiting, Parinaud's syndrome, and diplopia.

The first clinical symptoms were headache, nausea and/or vomiting in 4 patients, diplopia in 2 patients and Parinaud's syndrome in 1 patient. Four patients showed other symptoms as detailed in table 1. Cranial computed tomography (CT) scanning was performed in all patients. Signal characteristics before and after contrast enhancement are shown in table 2.

Magnetic resonance (MR) images were obtained in all cases and consistently demonstrated the morphology of the tumor and its anatomical relationships. MR T_2-weighted and

Table 1. Pretherapy findings

Patient age/sex	First sign and symptom	Hydrocephalus treatment	CSF/plasma markers	Biopsy, diagnosis	Other treatment
(1) 32/F	fortuitous	yes: VPS before biopsy	negative	SB, pinealoblastoma	chemotherapy
(2) 72/F	gait ataxia – behavioral disturbance	yes: vertriculocister-nostomy before RS	negative	no, meningioma	no
(3) 37/M	ICH	yes: VPS before biopsy	negative	SB, germinoma	no
(4) 10/M	fourth-nerve palsy	no	negative	SB, astrocytoma	no
(5) 21/M	Parinaud's syndrome, fourth-nerve palsy	no	negative	no (germinoma?)	no
(6) 14/F	ICH, visual deterioration	yes: ventriculo-cisternostomy	negeative	microsurgery, pinealocytoma	microsurgery
(7) 26/M	ICH	yes: VPS before biopsy	negative	SB, pinealocytoma	no
(8) 17/F	endocrinopathy	no	negative	SB, pinealocytoma	chemotherapy
(9) 8/M	follow-up MRI: von Recklinghausen	no	negative	no (astrocytoma?)	no
(10) 20/F	diplopia	yes: VPS before RS	negative	no (astrocytoma?)	no
(11) 20/F	ICH	yes: ventriculocister-nostomy before RS	negative	CSF cytology, pinealoblastoma	chemotherapy

VPS = Ventriculoperitoneal shunt; SB = stereotactic biopsy; RS = radiosurgery; ICH = intracranial hypertension; MRI = magnetic resonance imaging.

T_1-weighted images before and after gadolinium enhancement are detailed in table 2. Angiography was used to visualize the deep venous system prior to biopsy in 5 cases.

Five tumors were homogeneous and 6 were nonhomogeneous. Nine patients had well-delimited round or ovoid masses. Two tumors were poorly delimited. Tumor size was variable, ranging from 1,008 mm^3 to 10,625 mm^3 (mean 3,304 mm^3). Cystic regions were found in 2 tumors and necrotic regions in 3. Calcification was present in 1 tumor. Hemorrhage was recognized only after surgery as a hypersignal in short repetition time (TR) images and combined hyper- and hyposignals in long TR images. No fat-typical signal was seen on the MR images. PRTs have a reputation for CSF seeding within both the cranium and the spinal canal. However, no patient in this series showed dissemination metastases in the cerebrospinal spaces.

Occlusive hydrocephalus was found in 7 cases (63%). To relieve this, ventriculoatrial shunts were implanted in 3 patients, and ventriculocisternostomy was performed in 2. Shunting was performed prior to stereotactic biopsy and/or radiosurgery. Two patients with asymptomatic hydrocephalus were followed by CT or MRI, without shunt or ventriculostomy.

Table 2. CT and MRI characteristics before radiosurgery

Patient	Pretreatment imaging		Tumor size mm
	CT	MRI	
1	heterogeneous/poorly delimited iso and hypo Iodo+	heterogeneous/poorly delimited T_1-w iso and hypo T_2-w iso and hypo Gd+	20 × 22 × 26
2	homogeneous/well delimited iso Iodo++	homogeneous/delimited T_1-w iso T_2-w hyper Gd++	34 × 25 × 25
3	homogeneous/well delimited hypo Iodo++	homogeneous/delimited T_1-w hypo T_2-w iso Gd+	12 × 15 × 12
4	homogeneous/well delimited iso Iodo+	homogeneous/delimited T_1-w hypo T_2-w iso Gd+	12 × 9 × 14
5	heterogeneous/well delimited (cyst) iso Iodo+	heterogeneous/delimited (cyst) T_1-w iso and hypo T_2-w iso and hyper	16 × 12 × 14
6	heterogeneous/poorly delimited (calcifications/blood) hypo Iodo+	heterogeneous/poorly delimited (calcifications/blood) T_1-w hypo and hyper T_2-w hypo and hyper Gd++	22 × 19 × 20
7	homogeneous/well delimited iso Iodo++	homogeneous/delimited T_1-w hypo T_2-w hyper Gd++	12 × 20 × 14
8	heterogeneous/well delimited (cyst) iso and hypo Iodo++	heterogeneous/delimited (cyst) T_1-w iso and hypo T_2-w iso and hyper Gd++	15 × 15 × 12
9	homogeneous/well delimited iso Iodo	homogeneous/delimited T_1-w iso T_2-w hyper Gd++	14 × 12 × 12
10	heterogeneous/well delimited iso and hypo Iodo+	heterogeneous/well delimited (necrosis?) T_1-w iso and hypo Gd++ (ring enhancement)	15 × 20 × 15
11	heterogeneous/well delimited (necrosis?) iso and hypo lodo+	heterogeneous/well delimited (necrosis?) T_1-w iso and hypo T_2-W iso and hypo Gd++	17 × 28 × 16

iso = Isosignal; hypo = hyposignal; Iodo = contrast; T_1-w = T_1-weighted; T_2-w = T_2-weighted; hyper = hypersignal.

Levels of α-fetoprotein (AFP), human chorionic gonadotropin (HCG) and carcinoembryonic antigen in the serum or CSF were measured, in all cases with a negative result. Histological diagnosis was performed by stereotactic biopsy through an orthogonal-lateral approach after stereotactic angiogram (Talairach method) in 5 cases. In another case, the pathological diagnosis was obtained from LCR cell analysis (pinealoblastoma).

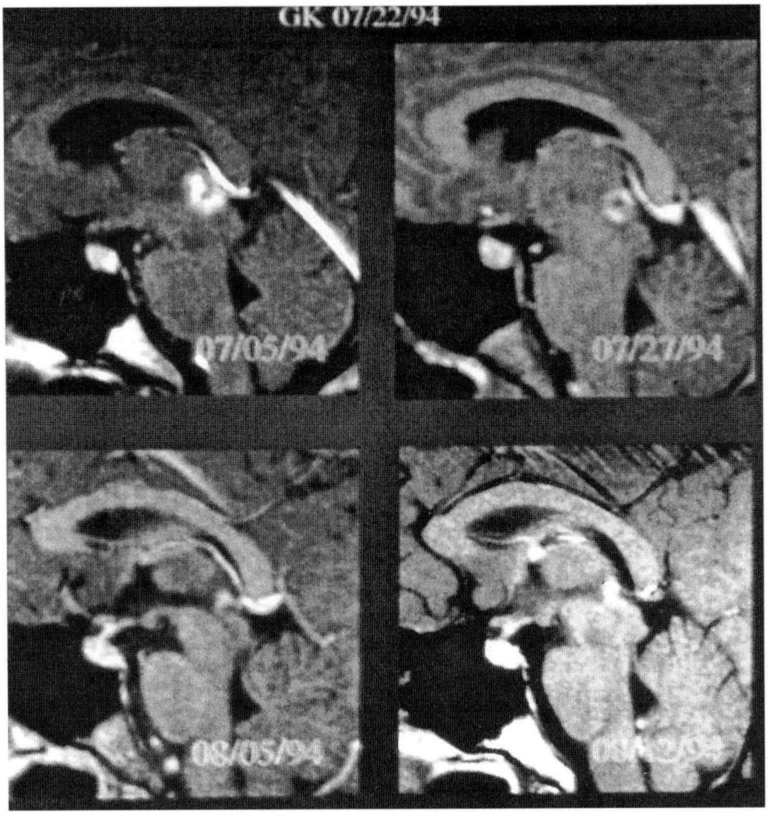

Fig. 1. MRI before and after radiosurgical treatment (on 22 July 1994) for a germinoma. **a** 5 July 1994. **b** 27 July 1994. **c** 5 August 1994. **d** 12 August 1994.

The pathological diagnosis was 3 pinealocytomas, 2 pinealoblastomas, 1 germinoma, and 1 astrocytoma. In 3 cases, tumor diagnosis was derived from radiological evidence. A round, well-defined, homogeneous tumor displacing the surrounding structures without invasion in an older woman was thought to most likely be a meningioma. Two tumors clearly originating from the upper part of the mesencephalon tectum in 2 young patients were most likely low-grade tectal gliomas. A very small pineal lesion in a young man, with MRI findings consistent with a germinoma and with no detectable markers (CSF, serum) and negative CSF cytology did not undergo stereotactic biopsy (fig. 1). The target was very small and very close to neighboring vascular structures. Microsurgical partial resection was performed previously in 1 patient of this series.

No patients received conventional external fractionated radiotherapy prior to radiosurgery. Chemotherapy was administered before radiosurgery to 3 patients (2 pinealoblastomas and 1 germinoma) and after radiosurgery in 1 patient (germinoma).

Table 3. Radiosurgical planning

Patient	Treatment date	Number of shots and collimator size	Peripheral isodose, %	Central dose, Gy	Radiosurgical protocol
1	Dec 7, 1992	2 – 14W/8	40	50	complementary (after chemotherapy)
2	Mar 8, 1993	5 – 18	50	24	initial
3	Jan 28, 1994	1 – 14E	50	14	initial
4	Jun 30, 1994	3 – 14/2 × 8	50	15	initial
5	Jul 22, 1994	5 – 14/3 × 8/4	50	12	initial
6	Aug 16, 1994	1 – 18	50	20	complementary (after surgery)
7	Oct 20, 1994	1 – 18	50	18	initial
8	Apr 18, 1995	3 – 14/8/4	50	20	sandwich (chemotherapy)
9	May 12, 1995	1 – 14	50	14	initial
10	Jun 20, 1995	2 – 14P	50	12	initial
11	Jul 8, 1995	1 – 18E	50	16	initial

All imaging was with CT and MRI.

Method

In 6 cases, Gamma Knife radiosurgery was the only treatment for PRT. Radiosurgical treatment was performed after microsurgery in 1 case. In 3 cases, radiosurgery followed chemotherapy, and in 1 case it was given before chemotherapy. The radiosurgical goal was tumor control in all patients. In 1 of these patients radiosurgical treatment was also performed as a 'therapeutic test' (germinoma).

The Leksell stereotactic frame type G (Elekta Instrument AB, Stockholm, Sweden) was used in all cases. The images for dose planning were obtained with a superconductive magnet MRI (Siemens, Magnetom 1.5 Tesla). Millimetric volumetric images in transverse and frontal orthogonal planes, before and after gadolinium enhancement were used. CT millimetric axial images were performed with a fourth-generation scanner (cGR GE 12000). The slice interval was 1 mm. Dose planning was performed with the KULA software (Elekta Instrument).

The radiosurgery treatment was performed using the Leksell Gamma Knife model B (Elekta Instrument AB). The margin dose was chosen principally as a function of the histological type of PRT and the tumor volume. The isocenter number, the marginal isodose and the marginal dose to the tumor are shown in table 3.

Table 4. Follow-up results after radiosurgical treatment

Patient	Tumor type	Follow-up months	Tumor disappearance	Tumor size control	No changes	Central tumor low-signal-intensity area
1	pinealoblastoma	33	6 months			
2	meningioma	30		6/9 months		yes
3	germinoma	19	7 days			yes
4	astrocytoma	14		6/9 months		
5	germinoma	13	15 days			yes
6	pinealocytoma	12			6 months	
7	pinealocytoma	10		6 months		yes
8	pinealocytoma	4			2 months	
9	astrocytoma	3		2 months		yes
10	astrocytoma	2				
11	pinealoblastoma	1		2 months		

Results

All patients were discharged from the hospital the day after radiosurgery. There was no treatment-related mortality or acute morbidity. After radiosurgery, clinical and neuroradiological examinations were conducted with a 1-week interval for the germ cell tumors and pinealoblastomas and a 6-month interval for the other types of PRT: Follow-up results are summarized in table 4.

Eight tumors decreased dramatically in size, and in many cases this was detected as early as 7 days after radiosurgery (germinomas). In 3 patients, no evidence of tumor was seen on follow-up MRI performed 6 months after radiosurgery (2 germinomas and 1 pinealoblastoma). In these 2 germinomas, disappearnce was detected at 1 and 2 weeks, respectively. In 1 patient, reduction of the tumor volume and mass effect were confirmed by regression of ventricular dilatation caused by the tumor. In 1 patient with pinealoblastoma, shunt infection necessitated removal of the shunt system 7 days after Gamma Knife radiosurgery. Further alternative treatment was not necessary. Tumor volume was unchanged in 2 patients (pinealocytomas). For 1 recent patient (low-grade tectal astrocytoma), follow-up is not yet available.

Repeated MRI revealed that characteristic changes were found in the tumors. Most showed a delayed central low-intensity-signal area after radiosurgery. In 1 patient with an astrocytoma, there was clinical and radiological evidence of radiation-induced edema of the tectum and the adjacent thalamus 4 months after radiosurgical treatment, but these clinical and radiological signs rapidly resolved under steroid medication.

Discussion

The treatment strategy for PRT remains controversial. Optimal management must be adapted on a case-by-case basis and includes microsurgery, radiotherapy, and chemotherapy, alone or in combination. Specific management decisions depend mainly on the histology, age, size, and spread of the tumor.

Radiosurgery is now available worldwide and indications for the method are expanding. Even so, only a very small number of PRT Gamma Knife radiosurgery cases have been reported [3, 4, 6]. As long as the total resection of small benign tumors (like pinealocytoma or low-grade astrocytoma) remains difficult, and as long as conventional radiotherapy is not curative, it is clearly logical to propose Gamma Knife radiosurgery as an alternative primary treatment. The first report of Gamma Knife radiosurgery for pinealocytoma by Backlund et al. [4] in 1974 established that PRTs could be a standard radiosurgical indication. It seems logical [6] to consider this kind of benign, well-circumscribed tumor as suitable for radiosurgery. These tumors often produce few symptoms and they are difficult to remove microsurgically.

In 1992, the experience of the Pittsburgh team in this field was reported by Dempsey and Lunsford [6], who indicated that pinealocytoma was the only PRT tumor to be treated using Gamma Knife radiosurgery as the primary treatment method. More recently Kihlström et al. [5] reported seven cases of low-grade tectum gliomas with disappearance or cessation of growth without definitive clinical deterioration.

Our preliminary results with these two diagnoses confirm the reports in the literature. For germinomas, fractionated radiotherapy currently offers the best results, with a 10-year survival rate of 70%. Microsurgical resection offers little additional benefit and exposes the patient to the risk of anesthesia and craniotomy. In 1990, Casentini et al. [3] were the first to propose a combination of radiosurgery with whole-brain radiation (WBR), to avoid seeding of neoplastic cells. Even though the results of conventional radiotherapy have been excellent, these authors have proposed using radiosurgery to reduce the irradiation of healthy tissues. Five germinomas were followed for more than 1 year by these authors

(14–58 months), who observed total regression of the tumor on follow-up control images in all five patients, without local or general recurrence.

The effectiveness in germinomas of a new chemotherapy regimen (carbaplatin VP16) has been confirmed by several studies [7]. Taking the information outlined above into account, we planned to treat germinomas by a combination of radiosurgery and chemotherapy, without radiotherapy. This approach was applied to patients without tumor seeding (as assessed using gadolinium-enhanced MR images and CSF cytology). This strategy did not exclude a second-line treatment by conventional radiotherapy in case of recurrence. According to this protocol, 2 germinomas were treated with complete tumor disappearance at 7 and 15 days. No recurrence was observed with a follow-up of 13 and 19 months. The same protocol was used to treat 2 pinealoblastomas. One, with a follow-up of only 2 months, showed a partial response, while the other, with a 33-month follow-up, had disappeared completely after 6 months. There was also resolution of preexisting hydrocephalus, though this took longer than with the germinomas. The disappearance of tumors and the hydrocephalus within a few days means that shunting can be avoided in some cases.

It has previously been our principle to have systematic anatomical pathological confirmation before undertaking any kind of treatment in this region [7, 8]. However, it would seem that Gamma Knife radiosurgery can be performed without anatomical patholgoical confirmation in some selected cases. Stereotactic biopsy may be dangerous, especially for smaller targets, due to the proximity of vital neural and vascular structures. Moreover, a 'radiosurgical test' can be proposed in these cases if the clinical context, MRI and CSF markers provide strong evidence for a radiosurgery-responsive tumor type.

In conclusion, in this study we have confirmed that radiosurgery can be an effective and safe alternative for the treatment of pinealocytomas and low-grade tectal gliomas, as previously reported by Backlund et al. [4] and Kihlström et al. [5]. For the first time we have reported treatment of pineal region germinomas by Gamma Knife radiosurgery and chemotherapy without WBR. We consider that the role of radiosurgery (without radiotherapy) should be evaluated for the treatment of malignant PRTs. This preliminary experience provides us with arguments for considering that radiosurgery has a specific place in the treatment of PRTs. More patients and longer follow-ups are required to improve the definition of that place.

References

1 Jooma R, Kendall B: Diagnosis and management of pineal tumors. J Neurosurg 1983;58:654–665.
2 Sano K: Pineal region and posterior ventricular tumors: A surgical overview; in Apuzzo MLJ (ed): Surgery of the Third Ventricle. Baltimore, Williams and Wilkins, 1992, pp 663–683.
3 Casentini L, Colombo F, Pozza F, Benedetti A: Combined radiosurgery and external radiotherapy of intracranial germinomas. Surg Neurol 1990;34:79–86.
4 Backlund EO, Rabin T, Sarby B: Treatment of pinealomas by stereotactic radiation surgery. Acta Radiol Ther Phys Biol 1974;13:368–376.
5 Kihlström L, Lindquist C, Lindquist M, Karlsson B: Stereotactic radiosurgery for tectal low-grade glioma. Acta Neurochir (Suppl) 1994;62:55–57.
6 Dempsey P, Lunsford D: Stereotactic radiosurgery for pineal region tumors. Neurosurg Clin North Am 1992;3:245–253.
7 Peragut JC, Dupard T, Graziani N, Sedan R: De la prévention des risques de la biopsie stéréotaxique de certaines tumeurs de la région pinéale. Neurochirurgie 1987;33:23–27.
8 Régis J, Bouillot P, Figarella-Branger D, Dufour H, Levrier O, Farnarier P, Peragut JC: Les biopsies stéréotaxiques des tumeurs de la région pinéale. Neurochirurgie 1994;40:3–9.

Proc 7th Int Meeting Leksell Gamma Knife® Society,
Island of Lana'i, Hawaii, November 1995
Stereotact Funct Neurosurg 1996;66(suppl 1):174–183

Stereotactic and Functional Neurosurgery

Two Cases of Gamma Knife Radiosurgery for Low-Grade Optic Chiasm Glioma

Y.J. Lim, W. Leem

Department of Neurosurgery, School of Medicine, Kyung Hee University, Seoul, Korea

Key Words

Optic glioma · Neoplasm · Astrocytoma · Optic chiasm · Low-grade optic glioma · Gamma Knife · Radiosurgery · Dose planning

Abstract

The effect of radiosurgery on optic gliomas is uncertain. We report two cases of low-grade glioma of the optic nerve and chiasm treated by transcranial subtotal removal and Gamma Knife radiosurgery. The first case was a 2-year-old boy, admitted with visual disturbance and nystagmus. Histopathological examination showed a pilocytic astrocytoma. The tumor volume was 14.4 cm^3. Dose planning was performed using axial and coronal T_1-weighted enhanced images. The marginal dose was 12 Gy at the 40% isodose line. The dose to the optic apparatus was less then 9 Gy. The second case was a 47-year-old woman, admitted to our hospital with headache and visual disturbance. The histopathological findings showed a fibrillary astrocytoma. The tumor volume was 12.3 cm^3. The marginal dose was 14.4 Gy at the 40% isodose curve. The follow-up periods for the two cases were 24 and 43 months, respectively. In both cases the most recent follow-up magnetic resonance scan showed a marked decrease in tumor size, and visual symptoms were improved. No postradiosurgical complications have developed to date. Gamma Knife radiosurgery could be an effective adjuvant therapy for low-grade optic glioma. However, long-term follow-up is required for further evaluation of the efficacy and potential side effects.

KARGER

E-Mail karger@karger.ch
Fax + 41 61 306 12 34
http://www.karger.ch

1011–6125/96/0665–0174$10.00/0

Young Jin Lim, MD
Department of Neurosurgery
KyungHee University Hospital
No. 1, Hoeki-Dong, Dongdaemun-Gu
Seoul, 131 (Korea)

Introduction

Optic gliomas are relatively infrequent tumors that can be seen in all age groups, but they occur most commonly in childhood. Optic nerve gliomas represent about 0.6–1.2% of primary intracranial tumors. Lesions confined to the optic nerve occur most frequently in children, while chiasm gliomas are more commonly seen in adolescents [1]. The majority of these tumors are low-grade astrocytomas. Nonetheless, the clinical course of these tumors is not benign. It may lead to blindness or death from tumor progression in a significant number of patients. Tumors involving the optic chiasm and the hypothalamus tend to be more aggressive than tumors involving the optic nerve alone. Moreover, the surgical management of chiasm gliomas carries a risk of serious morbidity [2]. The treatment of optic gliomas remains controversial. Subtotal excision, subtotal excision followed by irradiation, radiation therapy alone, chemotherapy, and no treatment at all have all been recommended [3]. Recently, stereotactic radiosurgery has been attempted for these tumors instead of conventional radiotherapy, both as primary and adjuvant therapy [4]. Stereotactic radiosurgery with the Leksell Gamma Knife makes possible delivery of a tumoricidal dose to the lesion and has an established role in the treatment of some brain tumors [5]. We present our experience with two patients who received Gamma Knife radiosurgery for chiasm gliomas.

Case Reports

Case 1

This 2-year-old boy presented with a 3-month history of nystagmus of the left eye. Fundoscopic examination showed little, but it seemed that his visual function was very poor, as judged by the preferential-looking test. Magnetic resonance imaging (MRI) at the time of admission demonstrated a lobulated mass with marked homogeneous contrast enhancement (on T_1-weighted images with gadolinium), located in the parasellar and suprasellar region. The mass extended to the hypothalamus and the optic chiasm. In September 1991, the patient underwent biopsy and partial excision of the tumor. Operative findings were compatible with an optic glioma. The large, thick, encapsulated mass was located between the left optic nerve and optic chiasm, extending to the hypothalamus. Histopathological examination showed a pilocytic astrocytoma (fig. 1). Visual evoked potentials were evaluated 15 days after surgery. The wave was flat on both sides. Six months after the operation, Gamma Knife radiosurgery was performed. The radiosurgical dosimetry is summarized in table 1.

Eight months after radiosurgery, MRI scanning showed a marked decrease in tumor volume. The last follow-up MRI scan showed a small residual mass at the anterior portion of the optic chiasm. The tumor had decreased to 8% of its initial volume (fig. 2). Moreover, the follow-up visual evoked potentials showed a normal wave form (fig. 3).

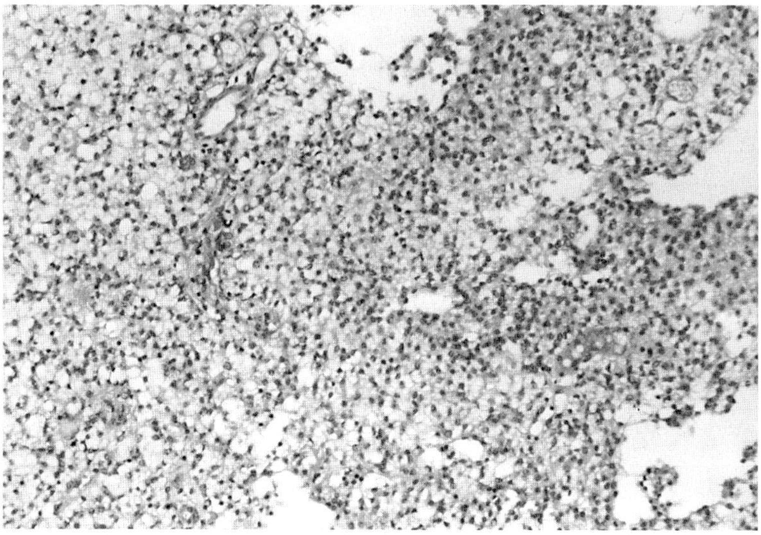

Fig. 1. Case 1. Photomicrograph depicting tumor tissue composed of relatively compact and moderately well differentiated astrocytes with vascular proliferation having prominent endothelial cells. HE. Original magnification × 100.

Table 1. Radiosurgical dosimetry

Case No.	Tumor volume, cm^3		Isocenters n	Collimator size, mm	Isodose curve, %	Marginal dose, Gy	Dose to optic nerve, Gy
	initial	last					
1	14.4	1.1	2	8, 18	50	15.0	6.0–9.0
2	12.3	7.0	6	14	45	16.2	7.2–10.8

Case 2

A 47-year-old woman was referred to our department for neurological assessment in September 1993. She had a 3-year history of headache and visual disturbance. During the previous 2 months, the symptoms had become worse. Ophthalmological examination at the time of the initial evaluation documented a normal visual field and unremarkable fundoscopic findings. However, visual acuity was decreased; OD 20/60 and OS 20/40. An MRI scan revealed an irregular shaped highly enhancing mass in the suprasellar region. A right frontal craniotomy was performed in October 1993. A large tumor was attached to the right optic nerve and the internal carotid artery. Intratumoral subtotal removal was performed.

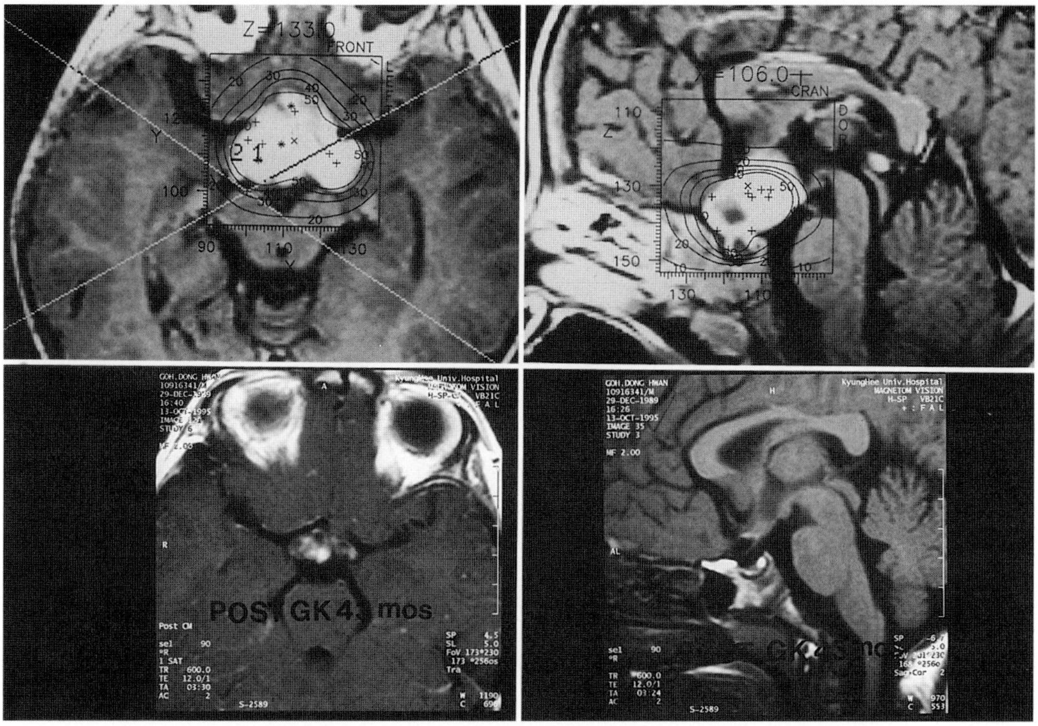

a b c d

Fig. 2. Case 1. **a, b** Stereotactic T_1-weighted MRI scan with gadolinium enhancement during Gamma Knife radiosurgery of a pilocytic astrocytoma after excision biopsy. **c, d** Forty-three months after radiosurgery, follow-up MRI scan revealed a marked decrease in tumor size.

Histopathological examination revealed fibrillary astrocytoma (fig. 4). Headache improved gradually, but visual acuity remained unchanged after operation. Visual field testing showed a right temporal hemianopsia. Gamma Knife radiosurgery was performed 17 days after the operation. The dosimetry is summarized in table 1. Five months after radiosurgery, the patient complained of a deterioration in visual acuity, but ophthalmological examination demonstrated the same visual acuity and visual field as previous evaluations. An MRI scan showed no change of tumor volume. Symptoms were relieved after steroid therapy.

The last MRI scan, 24 months after radiosurgery, showed that the tumor had decreased to 57% of its initial volume (fig. 5). The visual field was much improved, compared to that prior to radiosurgery (fig. 6).

3

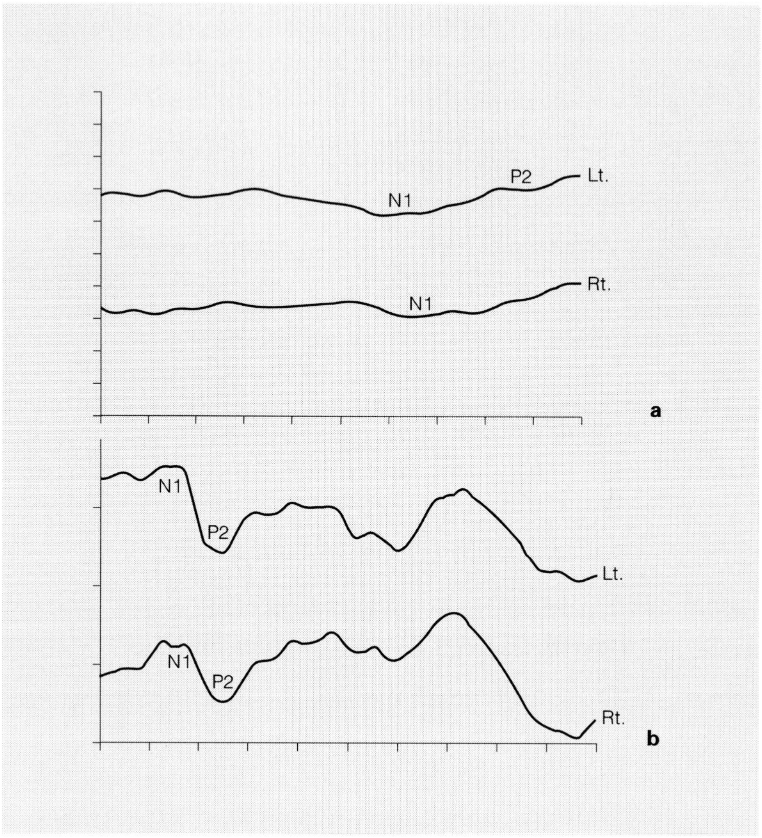

4

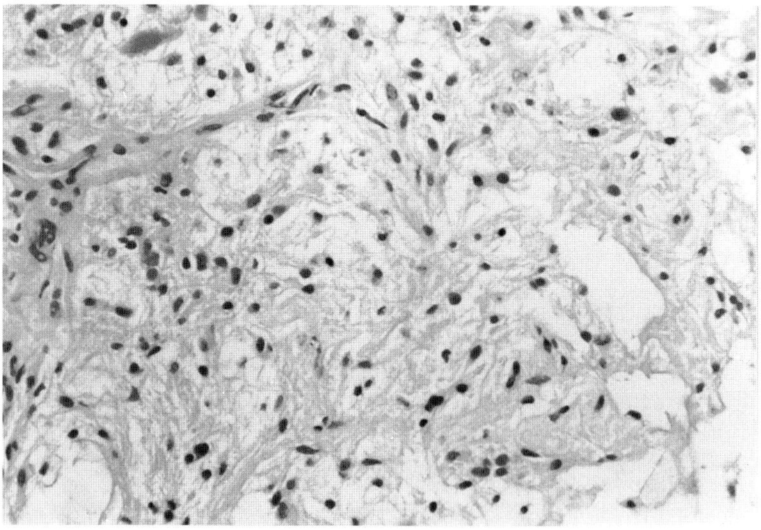

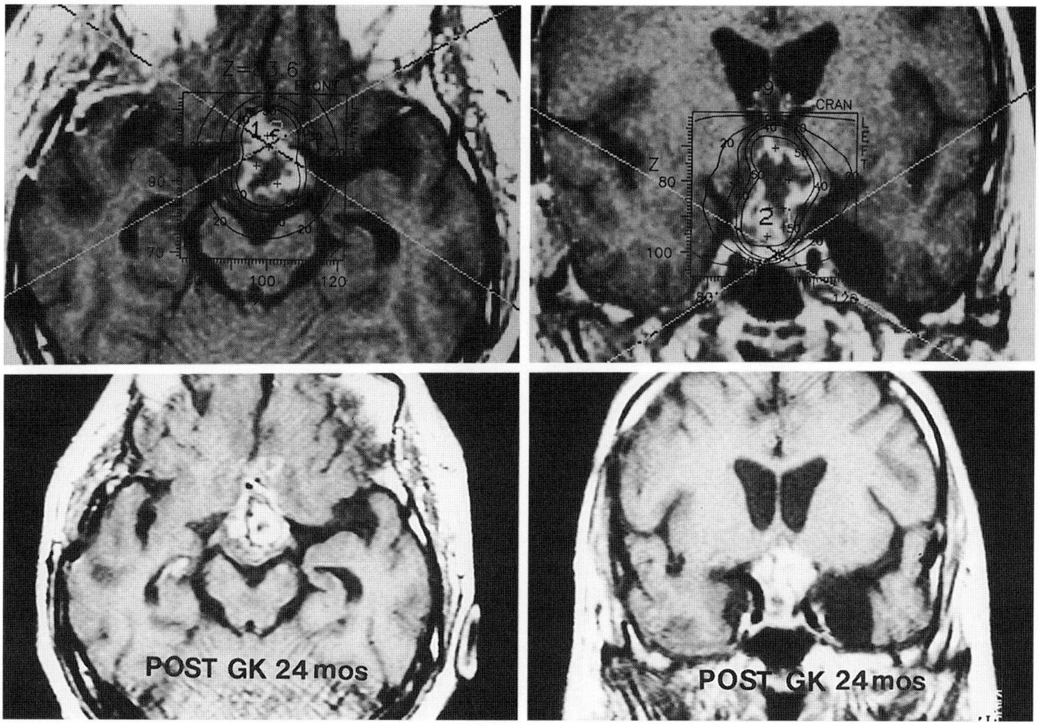

a b c d

Fig. 5. Case 2. **a, b** Stereotactic T_1-weighted MRI scan with gadolinium enhancement during Gamma Knife radiosurgery for a fibrillary astrocytoma after intratumoral subtotal removal. **c, d** Twenty-four months after radiosurgery, follow-up MRI scan shows the tumor has decreased to 57% of the initial volume.

Fig. 3. Visual evoked potentials (VEPs) in case 1. **a** Preoperative VEP shows flat waves on both sides. **b** Forty-three months after radiosurgery, VEP wave form is nearly normalized.

Fig. 4. Case 2. Photomicrograph of tumor tissue consisting of mature astrocytes with fibrillary background and mild nuclear pleomorphism. HE. Original magnification ×200.

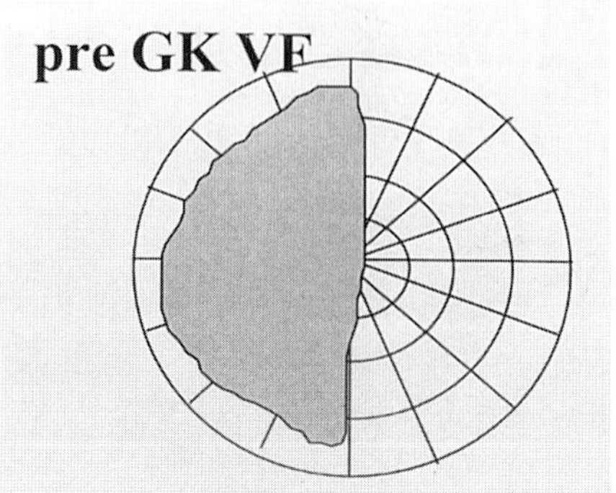

a

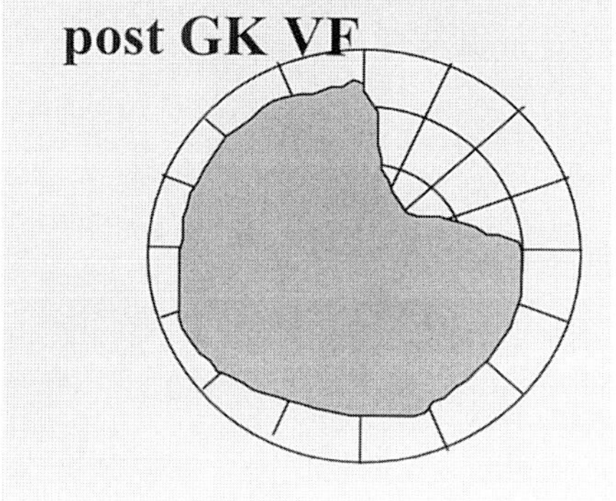

b

Fig. 6. Case 2. **a** Visual field test before radiosurgery shows right temporal hemianopsia. **b** The visual field defect was improved at 24 months.

Discussion

Optic gliomas are relatively uncommon tumors. Arkangelsky [6] estimated their frequency as 1 in 100,000 patients. Chiasm optic gliomas are more commonly seen in young adults and represent 2–5% of all childhood brain tumors [7]. Lesions affecting the optic nerve tend to have a female predominance, and chiasm lesions have an equal sex distribution. The distribution of optic nerve lesions is such that 26–36% of the tumors involve the prechiasmatic part of the optic system and 64–73% of the lesions involve the optic chiasm, optic tract and anterior third ventricle. They are generally considered surgically unresectable [1]. These tumors usually appear histologically as low-grade astrocytomas, those in the optic nerve invading the leptomeninges and evoking a dense fibroblastic reaction and frequently having an oligodendroglial component [8].

Despite the straightforward approach to the treatment of primary tumors of the optic nerve presented by Wishart in 1833, the problems managing these lesions have become more complex as medical knowledge has advanced [1]. The controversy in the management of this tumor is primarily due to the difficulty of analyzing treatment results because of the uncertain natural history of the tumor, which has been much debated, some investigators [9, 10] believing that they are not neoplasms but hamartomas, since they are usually slow growing. Nevertheless, tumors which are left untreated are associated with significant morbidity and mortality. Visual loss, hypothalamic signs, hydrocephalus and proptosis are common findings [10, 11]. Those authors who recommend nontreatment for this disease still report death and blindness in their series [12–14].

Surgical extirpation can effectivly control the disease, but is associated with an obvious visual morbidity. Surgical management appears to be successful in patients who have tumors in the optic nerve with a clear margin between the tumor mass and the chiasm, and complete excision gives excellent control of the disease in almost all patients [15, 16]. However, surgical mortality and postoperative morbidity may develop in patients with chiasm glioma. Bynke et al. [17] reported that two of eight patients who underwent partial resections had immediate postoperative complete loss of vision in one eye. Wong and Lubow [18] showed that in 9 of 12 patients who had partial resection, vision deteriorated after the operation. Other major complications, such as panhypopituitarism, diabetes insipidus and cranial nerve palsy, may develop after surgery, particularly when resection of a chiasmal tumor is attempted [13, 18].

The role of radiation therapy in the management of these tumors is not universally defined. Montgomery et al. [3] reported results of treatment of optic gliomas with irradiation following biopsy. Of three patients whose vision improved following treatment, two had normal vision. Nine of 15 patients have remained stable since the treatment. No patient who received a dose of 5,000 rad or more died of the tumor. Dosoretz et al. [15] reported that radiation therapy was effective in controlling disease in seven of nine patients. Although most of the patients treated by irradiation had severely compromised vision at the beginning of treatment, in two vision improved, and remained stable in the rest. Regression of the tumor visualized radiologically was evident in two patients. The optimum dose for controlling glioma involving the optic chiasm and avoiding serious complications appears to be 45–50 Gy to the 95% isodose line using 180 cGy fractions [2, 19]. Some investigators have been unable to correlate radiation therapy consistently with improvement in visual status [20–22]. Unfortunately, intellectual deficits and endocrinopathies have developed after radiation therapy, especially in young children [23].

Chemotherapy has been used in the treatment of young children with optic glioma with some success. Rosenstock et al. [7] demonstrated tumor control in 8 of 12 children with optic glioma and shrinkage of tumor on computed tomography scan in 6 of 12 children using actinomycin D and vincristine. They concluded that an initial trial of chemotherapy may serve as an alternative to initial radiation therapy in young children.

Several authors have reported results of stereotactic radiosurgery for low-grade glioma [5, 24]. Stereotactic radiosurgery provides a means of giving higher doses than with conventional radiotherapy within the small volume of the tumor, while sparing the surrounding structures, and thus could be a more effective way to deliver the radiation than conventional radiotherapy [24]. Ganz et al. [25] reported that pilocytic astrocytomas are suitable targets for Gamma Knife treatment. The appropriateness of radiosurgery for pilocytic astrocytomas as opposed to other gliomas is related to differences in their biology. The extent of pilocytic astrocytomas demonstrated on the images is far closer to the true extent of the tumor than with other gliomas. We have treated two cases of chiasm glioma with Gamma Knife radiosurgery. Tumor size was markedly decreased and visual symptoms were improved during the 24- and 43-month follow-up periods. We believe that surgery should be considered for optic gliomas as the primary treatment method. However, Gamma Knife radiosurgery may represent a useful therapeutic modality in selected cases of small tumors or when the optic chiasm is involved. Dose planning should be guided by stereotactic MRI and dose selection should be performed very carefully in these cases.

References

1 Tenny RT, Laws ER, Younge BR, Rush JA: The neurosurgical management of optic glioma. J Neurosurg 1982;57:452–458.

2 Flickinger JC, Torres C, Deutsach M: Management of low-grade gliomas of the optic nerve and chiasm. Cancer 1988;61:635–642.

3 Montgomery AB, Griffin T, Parker RG, Gerdes AJ: Optic nerve glioma: The role of radiation therapy. Cancer 1977;40:2079–2080.

4 Kobayashi T, Tanaka T, Kida Y: The effects of Gamma Knife treatment of neuroectodermal tumors. Acta Neurochir 1993;122:157.

5 Kihlström L, Lindquist C, Lindqvist M, Karlsson B: Stereotactic radiosurgery for tectal low-grade gliomas. Acta Neurochir 1994;62(suppl):55–57.

6 Arkangelsky VN: Neoplasm of the optic nerve. Ophthalmologica 1970;151:260–271.

7 Rosenstock JG, Packer RP, Bilaniuk L, Bruce DA, Radcliffe JL, Savino P: Chiasmatic optic glioma treated with chemotherapy. J Neurosurg 1985;63:862–866.

8 Alvord EC, Lofton S: Gliomas of the optic nerve or chiasm. J Neurosurg 1988;68:85–98.

9 Hudson AC: Primary tumours of the optic nerve. R Lond Ophthalmol Hosp Res 1912;18:317–439.

10 Miller NR, Iliff WJ, Green WR: Evaluation and management of gliomas of the anterior visual pathways. Brain 1974;97:743–754.

11 Marsa GW, Probert JC, Rubinstein LJ, Bagshaw MA: Radiation therapy in the treatment of childhood astrocytic gliomas. Cancer 1973;32:646–655.

12 Housepian EM: Surgical treatment of unilateral optic nerve gliomas. J Neurosurg 1963;31:604–607.

13 Hoyt WF, Baghdassarian SA: Optic glioma in childhood: Natural history and rationale for conservative management. Br J Ophthalmol 1969;53:793.
14 Hout WF, Meshel LG, Lessell S, Schatz NJ, Suckling RD: Malignant optic glioma of adulthood. Brain 1973;96:121–131.
15 Dosoretz DE, Blitzer PH, Wang CC, Liggood RM: Management of glioma of the optic nerve and/or chiasm (an analysis of 20 cases). Cancer 1980;45:1467–1471.
16 MacCarty CS, Boyd AS, Childs DS: Tumors of the optic nerve and optic chiasm. J Neurosurg 1970; 33:439–444.
17 Bynke H, Kagstrom E, Tjernstrom K: Aspects of the treatment of gliomas of the anterior visual pathway. Acta Ophthalmol 1977;55:269–280.
18 Wong IG, Lubow M: Management of optic glioma of childhood: A review of 42 cases. Neuroophthalmology Symp Univ Miami and Bascom Palmer Inst, vol 6. St. Louis, Mosby, 1971, pp 51–60.
19 Weiss L, Lagerman RH, King GA, Chung CT, Dubowy RL: Controversy in the management of optic nerve glioma. Cancer 1987;59:1000–1004.
20 Glaser JS, Hoyt WF, Corbett J: Visual morbidity with chiasmal glioma: Long-term studies of visual fields in untreated and irradiated cases. Arch Ophthalmol 1971;85:3–12.
21 Taveras JM, Mount LA, Wood EH: The value of radiation therapy in the management of glioma of the optic nerves and chiasm. Radiology 1956;66:518–528.
22 Rush JA, Younge BR, Campbell RJ: Optic glioma: Long-term follow-up of 85 histopathologically verified cases. Ophthalmology 1982;89:1213–1219.
23 Myles ST, Murphy SB: Gliomas of the optic nerve and chiasm. Can J Ophthalmol 1973;8:508–514.
24 Barcia JA, Barcia-Salorio L, Ferrer C, Algas R, Hernandes G: Stereotactic radiosurgery of deeply seated low grade gliomas. Acta Neurochir 1994;62(suppl):58–61.
25 Ganz JC, Smievoll AI, Thorsen F: Radiosurgical treatment of gliomas of the diencephalon. Acta Neurochir 1994;62(suppl):62–66.

Proc 7th Int Meeting Leksell Gamma Knife® Society,
Island of Lana'i, Hawaii, November 1995
Stereotact Funct Neurosurg 1996;66(suppl 1):184–192

Stereotactic and Functional Neurosurgery

Gamma Knife Radiosurgery for Intracranial Metastases: From Local Tumor Control to Increased Survival

M. Gerosa, A. Nicolato, F. Severi, P. Ferraresi, B. Masotto, G. Barone, R. Foroni, E. Piovan, A. Pasoli, A. Bricolo

Department of Neurosurgery, University Hospital, Verona, Italy

Key Words

Gamma Knife · Radiosurgery · Brain tumors · Metastases

Abstract

We have analyzed a series of 225 patients with intracranial metastases (343 lesions), treated in our department by Gamma Knife radiosurgery over a 30-month period. We have used a modified Pittsburgh protocol and performed 242 procedures on 164 single/78 multiple lesions. Primary tumors were mostly carcinomas of the lung (52%) and breast (11.6%). Neuroradiological localization of the target was usually performed by stereotactic computed tomography. Magnetic resonance imaging was only used in special circumstances. Routine dose planning was assisted by three-dimensional reconstruction programs. Mean tumor volume was larger than expected (5.7 ml). Mean prescription dose and average dose were 21.1 and 29.9 Gy, respectively. Middle- and long-term results were evaluated in a subset of 152 patients (236 lesions) with adequate (>4 months) follow-up. Mean follow-up was 53.1 weeks with 61/152 patients still living. There was a predominance of retrospectively classified 'not fully eligible cases' among the survivors, mainly because of uncontrolled primary tumor. The 1-year local tumor control rate was 88.2%. Treatment-related radiological (3.9%) and clinical (1.6%) sequelae were minimal. Overall mean survival in these patients (40 weeks) turned out to be higher than that commonly reported after conventional surgical-radiation treatments. It was encouraging that the mean survival of 'fully' eligible patients was 51 weeks. Karnofsky perfomance status and neurological (Order Grading) performance scores were consistently high for most of the follow-up period. Functional Independence and the Palliative Index were not far from the value of mean survival. The main cause of death remains uncontrolled systemic disease (64.8%). On the other hand, the relative incidence of intracranial tumor progression was considerably decreased. This indicated that these patients should perhaps be treated more aggressively and underlines the need for randomized trials to determine the optimal treatment.

KARGER

E-Mail karger@karger.ch
Fax + 41 61 306 12 34
http://www.karger.ch

1011–6125/96/0665–0184$10.00/0

Massimo Gerosa, MD
Department of Neurosurgery
University Hospital
Piazzale Stefani 1
I–37126 Verona (Italy)

Introduction

Stereotactic radiosurgery has recently gained considerable momentum as a major therapeutic option for patients harboring intracranial parenchymal metastases [1–8]. Local tumor control (LTC) has been reported with encouraging results after treating single [6, 7, 9] or multiple [1–5, 7, 8] brain metastases. Treatment has been undertaken either at presentation, at recurrence or after prior surgery and radiotherapy. The incidence of treatment-related morbidity has been minor [1–5, 7–9]. A further improvement in the LTC rate has been observed whenever radiosurgical boosts have been associated with adjuvant, fractionated, large-field irradiation [6, 10].

It has been reported that tumor control rates for radiosurgery in these patients are probably higher [4–12] than those obtained with surgical resection and conventional radiotherapy in specifically selected series [13–16]. However, randomized studies of such cases are still scant [14–18], and treatment optimization parameters, particularly for multifocal lesions, need to be defined [6, 7, 13, 16].

Until the last decade, intracranial tumor progression was generally considered as the main cause of death in nearly 50% of patients with cerebral metastases [1, 5, 6, 13, 19]. To date, the vast majority of radiosurgically treated cases are reported to die because of uncontrolled systemic disease with neurologic deaths currently accounting for 17–29% of all cases [7, 9]. There is increasing evidence that future investigations should examine not only the effectiveness of radiosurgery in focal intracranial tumor control, but also its real influence on the quality of life and expected survival.

Material and Methods

Between February 1993 and September 1995, a total of 225 patients, 158 males/67 females, mean age 58.1 years (24–79), harboring 343 brain metastases (242 procedures, 164 solitary-single/78 multiple) were treated by Leksell Gamma Knife stereotactic radiosurgery in our department. A modified Pittsburgh protocol was used, the details of which have already been published [12].

The main eligibility criteria are summarized in table 1. Patients meeting these conditions were subsequently evaluated separately from other cases treated for palliative purposes, even though they did not fulfill the protocol requirements. By far the major difference between the groups of eligible and noneligible patients was the absence/presence of controlled primary tumor.

End points of the protocol were represented by: (1) real effectiveness of radiosurgery in terms of LTC rate versus incidence of focal recurrences; (2) clinical and radiological impact of treatment sequelae (particularly radiation necrosis) evaluated according to Radiation Therapy Oncology Group criteria [20, 21]; (3) quality of life, as analyzed using international-

Table 1. Main eligibility criteria

Number of endocranial lesions: ≤3
Total target volume: ≤20 ml
Biopsy: whenever indicated
Timing of associated whole-brain radiation therapy: within 6 weeks
Primary tumor: absent or under control

Table 2. Intracranial location (343 lesions)

Location	n	%
Frontal	131	38.2
Parietal	65	19.0
Temporal	31	9.0
Occipital	41	12.0
Cerebellar	43	12.5
Other (corpus callosum, carr.)	32	9.3

ly acknowledged clinical and neurological performance scores (Karnofsky, Order Grading, Palliative Index and Functional Independence Index) [20, 21], and (4) life expectancy with actuarial survival rate examined by routine statistical procedures (Kaplan-Meier curves).

Neuroradiological localization of the target was mostly performed using stereotactic computed tomography, double-contrast and thin-slice procedures. Stereotactic magnetic resonance imaging was performed only in selected cases where critical regions of the brain needed to be avoided.

Routine radiosurgical dose planning was implemented by three-dimensional computerized reconstruction of both tumor and isodose volumes, with matching of the resulting contours.

The intracranial localization of the lesions is summarized in table 2. Primary tumors (table 3) were mostly represented by non-small-cell lung cancers (52%), mainly adenocarcinomas. As shown in table 4, the mean prescription dose on each lesion (21.1 Gy) was rather close to the maximum accepted edge dose (25 Gy) even though the average target volumes were probably larger (5.7 ml) than expected. The follow-up schedule included periodical (12–14 weeks) clinical and neuroradiological examination, with assessment of the appropriate scores.

Table 3. Primary tumor sites (225 patients)

Tumor type	Patients	%
Lung	117	52.0
Adenocarcinoma	41	18.2
Squamous-cell carcinoma	35	15.6
Large cell	8	3.5
Small-cell lung cancer	7	3.1
Other (e.g., undifferentiated)	26	11.6
Breast	26	11.6
Kidney	19	8.4
Gastrointestinal tract	15	6.7
Melanoma	13	5.8
Unknown	23	10.2
Others	12	5.3

Table 4. Treatment parameters (225 patients/343 lesions)

Mean tumor volume: 5.7 ml
Mean prescription dose: 21.1 Gy
Average dose: 29.9 Gy
Mean number of targets: 2.5

Table 5. AFG

Number of patients: 152
Number of lesions: 236
Fully eligible/noneligible patients: 51/101
Mean follow-up
Overall: 53.1 weeks (16–140)
Fully eligible patients: 59.4 weeks
Noneligible patients: 47.3 weeks
Living/died: 61/91

Results

For the purpose of this study, results were evaluated only in the series of patients treated up to June 1995, to ensure an adequate (≥16 weeks) follow-up period (adequate follow-up group; AFG; table 5). In this selected AFG group, retrospective analysis showed a prevalence of not fully eligible cases. The presence of primary tumor control was the main discriminating factor underlying the definition of a not fully eligible case. Indeed several patients who had been treated under the criterion of an appropriate primary tumor control turned out to show unexpected short-term extracranial disease progression.

Mean target volumes and dosimetry parameters (table 6) were quite similar to those shown in the overall series. LTC (88.2% with >1 year mean follow-up)

Table 6. AFG: radiosurgical treatment (236 lesions)

Mean tumor volume: 5.7 cm^3
Mean prescription dose: 21.2 Gy
Average dose: 30.2 Gy

Table 7. AFG: tumor control (152 patients, 236 lesions, 1-year follow-up)

	%
LTC	88.2
Focal recurrence	11.8
Radiation injury	
Radiological	3.9
Clinical	1.6

Table 8. AFG: clinical results (152 patients)

	Overall	Fully eligible patients	Noneligible patients
Mean survival time, weeks	40	51	32.3
Mean palliative index, weeks	28.5	34.4	25.5
Functional independence index, weeks	24	36.5	17.5

was extremely gratifying (table 7), even if it was slightly less than we found at an earlier evaluation [12].

Focal recurrence was observed in 11.8% of the cases. Most of these patients were operated upon. Some were retreated by Gamma Knife radiosurgery or conventional radiation techniques with satisfactory results. It is worth stressing that 4 of the operated cases, with substantial histologically documented tumor regrowth, had been submitted to a positron emission tomography scan for 6-deoxyglucose uptake, with surprisingly negative results in 2/4 cases.

The incidence of treatment-related sequelae was quite limited, and mostly confined to imaging pictures of radiation-induced perilesional edema or focal radionecrosis with minor or no clinical deficit.

Clinical results (table 8) have been encouraging. Overall mean survival is certainly appreciable (40 weeks) and particularly high in the group of fully eligible patients (51 weeks). However, it was lower in palliative treatments (34 weeks), as emphasized by actuarial curves (fig. 1). Furthermore, there was evidence of an improved quality of life. Both the Karnofsky performance scores and the Order Grading were consistently improved or stable for most of the survival time, as

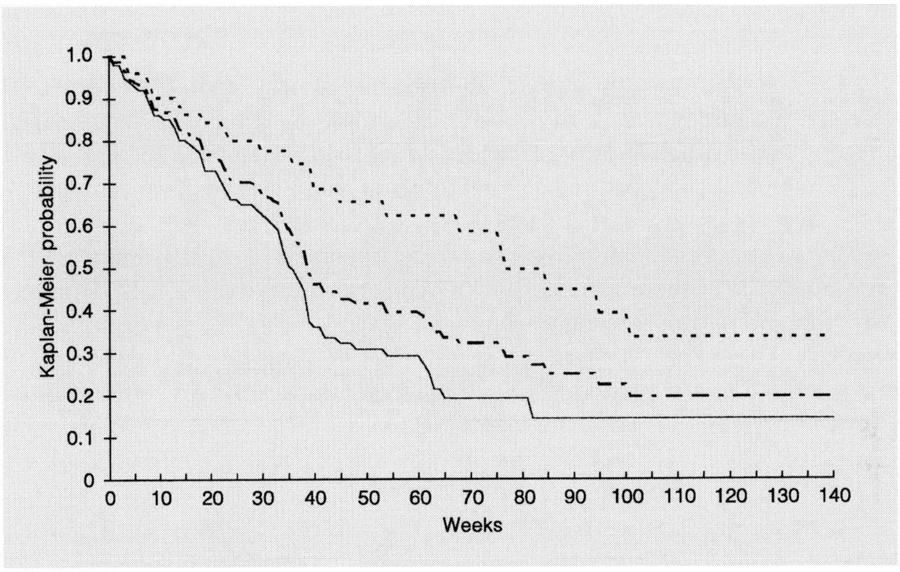

Fig. 1. Actuarial survival analysis showed an overall (– – –) 50% life expectancy of 39 weeks, with 77 weeks for fully eligible patients (······) and 36 weeks for noneligible patients (——). χ^2 for eligible vs. noneligible = 12.445, $p < 0.001$.

Table 9. AFG: causes of death (91 patients)

	n	%
Systemic disease progression	59	64.8
Local tumor recurrence	13	14.3
New brain metastases	14	15.4
Other	5	5.5

confirmed by the sustained mean Palliative Index (overall 28.5 weeks) and Functional Independence Index (24 weeks).

Finally, the main cause of death in these patients (table 9) was systemic disease progression (64.8%) with 'neurological deaths' (local recurrences + new intracranial metastases) accounting for only 29.7% of the total.

Discussion

Despite discrepancies between autopsy and clinical reports, it is generally accepted that the incidence of intracranial metastases remains extremely high, affecting approximately 50% of cancer patients [1–7, 13, 16, 20, 21]. These lesions represent the most frequent neurological complication of cancer and one of the most common causes of death [1, 7, 13, 16, 20–23].

In the last decade, multidisciplinary treatments have slightly improved the grim prognosis of these patients, and stereotactic radiosurgery might definitely play a major role in integrated combined surgery/radiotherapy/chemotherapy protocols. The therapeutic goal entails a variety of aims: (a) effective control of intracranial tumor growth; (b) minimizing treatment-related side effects on the surrounding brain; (c) adequate quality of life, and (d) extended survival. Our preliminary experience seems to confirm the role of Gamma Knife radiosurgery as a promising, reliable approach to this demanding task.

In this series of patients, the 1-year LTC rate is close to 90%, which is higher than that reported with conventional surgical-radiation techniques [13–15, 17–19, 22, 23]. Moreover, differences between 6- [12] and 12-month tumor control rates were slender.

The overall frequency of focal recurrence was reasonably low, even in the putatively 'radioresistant' oncotypes. This confirms the specific therapeutic advantage of the procedure [6–9, 11]. Moreover, in most cases where the treatment has been less effective, surgery or repeated radiosurgery was able to provide further treatment options.

The questionable pictures obtained by positron emission tomography evaluation of the suspected tumor regrowth might suggest the need for a more appropriate diagnostic technique to discriminate real neoplastic recurrence from radiation necrosis. At all events, the radiological or clinical relevance of undue radiation effects has been minimal. This has applied even though the average target volume was large enough to imply some risk. Moreover, the complications (mostly edema) have mostly been pharmacologically manageable.

As regards life quality, all the parameters investigated turned out to be quite encouraging with the values for both Functional Independence and the Palliative Index being fairly close to the value of mean survival.

The increased life expectancy observed in this study may stress the therapeutic role of radiosurgery in these patients [7, 9, 13], but might also be related to an intrinsic bias in selecting eligible candidates for the treatment protocol. However, the considerable fraction of palliative cases registered at later follow-up evaluations, together with the overall reduction in neurological deaths, seem to validate the results of this approach, even in terms of survival.

Finally, considering the main causes of death, the relative incidence of systemic disease progression is definitely increased in our study. This lends support to the notion that a more aggressive therapeutic attitude toward primary tumors in these patients is indicated. Thus, the development of large-scale randomized trials for treatment optimization are badly needed.

References

1 Loeffler JS, Alexander E III, Wen PY, Fine HA, Kooy HM, Black P: Radiosurgery for brain metastases: Five-year experience of the Brigham and Women's Hospital; in Lunsford LD (ed): Stereotactic Radiosurgery Update. Amsterdam, Elsevier, 1992, pp 383–392.

2 Kihlström L, Karlsson B, Lindquist C: Gamma Knife surgery in brain metastases; in Lunsford LD (ed): Stereotactic Radiosurgery Update. Amsterdam, Elsevier, 1992, pp 429–434.

3 Sturm V, Kimmig B, Wowra B, Voges J, Shabbert S, Schlegger W, Pastyr O, Trever H, Lorenz WJ: Radiosurgery in malignant intracranial tumors; in Steiner L (ed): Radiosurgery – Baseline and Trends. New York, Raven Press, 1992, pp 155–160.

4 Adler JR, Cox RS, Kaplan I, Martin DP: Stereotactic radiosurgical treatment of brain metastases. J Neurosurg 1992;76:444–449.

5 Loeffler JS, Alexander E III: Radiosurgery for the treatment of intracranial metastases; in Alexander E III, Loeffler JS, Lunsford LD (eds): Stereotactic Radiosurgery. New York, McGraw-Hill, 1993, pp 197–206.

6 Flickinger JC, Kondziolka D, Lunsford LD, Coffey RJ, Goodman ML, Shaw EG, Hudgins WR, Weiner R, Harsh GR IV, Sneed PK, Larson DA: A multi-institutional experience with stereotactic radiosurgery for solitary brain metastases. Int J Radiat Oncol Biol Phys 1992;23:413–418.

7 Black P, Alexander E III, Loeffler JS: New treatment for metastatic brain tumors; in Salcman M (ed): Current Techniques in Neurosurgery. Philadelphia, Current Medicine, 1995, pp 151–156.

8 Kihlström L, Karlsson B, Lindquist C: Stereotactic radiosurgery for single and multiple cerebral metastases. Acta Neurochir 1993;122:158–164.

9 Loeffler JS, Flickinger JC, Larson DA, Shrieve DC: Radiosurgery for the treatment of intracranial lesions. Important Adv Oncol 1995;11:141–156.

10 Fuller BG, Kaplan ID, Adler J, Cox RS, Bagshaw MA: Stereotactic radiosurgery for brain metastases: The importance of adjuvant whole brain irradiation. Int J Radiat Oncol Biol Phys 1992;23: 413–418.

11 Phillips MH, Stelzer KJ, Griffin TW, Mayberg MR, Winn HR: Stereotactic radiosurgery: A review and comparison of methods. J Clin Oncol 1994;12:1085–1099.

12 Gerosa M, Nicolato A, Berlucchi S, Piovan E, Zampieri P, Pasoli A, Foroni R, Giri MG, Marchini G, Babighian S, Bricolo A: Gamma Knife radiosurgery of primary and metastatic malignant brain tumors: A preliminary report. Stereotact Funct Neurosurg 1995;64(suppl 1):56–66.

13 Aarbit E, Wronski M: The treatment of brain metastases. Neurosurg Q 1995;5:1–17.

14 Mandell L, Hilaris B, Sullivan M, Sundaresan N, Nori D, Kim JH, Martini N, Fuks Z: The treatment of single brain metastasis from non-oat cell lung carcinoma: Surgery and radiation vs. radiation alone. Cancer 1986;58:641–649.

15 Patchell RA, Tibbs PA, Walsh JW, Dempstey R, Maryuama Y, Krycio R, Markesberg W, Macdonald J, Young B: A randomized trial of surgery in the treatment of single metastases to the brain. N Engl J Med 1990;322:494–500.

16 Smalley SR, Laws ER, O'Tallon JR, Shaw EG, Schray MF: Resection for solitary brain metastases. J Neurosurg 1992;77:531–540.

17 Moser RP, Johnson ML, Yung A IV: Metastatic brain cancer in patients with no known primary site. Cancer Bull 1989;41:173–177.

18 Vecht CJ, Haaxima-Reiche H, Noordijk EM: Treatment of single brain metastasis: Radiotherapy alone or combined with neurosurgery? Ann Neurol 1993;33:583–590.

19 Sano K: Intracranial metastatic tumors – An overview; in Paoletti P, Takakura K, Walker MD, Butti G, Pezzotta S (eds): Neuro-oncology. Dordrecht, Kluwer, 1991, pp 309–319.
20 Borgelt B, Gelbert R, Kramer S, Brady LW, Chang CH, Davis LW, Perez CA, Hendrickson ER: The palliation of brain metastases: Final results of the first two studies by Radiation Therapy Oncology Group. Int J Radiat Oncol Biol Phys 1980;6:1–9.
21 Diener-West M, Dobbins T, Phillips T, Nelson D: Identification of an optimal subgroup for treatment evaluation of patients with brain metastases using RTOG study 7916. Int J Radiat Oncol Biol Phys 1989;16:669–673.
22 Posner JB: Management of brain metastases. Rev Neurol (Paris) 1992;148:477–487.
23 Coia LR: The role of radiation therapy in the treatment of brain metastases. Int J Radiat Biol Phys 1992;23:229–238.

Proc 7th Int Meeting Leksell Gamma Knife® Society,
Island of Lana'i, Hawaii, November 1995
Stereotact Funct Neurosurg 1996;66(suppl 1):193–200

Stereotactic and Functional Neurosurgery

Radiosurgery of Brain Metastases with the Gamma Knife

S. Fukuoka, Y. Seo, M. Takanashi, S. Takahashi, K. Suematsu, J. Nakamura

Department of Neurosurgery, Nakamura Memorial Hospital, Hokkaido Brain Research Foundation, Sapporo, Japan

Key Words

Radiosurgery · Gamma Knife · Brain neoplasm · Metastasis

Abstract

A total of 130 patients with metastatic brain tumors were treated with the Gamma Knife; 85 had multiple lesions. The marginal dose was 14–30 Gy for the initial 20 cases during the first 6 months. Thereafter, we increased the marginal dose to between 25 and 30 Gy for the last 110 cases. The follow-up period ranged from 1 to 49 months (mean 9 months). The recurrence rate fell from 20% for the early low-dose cases to 4.6% for the later 110 higher-dose cases ($p = 0.043$). Transient neurological deterioration developed in 7 cases (5.4%), and permanent neurological deficits were recognized in a further 6 cases (4.6%). The relatively high prescription dose of 25–30 Gy at the margin of brain metastases treated with the Gamma Knife resulted in an acceptably high control rate with a low rate of complications.

Introduction

Radiosurgery has recently provided an alternative to conventional therapy for the treatment of brain metastases. It assists in attaining local control with low risk, even in multiple lesions [1, 2]. The main aim of treatment for brain metastases is to obtain better quality of life for a group of patients with a limited life expectancy. Recurrence or radiation injury may impair that quality of life. However, the optimal dose which controls the tumor while minimizing the risk of complications is still controversial [3, 4]. In this report, we discuss how to determine this.

KARGER

E-Mail karger@karger.ch
Fax + 41 61 306 12 34
http://www.karger.ch

1011–6125/96/0665–0193$10.00/0

Seiji Fukuoka, MD
Department of Neurosurgery
Nakamura Memorial Hospital
West-14, South-1, Chuo-ku
Sapporo 060 (Japan)

Materials and Methods

We analyzed 130 cases of brain metastases treated with the Gamma Knife. There were 92 males and 38 females ranging in age from 19 to 80 years (mean 60). Of these, 85 cases (65%) had multiple lesions. Prior to Gamma Knife radiosurgery, each patient underwent magnetic resonance imaging (MRI) examination with contrast enhancement, using 3-mm axial scans. The tumor volume ranged from 0.01 to 36.4 ml; the mean was 5.5 ml. The primary malignancies were from the lung in 81 cases (62.3%), the gastrointestinal tract in 24 cases (18.5%), the breast in 9 cases (6.9%), the kidney in 6 cases (4.6%), the thyroid and the uterus in 2 cases. There were also single cases originating in the liver, the pharynx, the ovary, the prostate, the thymus, and the bladder. Three cases had tumors of unknown origin.

Gamma Knife Technique

All patients underwent application of the Leksell stereotactic frame under local anesthesia, and all tumors were visualized by contrast-enhanced MRI scans. In selected cases where the lesions were far from the center of the MRI head coil, enhanced computed tomography (CT) imaging was used to verify the coordinates.

Results

Rate of Recurrence

The patients were divided into two groups, based on when they were treated. The first group included the initial 20 cases treated during the first 6 months after the start of Gamma Knife radiosurgery at Nakamura Memorial Hospital in May 1991. The second group consists of the subsequent 110 cases treated with Gamma Knife radiosurgery after November 1991. The first group was treated with a marginal dose of 14–30 Gy, which varied according to the location or size of tumors. Recurrences were recognized in 4 cases (20%) during a follow-up period of 3–5 months (mean 4.3 months). The tumor volumes of these 4 cases ranged from 2.1 to 22 ml (mean 8.4 ml). The tumors in 2 cases were located very near to the brain stem, so the marginal doses were set at 14 and 20 Gy (fig. 1). The third and fourth cases received 19 and 20 Gy at the margin. We analyzed the cause of recurrence, and we theorized that a higher marginal dose and more precise dose planning might be necessary to achieve better control of metastatic tumors. None of the other 16 cases treated with 25–30 Gy at the margin showed any recurrence.

The second group was treated with 25–30 Gy at the tumor margin and the rate of recurrence was 4.6%. The difference in recurrence rates between the two groups was statistically significant ($p = 0.043$). Five cases in group 2 recurred from 5 to 13 months (mean 7.8 months) after radiosurgery. The tumor volumes ranged from 1.0 to 29 ml (mean 14 ml). The time from treatment to recurrence was longer in group 2 and the difference between groups 1 and 2 was significant ($p = 0.046$).

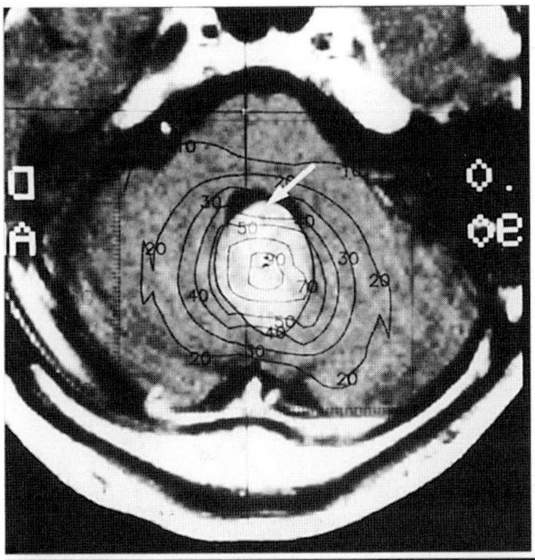

a

Fig. 1. Transaxial enhanced MRI images of a 46-year-old patient with metastatic lung adenocarcinoma. **a** Isodose curve distributions. The arrow indicates the tumor margin irradiated at 14 Gy. **b, c** Before (**b**) and 4 months after (**c**) Gamma Knife radiosurgery. Note the expansion of the tumor. This patient was retreated with Gamma Knife surgery with a 20 Gy marginal dose, and then a third treatment was performed for recurrence.

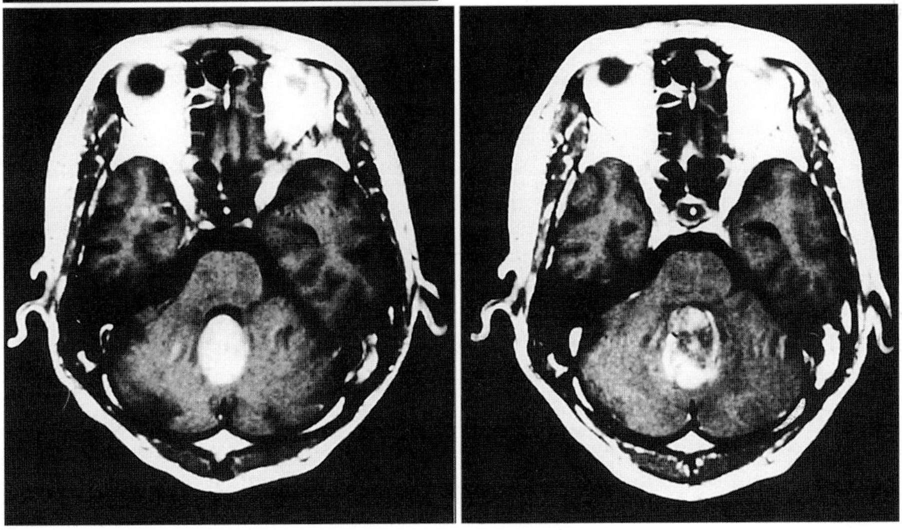

b c

Factors which might influence the rate of recurrence were analyzed. The size of the recurrent tumors was compared with the largest lesion found in each of the 130 patients. There was no statistical difference in tumor size. The marginal dose was the only factor found to influence the risk of recurrence. There was no significant difference in the distribution of primary tumors between the two groups (table 1).

Over the follow-up period, ranging from 1 to 49 months (mean 9 months), new distant lesions were recognized in 35 of the 130 patients (27%). Eleven cases

Table 1. Summary of cases with recurrence after Gamma Knife radiosurgery

Case	Primary tumor	Time to recurrence months	Margin dose Gy	Tumor volume ml	Second treatment
1	lung (adenocarcinoma)	4	14	2.4	Gamma Knife (20 Gy) followed by surgery
2	colon	5	20	2.1	Gamma Knife
3	kidney	5	19	7.2	Gamma Knife
4	uterus	3	20	22.0	
5	lung (adenocarcinoma)	7	30	28.8	surgery
6	prostate	6	30	29.0	
7	ovary	13	30	2.7	
8	lung (adenocarcinoma)	9	30	9.1	surgery
9	colon	5	30	1.0	surgery

(24%) had a single initial lesion and 24 cases (28%) presented initially with multiple lesions. Of these 35 patients, 30 (86%) were subsequently retreated with the Gamma Knife.

Complications

Radiation-Induced Edema or Radiation Injury. Over the follow-up period, perifocal edema occurred in 14 cases (10.8%) and was detected by MRI or CT scans. The tumor volume in these cases ranged from 1.0 to 22 ml (mean 7.6 ml) and they were irradiated at 25–30 Gy peripheral dose. There was no statistical difference in tumor volume or marginal dose between patients who developed edema and those who did not. Transient expansion of tumors with increased perifocal edema was observed in an additional 5 cases. Among these 19 cases with edema, transient hemiparesis developed in 7 cases, and disappeared within 1 week to 1 month. Permanent deficits developed in 4 cases due to radiation injury. Three of these patients suffered hemiparesis and the fourth exhibited a change in mental status. In 1 further case, the lesion (small-cell carcinoma of the lung) with a volume of 9 ml was located in the cerebellar hemisphere and was treated with 30 Gy to the margin. The lesion subsequently swelled and the preexisting perifocal edema increased, requiring surgical resection the day after Gamma Knife surgery. The patient was able to walk without assistance 2 months after surgery.

Bleeding. One case (renal cell carcinoma origin) developed hemiplegia 3 days after Gamma Knife surgery due to intratumoral bleeding, but recovered with minimal hemiparesis. The tumor size was 1.4 ml and was irradiated with 30 Gy to the margin. In another case of metastasis from thyroid cancer, surgical removal was performed for a massive perifocal hematoma 14 days after Gamma Knife surgery. The volume of this lesion, located in the cerebellar hemisphere, was 19 ml and it received 30 Gy to the margin. It is hard to determine whether or not this bleeding was related to Gamma Knife surgery.

In summary, complications with permanent neurological deficit developed in 6 cases (4.6%), of which 4 were related to radiation injury and 2 to bleeding.

Survival

Survival data are shown in figure 2. The median survival of patients with single and multiple metastases was 8 months, and survival rates at 1 and 2 years were 30 and 26%, respectively, in cases with a single lesion, and 39 and 7%, respectively, in cases with multiple lesions. These data suggest that patients with multiple metastases tended to enjoy almost the same life expectancy as those with a single lesion, in this material.

Histopathology

Figure 3 shows the pathological findings of a metastatic tumor originating from a uterine adenocarcinoma. The patient was treated with 30 Gy to the margin, but died from a heart attack 1 month after Gamma Knife surgery. Microscopic examination revealed a glial layer covering necrotic tissue, which included some islands of bizarre giant cells that seemed to be unable to proliferate. No viable tumor cells were found inside or outside the glial layer.

Discussion

Survival rates of patients with single and multiple metastases were almost the same in our series. These results are comparable with those of other patients treated by radiosurgery plus whole-brain radiotherapy [5, 6]. This may indicate that even multiple metastatic tumors can be treated by radiosurgery alone if all the tumors are successfully treated [2]. Moreover, the incidence of new distant lesions in cases with single and multiple metastases was also similar (24 and 28%, respectively). This implies the importance of thin-slice whole-brain enhanced MRI scanning prior to treatment for detecting small lesions of a few millimeters in diameter.

Others have shown that radiosurgery alone for cerebral metastases has been associated with a low recurrence rate where the margin dose has been from 25 to 30 Gy [1, 2, 7]. However, the optimal dose remains an unresolved issue. In general, the important factors in deciding the appropriate marginal dose for intracranial tumors are the histology, size, and location of the tumors. However, in cases of malignancy such as brain metastases, an inadequate dose may be associated with recurrence after a short latency interval. Recurrences usually need a second treatment, such as further radiosurgery or surgical removal.

It is now obvious that the goals of the treatment of brain metastases are control of the intracranial lesions and prolongation of the useful life of patients whose

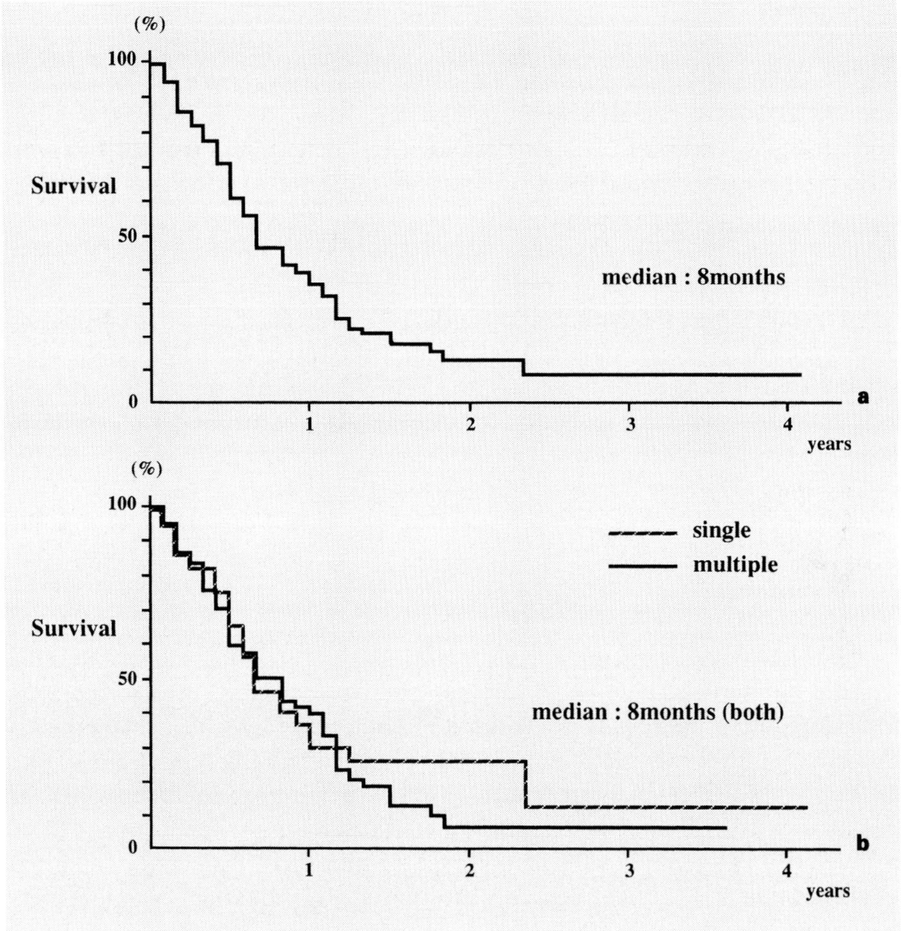

2

Fig. 2. **a** Survival (Kaplan-Meier) of all patients. **b** Survival of patients with single and multiple metastases.

Fig. 3. Photomicrographs of sections after radiosurgery. **a** The glial layer covers necrotic tissue, which includes some islands. HE. × 40. **b** The island consists of bizarre giant cells, which seem to be unable to proliferate. HE. × 200.

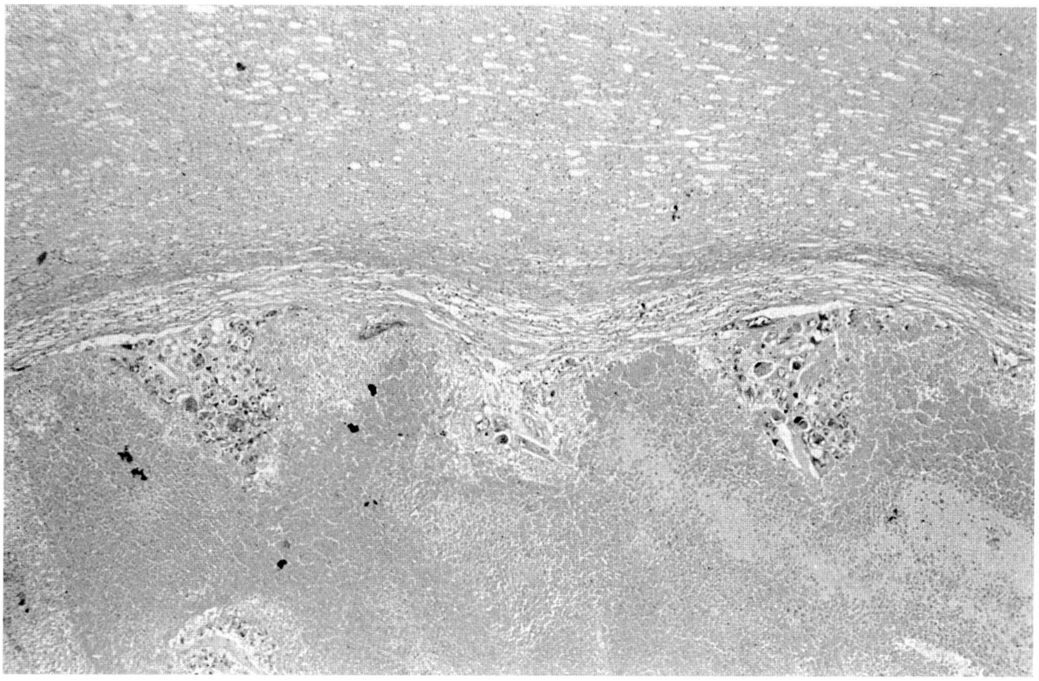

3a

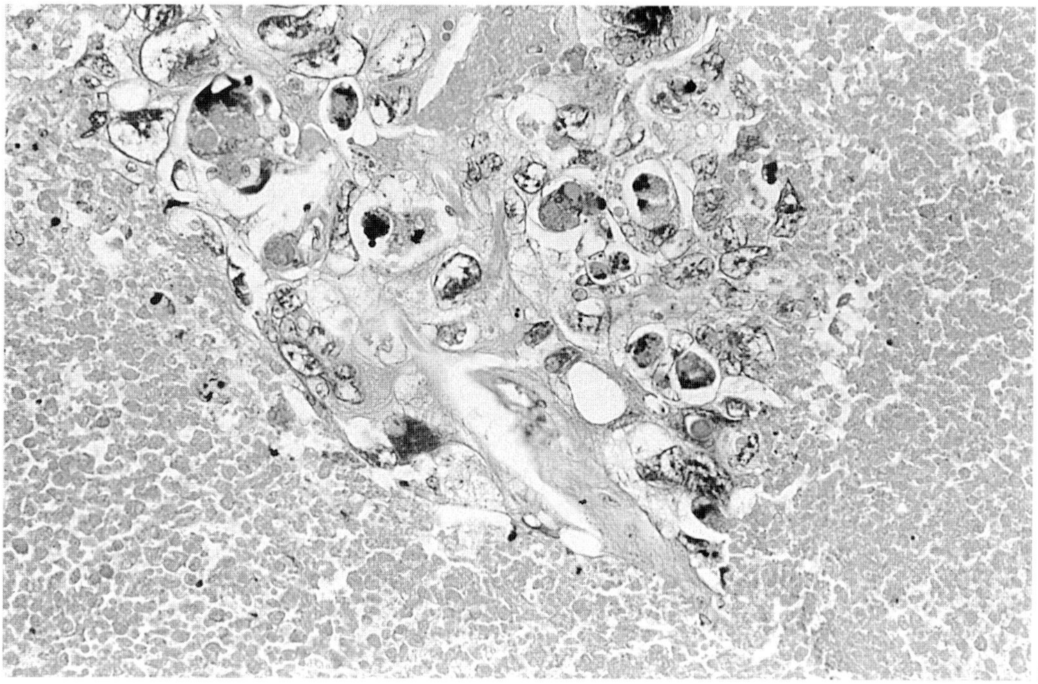

3b

life expectancy is limited. To achieve these aims, both a low rate of recurrence and a low rate of complications need to be achieved. All of our initial patients who were treated with under 20 Gy at the margin suffered some recurrence, which led us to conclude that the marginal dose for the metastatic tumors should be more than 25 Gy. This dose strategy differs from that used for benign intracranial disease, due to the malignancy of metastatic tumors and the short life expectancy of patients with systemic cancer. The incidence of recurrence and permanent deficit in our study seems to be acceptable, and a marginal dose of 25–30 Gy seems to be reasonable for treating brain metastases with the Gamma Knife. However, we have to reflect on 2 cases which needed surgical intervention after radiosurgery. The tumors were large, located in the posterior fossa, and were treated with 30 Gy to the margin. This relatively high irradiation dose to a large volume in the posterior fossa in a single procedure might be related to these rare complications. Sturm et al. [8] reported a similar case. In such cases, a lower marginal dose in addition to fractionated radiotherapy [9] may be a preferable, safer treatment.

Acknowledgments

We wish to express our warm thanks to Mr. Masafumi Nakamura, Miss Akiko Kawamura, Miss Chiyoko Suzuki, and Mr. Simon Thollar for preparation of the manuscript.

References

1 Lindquist C: Gamma Knife surgery for recurrent solitary metastasis of a cerebral hypernephroma: Case report. Neurosurgery 1989;25:802–804.
2 Kihlström L, Carlsson B, Lindquist C: Gamma Knife surgery in brain metastases; in Lunsford LD (ed): Stereotactic Rdiosurgery Update. Amsterdam, Elsevier, 1992, pp 429–434.
3 Rand RW, Jacques DB, Melbye RW, Copcutt BG, Irwin L: Gamma Knife radiosurgery for metastatic brain tumors. Acta Neurochir 1995;63:85–88.
4 Kida Y, Kobayashi T, Tanaka T: Radiosurgery of the metastatic brain tumors with Gamma Knife. Acta Neurochir 1995;63(suppl):89–94.
5 Coffey RJ, Flickinger JC, Bissonette DJ, Lunsford LD: Radiosurgery for solitary brain metastases using the cobalt-60 gamma unit: Methods and results in 24 patients. Int J Radiat Oncol Biol Phys 1991;20:1287–1295.
6 Mehta MP, Rozental JM, Levin AB, Mackie TR, Kubsad SS, Gehring MA, Kinsella TJ: Defining the role of radiosurgery in the management of brain metastases. Int J Radiat Oncol Biol Phys 1992; 24:619–625.
7 Jokura H, Takahashi K, Kayama T, Yoshimoto T: Gamma Knife radiosurgery of a series of only minimally selected metastatic brain tumours. Acta Neurochir 1994;62:77–82.
8 Sturm V, Kober B, Hover KH, Schlegel W, Boesecke R, Pastyr O, Hartmann GH, Schabbert S, zum Winkel K, Kunze S: Stereotactic percutaneous single dose irradiation of brain metastases with a linear accelerator. Int J Radiat Oncol Biol Phys 1987;13:279–282.
9 Lunsford LD, Flickinger J, Coffey RJ: Stereotactic Gamma Knife radiosurgery. Arch Neurol 1990; 47:169–175.

Proc 7th Int Meeting Leksell Gamma Knife® Society,
Island of Lana'i, Hawaii, November 1995
Stereotact Funct Neurosurg 1996;66(suppl 1):201–207

Stereotactic and Functional Neurosurgery

Preliminary Application of Gamma Knife in the Treatment of Nasopharyngeal Carcinoma

Ren-He Dong[a], *Zi-wei Gao*[a], *Zheng-qing Hu*[a], *Wei-ming Xu*[b], *Li Pan*[b]

[a] ENT Department and [b] Neurosurgery Department, Huashan Hospital, Shanghai Medical University, Shanghai, P.R. China

Key Words

Nasopharyngeal carcinoma · Radiotherapy · Stereotactic radiosurgery · Gamma Knife

Abstract

Nasopharyngeal carcinoma is a malignant tumor which occurs frequently in China. Currently, radiotherapy using ^{60}Co is the main method of treatment. However, the 5-year survival rate is only 49.5%. There is no effective method today for treating residual or recurrent tumor following radiotherapy. In principle, the Leksell Gamma Knife could contribute to better results. Since December 1993, we have treated 36 patients suffering from nasopharyngeal carcinoma with the Gamma Knife: 32 were relapses after radiotherapy and 4 were primary cases. Treatment was very effective for a short period. The rate of improvement of such symptoms as headache, facial paralysis, reduced vision, nasal obstruction and nasal bleeding was 70–100%. After treatment, tumors became smaller or even disappeared. A new nasopharyngeal biopsy was performed in 12 patients and demonstrated that the pathological tissue had returned to normal. The short duration of the survey precludes conclusions about the long-term effects of the treatment.

Introduction

Nasopharyngeal carcinoma is an extremely common malignant tumor in China. It is estimated that 80% of nasopharyngeal carcinomas in the world occur in the southern provinces of China. The prevalence for males in Guandong province in the south is the highest, approaching $30–50 \times 10^{-5}$ [1]. The prevalence in

KARGER

E-Mail karger@karger.ch
Fax +41 61 306 12 34
http://www.karger.ch

1011–6125/96/0665–0201$10.00/0

Li Pan, MD, PhD
Department of Neurosurgery, Huashan Hospital
Shanghai Medical University
Shanghai 200040 (P.R. China)

the northern part of China is only 2–3 × 10^{-5}. The prevalence in the rest of the world is less than 1 × 10^{-5} [2, 3]. The incidence rises rapidly from the age of 20 years and reaches a peak at 50–59 years. The disease is commoner in males, with a male:female ratio of 2.5–4:1. It is also common across southeast Asia, though it seldom occurs in Caucasians.

The site of nasopharyngeal carcinoma is occult. However, it is situated close to important structures such as the eye, nose, ear, base of the skull and cranial nerves. It readily infiltrates nearby structures directly, via a submucosal route, and also often metastasizes to lymph nodes. The presenting symptoms of the tumor are so variable and nonspecific that it is most often ignored by both patients and their doctors. These symptoms include epistaxis, nasal obstruction, tinnitus, hearing loss, headache and cranial nerve deficits. Of the tumors, 95% are poorly differentiated squamous cell carcinomas or undifferentiated carcinomas of high malignancy. They develop rapidly with a tendency to early intracranial infiltration and distant metastasis to the cervical lymph nodes. The mean survival period for nasopharyngeal carcinoma is about 18.7 months. It is only 7–9 months if a fourth-stage case remains untreated.

The most popular treatment currently is radiotherapy. Initially, high-dose external beam (>70 Gy) therapy is employed. In some cases this may be combined with intracavitary brachytherapy. In 10–30% of patients with nasopharyngeal carcinoma, the tumor recurs. Two-thirds of the recurrences are limited to the region of origin [4, 5]. After radiotherapy, 20–36% of patients suffer metastases. The morbidity is high, and the 5-year survival rate is only 49.5%. The risk of side effects of radiotherapy is high and the complications can be severe. Forty percent of patients are seriously thirsty. Mouth opening may be restricted.

Radiation damage to the brain and spinal cord occurs in 1.7–4% of patients. Thus, it is necessary to find new methods of treatment which are effective and which have a lower rate of complications.

Stereotactic radiosurgery represents a method of delivering a high radiation dose to a sharply defined tumor volume while limiting the dose to surrounding tissues. To date, one case of recurrent nasopharyngeal carcinoma treated with the Gamma Knife has been reported [6]. Thus, in this study we report our experience with this condition at Hua Shan Hospital, where 36 cases suffering from nasopharyngeal carcinoma have been treated with the Gamma Knife since December 1993.

Materials and Methods

There were 36 patients (33 males and 3 females) aged from 34 to 69 years (average 52.2 years). Thirty-two cases had recurrences after fractionated radiotherapy. The other 4 cases had primary tumors. Twenty-seven cases had poorly differentiated squamous cell carcino-

Table 1. Symptom improvement

Symptom	Cases before Gamma Knife	Cases after Gamma Knife	Improvement rate, %
Epistaxis	25	0	100
Nasal obstruction	19	0	100
Tinnitus	27	8	70.3
Headache	10	1	90
Reduced visual acuity	4	1	75
Facial paralysis	5	4	80
Restriction in opening mouth	13	5	38
Dermatomyositis	1	0	100

Table 2. Clinical follow-up

Cases	Recurrence group	Primary group
Total	32	4
Survival	28	4
Dead	4	4
Symptomatolytic	24	3
Relapse	4	1
Metastasis	3	0

mas, 2 cases had well-differentiated squamous cell carcinoma, 4 cases had undifferentiated carcinoma, 2 cases had vesicular nucleus cell carcinomas and the remaining case had a leiomyosarcoma.

Dose planning was based on contrast-enhanced computed tomography (CT) or magnetic resonance imaging (MRI) using the KULA dose planning system. We used 4–12 shots. The 40% or the 50% isodose was placed at the tumor margin. The edge dose was 18–20 Gy.

Results

An excellent initial effect was seen in all 36 cases (table 1). The patients were followed regularly with clinical examinations every month for 1.5 years. The results of these examinations are summarized in table 2. Regular imaging follow-up was performed every 1–3 months. Tumor shrinkage or even disappearance was observed in 30 cases.

1

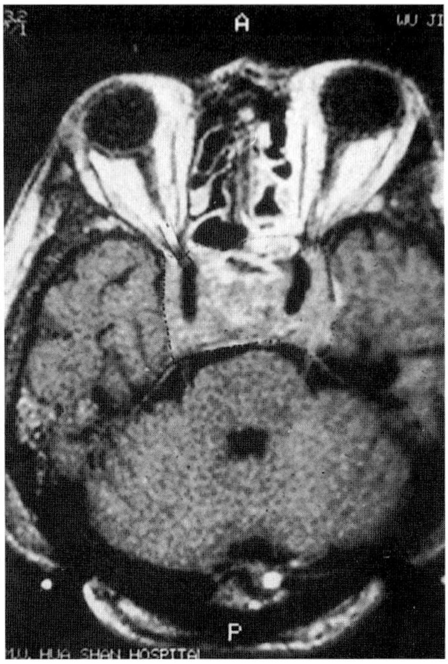

2

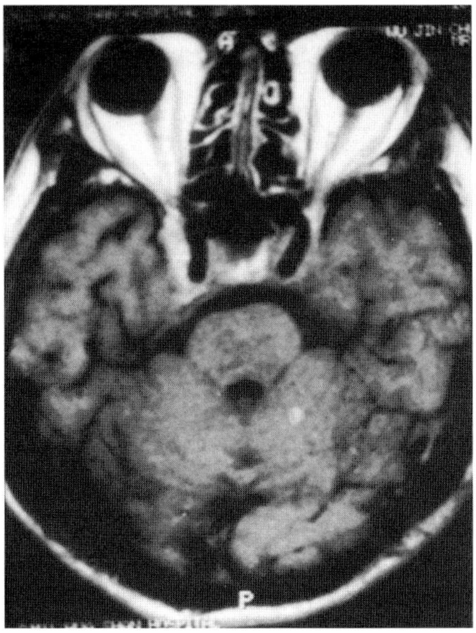

Fig. 1. Patient 1. MRI scan showing a mass in the sphenoid sinuses and infiltration both sides of the optic nerves.

Fig. 2. Patient 1. MRI scan showing the mass shrinkage.

Typical Case Reports

Patient 1. This 57-year-old man had a poorly differentiated squamous cell carcinoma. He suffered clinical deterioration 6 months after external beam radiotherapy. The left eye became blind over 1 month, and visual acuity on the right side decreased rapidly over about a week. MRI scans showed evidence of a mass in the nasopharynx and sphenoid sinuses with bilateral infiltration of the optic nerves (fig. 1). At Gamma Knife radiosurgery, ten 18-mm shots were given. Most of the tumor volume as shown on MRI was encompassed in the 50% isodose line. The margin dose was 18 Gy. The dose to the optic fibers was less than 8–10 Gy. The next day, the patient's eyesight on both sides had recovered to the levels prior to the recent deterioration. MRI scans showed tumor shrinkage (fig. 2). Biopsy of the nasopharynx was normal 3 months later.

Patient 2. This 34-year-old man presented with symptoms of nasal obstruction and epistaxis. The MRI scan showed evidence of a mass in the left nasopharynx and choanae (fig. 3). Biopsy was performed and histologic examination revealed a poorly differentiated squamous cell carcinoma. The patient was treated with the Gamma Knife. Three and 5 days later, two pieces of tissue detached themselves spontaneously from the tumor. The first was 1.2 × 1.5 × 2.5 cm, the second was 1.0 × 1.2 × 2.0 cm. Histological examination showed

3

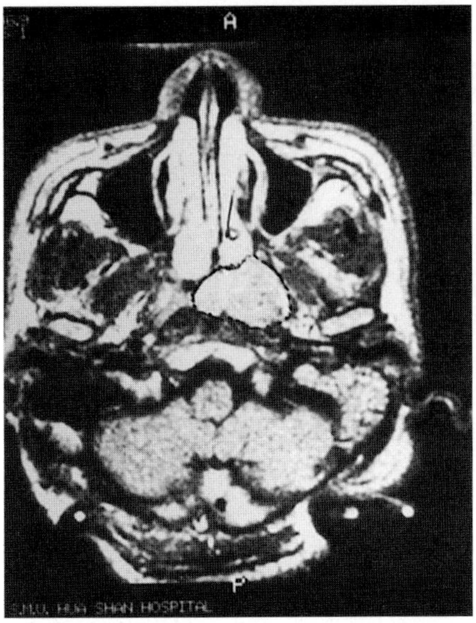

4

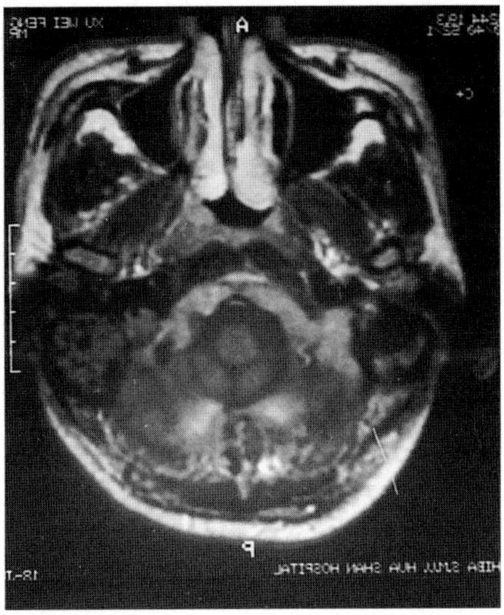

Fig. 3. Patient 2. MRI scan showing a mass in the left side of the nasopharynx and choanae.

Fig. 4. Patient 2. MRI scan showing the mass shrinkage.

necrotic tumor tissue (fig. 5). The patient is now symptom free. The mucosa of the nasopharynx is smooth. Histologic examination has become normal (fig. 4, 6).

Patient 3. This 60-year-old man had received high-dose radiotherapy, 86 Gy 1 year previously. Four months after radiotherapy, the upper part of the nasopharynx was seen to be bulging. A vesicular nucleus cell carcinoma was reported following biopsy. Chemotherapy was attempted to no avail. A left facial palsy then developed. Mouth opening became restricted. Hearing in the left ear deteriorated. A CT scan showed tumor infiltration into the intracranial cavity, the middle ear and the mastoid region. The patient was treated with the Gamma Knife. Six 18-mm shots were given. The margin dose was 18 Gy. Most of the nasopharyngeal part of the tumor was enveloped with the 40% isodose line. However, the components of tumor in the intracranial cavity, the middle ear and the mastoid region fell outside this dose. The next day, the patient's left facial palsy improved. The left eye could close. The mouth could open more widely. Clinical examination showed tumor shrinkage. Two weeks later, histologic examination did not detect any tumor cells.

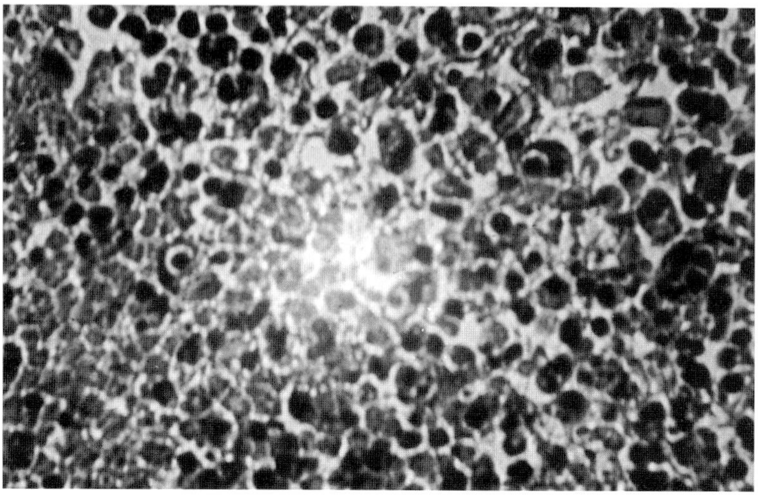

Fig. 5. Patient 2. Microscopic view showing the degeneration and pyknosis of the tumor cell. × 340.

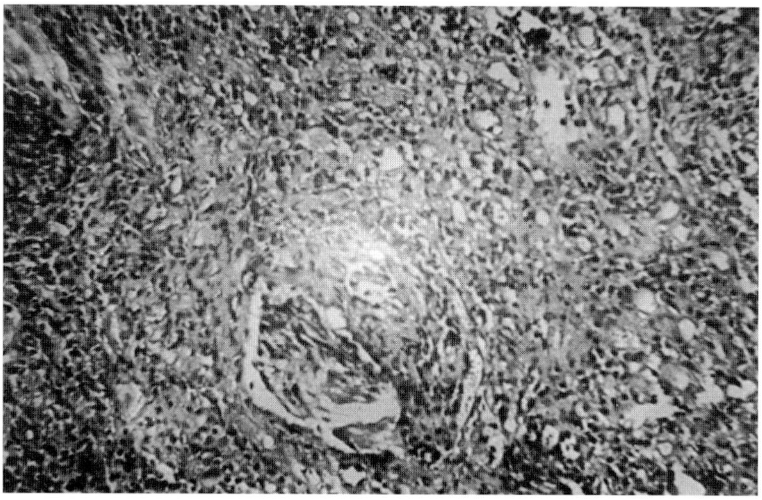

Fig. 6. Patients 2. Microscopic view showing fibrosis of the submucosa. × 85.

Discussion

It has been reported that stereotactic radiosurgery can be used to deliver a boost dose of radiation to recurrent nasopharyngeal carcinomas [7]. The technique is increasingly available and may offer some advantages over other treatment methods. Our preliminary application of the Gamma Knife in the treatment of nasopharyngeal carcinoma gave good short-term results.

In the absence of any appropriate alternative, use of the Gamma Knife for locally recurrent nasopharyngeal carcinoma is not controversial. It is clear that in more advanced cases with a large mass volume the application of the frame requires considerable attention to detail if treatment is to be successful. For tumor recurrence even with metastases, local radiosurgery may also be valuable and promote improved survival. The Gamma Knife is also useful for intracranial metastasis.

The use of the Gamma Knife for the primary treatment of nasopharyngeal carcinoma is more controversial. There is a sensible concern that invisible tumor may fall outside the high-dose therapeutic region. We selected the 4 cases who received primary Gamma-Knife treatment carefully. It would seem that the therapeutic effect on these primary tumors was better than the effect on recurrences. It is necessary to place the marginal dose outside the borders of the visible tumor. Moreover, prophylactic radiotherapy of the neck will be required. At present the long-term effects of Gamma Knife radiosurgery on the outcome of these patients are not established. Further work is required.

References

1 Chinese Health Department (ed): Diagnosis and Therapy of Malignant Tumor. Beijing, Beijing Medical University and Xiehe University, 1991, vol 6, pt 5, pp 1–41.

2 Ning JP, Yu MC, Wang QS: Consumption of salted fish and other risk factors for nasopharyngeal carcinoma in Tianjin. J Natl Cancer Inst 1990;82:291.

3 Tang Zhaoyou (ed): Modern Oncology. Shanghai, Shanghai Medical University, 1993, vol 6, pp 586–608.

4 Carlson LS, Fletcher GH, Oswald WJ: Guidelines for radiotherapeutic techniques for cervical metastasis from an unknown primary. Int J Radiat Oncol Biol Phys 1986;12:2101–2110.

5 Pryzant RM, Nendt CD, Delclos L, Peters LJ: Retreatment of nasopharyngeal carcinoma in 53 patiens. Int J Radiat Oncol Phys 1992;22:941–947.

6 Kondziolka D, Lunsford DL: Stereotactic radiosurgery for squamous cell carcinoma of the nasopharynx. Laryngoscope 1991;101:519–522.

7 Buatti JM, William A: LINAC radiosurgery for locally recurrent nasopharyngeal carcinoma: Rationale and technique. H N 1995;14:93.

Proc 7th Int Meeting Leksell Gamma Knife® Society,
Island of Lana'i, Hawaii, November 1995
Stereotact Funct Neurosurg 1996;66(suppl 1):208–213

Stereotactic and Functional Neurosurgery

Gamma Knife Stereotactic Radiosurgery for Uveal Melanoma: Clinical Results after 2 Years

G. Marchini, M. Gerosa, E. Piovan, A. Pasoli, S. Babighian, M. Rigotti, M. Rossato, L. Bonomi

University Hospital of Verona, Italy

Key Words
Uveal melanoma · Gamma Knife · Radiosurgery

Abstract

We report on 36 cases of uveal melanoma treated at our center between March 1993 and September 1995. There were 16 men and 20 women, aged 57 ± 11 years. The choroid was affected in 35 patients and the ciliary body in 1. The same preoperative and follow-up protocol was adopted for all cases. The procedure included fixation and positioning of the eye with a retrobulbar injection of long-lasting anesthetic and two extraocular muscle sutures, application of the frame, computed tomography scan localization, dose planning and treatment with the Gamma Knife. The patients were divided into three groups. Group A: 10 patients with a follow-up of 24 ± 4 months, treated with a high dose (surface dose 58 ± 9 Gy, maximum dose 81 ± 15 Gy, mean dose 66 ± 11 Gy). Group B: 9 patients with a follow-up of 16 ± 2 months, treated with a lower dose (surface dose 41 ± 3 Gy, maximum dose 76 ± 10 Gy, mean dose 53 ± 11 Gy). Group C: 17 patients with a follow-up of 6 ± 3 months, treated with a lower dose (surface dose 42 ± 3 Gy, maximum dose 72 ± 16 Gy, mean dose: 54 ± 6 Gy). In group A, we observed marked tumor regression in 9 cases, tumor recurrence in 1 case and severe complications in 5 cases (neovascular glacuoma and/ or radiation retinopathy and/or radiation optic neuropathy). In group B, significant local control of the tumor was obtained with minor complications (cotton wool spots, hard exudates, intraretinal hemorrhages). In group C, to date we have observed a regression of the tumor in 7 cases and 1 severe complication (neovascular glaucoma). Our data show that uveal melanomas may be adequately controlled by a high radiosurgical dosage (50–70 Gy), though there are significant side effects. Comparable levels of local tumor control may be obtainable using lower doses (40–45 Gy) which would hopefully reduce the rate of complications. However, a longer follow-up is needed for further validation of these results.

KARGER

E-Mail karger@karger.ch
Fax + 41 61 306 12 34
http://www.karger.ch

1011–6125/96/0665–0208$10.00/0

Dott. Giorgio Marchini
Clinica Oculistica dell'Università
Ospedale di Borgo Trento
I–37126 Verona (Italy)

Introduction

Most uveal melanomas are currently managed conservatively. Different options available for therapy include observation for small suspect tumors, laser photocoagulation, local surgical excision, brachytherapy with different radioactive scleral plaques, and proton beam irradiation [1]. Radiation therapy is effective for medium-sized to large tumors; but it is not known whether it achieves a better patient survival than enucleation [2]. Since there is no definitive treatment for large uveal melanomas, alternative therapies must be investigated.

Gamma Knife stereotactic radiosurgery allows a high dose of radiation to be delivered to an intracranial target with a very high spatial accuracy, and its use has been proposed for the treatment of ocular melanomas [3, 4]. In early 1993 at the Gamma Knife Stereotactic Radiosurgery Center of Verona University Hospital, we developed a specific protocol to treat the ocular melanoma. Preliminary results show that single, high-dose Gamma Knife radiosurgery is effective in the local control of uveal melanomas and achieves a significant shrinkage of the tumor [5].

In this clinical study, we report the results of 36 melanoma patients treated with the Gamma Knife, noting especially the dose response. The follow-up was 1–30 months.

Patients and Methods

Patients

We treated 36 cases of uveal melanoma between March 1993 and September 1995. They include 16 men and 20 women, 57 ± 11 years old, with choroidal (35 patients) and ciliary body (1 patient) melanomas. Follow-up was from 1 to 30 months. The choroidal tumor location was anterior to the equator in 5 eyes (14%), posterior to the equator in 21 eyes (58%) and in contact with the optic nerve in 9 eyes (25%). With ultrasonography, the maximum base diameter ranged from 8 to 21 mm and the maximum thickness from 3.5 to 14 mm. According to the TNM criteria, the tumor size was T2 in 4 patients (11%) and T3 in 32 patients (89%).

The same preoperative protocol was followed for each patient. It included opthalmological and systemic assessment. Complete ocular examination including fundus photography, fluorescein angiography and standardized ultrasonography, as well as computed tomography (CT) and magnetic resonance imaging, chest X-rays, liver echography and blood tests were performed. Follow-up was carried out every 6 months, with local (echography, fundus photography and fluorangiography) and systemic (liver echography and blood tests) examinations. At the time of diagnosis, only 1 patient had a suspected hepatic metastasis, which was confirmed by biopsy. There were no other metastases.

Procedure

The treatment is a standard Gamma Knife radiosurgery procedure modified for ocular therapy. There are five steps including fixation of the eye, application of the stereotactic frame, neuroradiological localization, dose planning and treatment with the Gamma Knife [5]. To achieve total immobilization and proper positioning of the globe, a retrobulbar injection of long-lasting anesthetic (a mixture of 4 ml Marcaine 0.5% and 1 ml Carbocaine 2%) was given and two extraocular muscle sutures were tied to the stereotactic frame. The frame must be set low, anterior and displaced to the side of the eye involved in order to place the tumor as close as possible to the center of the stereotactic system. Sometimes a rotation of the head is required to reach a useful compromise between X and Y coordinates. CT imaging is employed for neuroradiological localization.

Gamma Knife Treatment Parameters and Dose Planning

Single- or multi-isocentre conformational dose planning was performed, with the aim of covering the uveal melanoma and a 2-mm-wide margin around the tumor border. A surface dose between 38 and 70 Gy was delivered at the 45–90% isodose curve. The maximum dose at the center of the target ranged from 50 to 116 Gy. We used 4-, 8- and 14-mm collimators, and 1–6 shots were administered. Weighted fields were adopted in 3 cases.The gamma angle ranged between 45° and 90°, but most of the patients were treated with a gamma angle of 50–60°.

Clinical Evaluation Criteria

The patients were divided into three groups. Group A: 10 patients with a follow-up >1 year, treated with a high dose (surface dose between 50 and 70 Gy at the 60–90% isodose line). Group B: 9 patients with a follow-up >1 year, treated with a lower dose (surface dose between 40 and 45 Gy at the 50–65% isodose line). Group C: 17 patients with a follow-up <1 year, treated with a lower dose (surface dose between 38 and 50 Gy at the 45–85% isodose line).

Survival and globe retention rates were not considered, because of the short follow-up period. The evaluation criteria included local control of the tumor, complications of the treatment and visual acuity. The melanoma was considered locally controlled if its dimensions decreased or remained unchanged using ultrasonographic maximum-thickness measurements. Results were analyzed for all patients as well as within each individual group.

Results

Figure 1 shows the percentage reduction in echographic thickness of all tumors after Gamma Knife radiosurgery, compared with pretreatment values. The melanoma regressed in 17 out of 36 cases (47%) and remained unchanged in 18 our of 36 cases (50%). In a T3N0M0 melanoma patient, we observed a recurrence of the tumor after 18 months, so the eye was enucleated.

Severe complications such as neovascular glaucoma and/or radiation retinopathy and/or radiation optic neuropathy were observed in 6 out of 36 patients (17%). One eye affected by neovascular glaucoma was enucleated 1 year after the treatment. Other severe complications occurred after 6 months in 2 eyes, 12 months in 3 eyes and 24 months in 1 eye. In 10 out of 36 patients (28%), minor complications such as cotton wool spots, hard exudates and small intraretinal

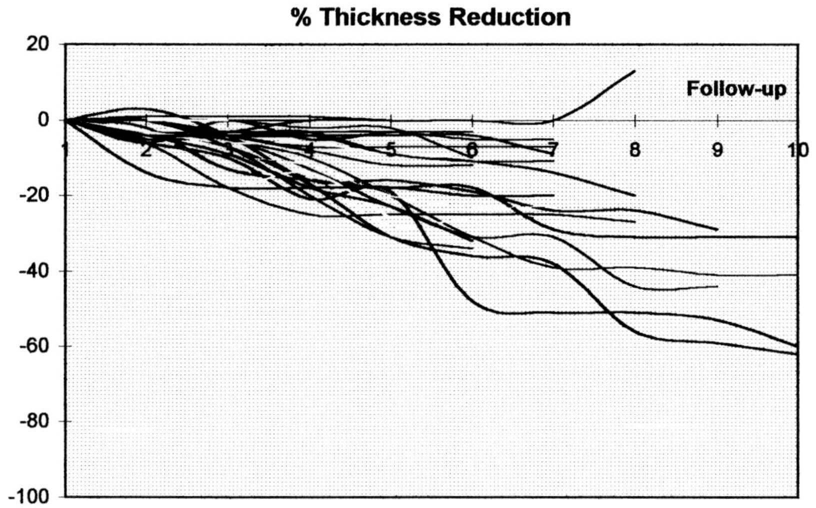

Fig. 1. Percent reduction in echographic thickness of 36 uveal melanomas after Gamma Knife stereotactic radiosurgery, compared with pretreatment values. Follow-up at 3-month intervals.

hemorrhages were observed. One eye developed hemovitreous and another posterior subcapsular cataract.

At the most recent follow-up, the visual acuity was 0.2–1 in 17 out of 34 cases (50%), hand motion to 0.1 in 12 out of 34 cases (35%), and no light perception in 5 out of 34 cases (15%). The results for each individual group are summarized in table 1.

Discussion

Conservative radiation therapies for large melanomas include ^{125}I scleral plaques [6], proton [7] and helium ion [8] irradiation. Clinical experience has shown that a very high radiation dose is essential for the local control of this uveal tumor. The treatments are usually divided over a 1-week period and surgical procedures are an integral part of the methods.

The Gamma Knife emits a high dose of radiation in a single procedure, without the requirement for surgery, and significantly reduces the size of ocular melanomas [5]. From a technical point of view, some issues may jeopardize the accuracy and/or the feasibility of the treatment, such as the size of the patient's head and the neuroradiological detection/localization of small tumors [5]. Furthermore,

Table 1. Results of three groups of uveal melanomas treated with Gamma Knife radiosurgery

Parameter	Group A	Group B	Group C
Number of patients	10	9	17
Follow-up, months	24±4	16±2	6±3
Dosage, Gy			
Surface	58±9	41±3	42±3
Maximum	81±15	76±10	72±16
Average	66±11	53±11	54±6
Local control of tumor			
Regression[a]	9/10 (–20 to –62%)	6/9 (–10 to –30%)	7/17 (–12 to –34%)
Unchanged	–	3/9	10/17
Recurrence	1/10 (enucleated)	–	–
Severe complications[b]	5/10 (1 enucleation)	–	1/17
Visual function[c]			
Before radiosurgery	0.5±0.3 (1 LP)	0.6±0.4 (1 HM, 1 CF)	0.4±0.4 (2 CF, 3 LP)
At last follow-up visit	0.1±0.2 (4 NLP)	0.4±0.4 (1 LP, 1 NLP)	0.3±0.3 (2 HM, 2 LP, 1 NLP)

[a] In parentheses, the range of percent reduction in echographic thickness compared with pretreatment values.

[b] Severe complications include neovascular glaucoma and/or radiation retinopathy and/or radiation optic neuropathy.

[c] HM = Hand motion; CF = counter finger; LP = light perception; NLP = no light perception.

ocular fixation is crucial for successful Gamma Knife radiosurgery. Different methods of ocular fixation have been proposed: minor conjunctival surgery with muscle sutures [3], a suction attachment [4], and extraocular muscle sutures only [5]. Currently, there is no best method for ocular immobilization.

The most important issue in Gamma Knife radiosurgery is the optimum radiation dosage. There is an association between dose, local control and complications. With other radiation therapies, the relative biologic effect and the dose rate seem to be important parameters in determining local control and complication rates. For instance, charged-particle helium ion irradiation achieves better tumor control than ^{125}I brachytherapy, but it is characterized by more severe complications, such as neovascular glaucoma [9]. Larger tumors are generally characterized by higher rates of complications [6] and recurrences [10].

Our study is mainly composed of large, posteriorly located melanomas [32/36 (89%) are T3N0M0 tumors; 9/36 (25%) are in contact with the optic nerve], so there is a higher risk of complications. The data in table 1 suggest that large uveal melanomas may be adequately controlled by higher single-session radiosurgical doses (surface dose of 50–70 Gy), even though side effects are severe. Lower doses (surface dose of 40–45 Gy) may reduce complications, while obtaining a satisfactory level of local tumor control. We achieved the best results with a surface dose of 40–45 Gy at the 50–60% isodose line (maximum dose of 75–80 Gy) delivered with 2–4 shots of the 8 mm collimator and conformational dose planning.

After 30 months, our data show that Gamma Knife radiosurgery may be considered an alternative technique for the treatment of large melanomas. However, a longer follow-up is needed to complete this phase of the clinical study and to validate our results.

References

1 Shields JA, Shields C, Donso LA: Management of posterior uveal melanoma. Surv Ophthalmol 1991;36:161–195.

2 Straatsma BR, Fine SL, Earle JD: The Collaborative Ocular Melanoma Study Research Group: Enucleation versus plaque irradiation for choroidal melanoma. Ophthalmology 1988;95:1000–1004.

3 Chinela AB, Zambrano A, Bunge HY, Guevara JA, Antico JC, Alva O, Artes C, Coscia G: Gamma Knife radiosurgery in uveal melanomas; in Steiner L (ed): Radiosurgery: Baseline and Trends. New York, Raven Press, 1992, pp 161–169.

4 Zehetmeyer M, Menapace R, Kitz K, Ertl A: Suction attachment for stereotactic radiosurgery of intraocular malignancies. Ophthalmologica 1994;208:119–121.

5 Marchini G, Babighian S, Tomazzoli L, Gerosa MA, Nicolato A, Bricolo A, Piovan E, Zampieri PG, Alessandrini F, Benati A, Foroni R, Giri MG, Pasoli A, Bonomi L: Stereotactic radiosurgery of uveal melanomas: Preliminary results with Gamma Knife treatment. Stereotact Funct Neurosurg 1995;64(suppl 1):72–79.

6 Packer S, Stoller S, Lesser ML, Mandel FS, Finger PT: Long-term results of iodine-125 irradiation of uveal melanoma. Ophthalmology 1992;99:767–774.

7 Gragoudas ES, Seddon JM, Egan K, Glynn R, Munzenrider J, Austin-Seymour M, Goitein M, Verhey L, Urie M, Koeler A: Long-term results of proton beam irradiated uveal melanomas. Ophthalmology 1987;94:349–353.

8 Char DH, Castro JR, Kroll SM, Irvine AR, Quivey JM, Stone RD: Five-year follow-up of helium ion therapy for uveal melanoma. Arch Ophthalmol 1990;108:209–214.

9 Char DH, Quivey JM, Castro JR, Kroll SM, Phillips T: Helium ions versus iodine-125 brachytherapy in the management of uveal melanoma: A prospective, randomised, dynamically balanced trial. Opthalmology 1993;100:1547–1554.

10 Gragoudas ES; Egan KM, Seddon JM, Walsh SM, Munzenrider JE: Intraocular recurrence of uveal melanoma after proton beam irradiation. Ophthalmology 1992;99:760–766.

Proc 7th Int Meeting Leksell Gamma Knife® Society,
Island of Lana'i, Hawaii, November 1995
Stereotact Funct Neurosurg 1996;66(suppl 1):214–224

Stereotactic and Functional Neurosurgery

Positron Emission Tomography Using ^{18}F-Fluorodeoxyglucose in Patients with Stereotactically Irradiated Brain Metastases

K. Ericson[a], *L. Kihlström*[b], *J. Mogard*[a], *B. Karlsson*[b], *C. Lindquist*[b], *L. Widén*[c], *V.P. Collins*[d], *S. Stone-Elander*[e]

Departments of
[a] Neuroradiology, [b] Neurosurgery, [c] Clinical Neurophysiology, [d] Pathology, and
[e] The Karolinska Pharmacy, Karolinska Hospital, Stockholm, Sweden

Key Words
Stereotactic radiosurgery · ^{18}F-Fluorodeoxyglucose · Positron emission tomography · Radiation necrosis/reaction · Tumor recurrence · Therapy

Abstract

Thirty-one patients with intracranial metastases were examined with positron emission tomography (PET) using ^{18}F-fluorodeoxyglucose (FDG) as a tracer. The PET study was prompted by growth of the tumor in spite of therapy, or regrowth after an initially favorable response. Increased accumulation of FDG was seen in 14 patients (group 1) and decreased in 17 (group 2). Patients in group 1 had verified tumor growth in 9 of 14 cases. The median survival after radiosurgery was 12.3 months. One patient in this group is still alive after open surgery of a recurrent metastasis. Six patients in group 2 are still alive. The median survival after radiosurgery was 19.9 months. Verified radiation reaction/necrosis was found in 5/17 and viable tumor tissue in 2. The survival time in group 2 was significantly longer than in group 1. PET is superior to computed tomography and magnetic resonance imaging in the differentiation between recurrence and radiation reaction/necrosis. However, temporary radiation effects may mask remaining tumor tissue, and repeat PET studies may sometimes be necessary.

KARGER
E-Mail karger@karger.ch
Fax + 41 61 306 12 34
http://www.karger.ch

1011–6125/96/0665–0214$10.00/0

Kaj Ericson, MD, PhD
Department of Neuroradiology
Karolinska Hospital
S–171 76 Stockholm (Sweden)

Introduction

It has been claimed that some 20–30% of patients with malignant disease develop intracranial metastases [1–3]. Untreated, patients with brain metastasis have a mean survival of 4 weeks [4, 5]. Treatment with steroids sometimes has a dramatic effect, increasing mean survival to 15 weeks [5]. Mean survival can also be prolonged with whole-brain radiation therapy (WBRT): previous authors state an increase in survival for solitary metastasis of 9–15 weeks [6–8], while surgery in combination with WBRT prolongs the median survival to 40 weeks. It appears that the combination of surgery and WBRT is superior to either surgery or WBRT alone, for solitary metastases [8].

Stereotactic irradiation with the Gamma Knife (Elekta, Stockholm, Sweden), has been called radiosurgery and has been used in the treatment of a number of different types of lesions, including intracranial metastases, for which it seems to be successful [9–15]. It is claimed that growth control, i.e., 'local tumor control,' is obtained in 94% of the patients [13]. Local tumor control means in this context that the treated tumor disappears or at least does not grow. Somaza et al. [14] even report 97% local control in a small series of patients with malignant melanoma. An advantage of radiosurgery over surgical treatment is the ease with which multiple metastases can be treated. However, the survival time for patients treated in this way is not overwhelmingly superior, which may be explained in part by the fact that only the intracranial manifestations are addressed by radiosurgery. Flickinger et al. [15] report a median survival of 48 weeks after treatment of 116 patients with a solitary cerebral metastasis. At Karolinska Hospital, the mean survival time of patients with a single metastasis was 48 weeks in a series of 198 patients treated between 1975 and 1993 [16]. In the total material, the mean survival time was 42 weeks and in patients treated for three or more metastases it was as short as 22 weeks.

The purpose of this study was a further analysis of the value of positron emission tomography (PET) with ^{18}F-fluorodeoxyglucose (FDG) in the evaluation of patients with radiosurgically treated intracranial metastases with lost local control.

Material and Methods

Between June 1991 and May 1994, 31 patients were selected for examination with PET. They had all been treated with radiosurgery for intracranial manifestations of verified malignant disease of known origin. An FDG-PET study was suggested when the radiosurgical treatment failed or when progression of an irradiated metastatic tumor was seen after an initial favorable response. Seventeen patients were females and 14 were males. The mean age at radiosurgery was 57 years (range 23–79 years). Eleven patients had primary lung tumors, 7 had mammary cancer, 4 had hypernephroma, 3 had malignant melanoma, 2 had colon cancer, 2 had rectal cancer, 1 had a sarcoma and 1 had choriocarcinoma. Seventeen patients had multiple metastases at the time of first treatment, and some patients developed new metastases during the follow-up period.

In each patient in the present study there was one particular metastasis that did not respond to treatment and it was this metastasis which prompted further evaluation with PET. Only the selected lesion was studied, and lesions that developed during follow-up in some patients were disregarded for the purposes of the current analysis. Fourteen patients had a solitary metastasis, 4 had two metastases, 5 had three and 8 had more than three. As a rule, patients with more than three metastases were not accepted for radiosurgery, except for social and humanitarian reasons.

The patients' clinical condition at the time of radiosurgery was reflected by a Karnofsky score of more than 70. All patients had an expected survival time of at least 3 months. Control of the primary malignancy was otherwise not required. Follow-up after PET was for a minimum of 2 years. One patient has now been followed for over 10 years.

Four patients were treated with WBRT prior to radiosurgery. Seven had been treated with cytostatic agents. The radiosurgical technique has been described elsewhere [17]. The maximal dose was 42–100 Gy and the margin dose was 18–50 Gy. The interval from radiosurgery to PET varied from 101 days to 8.6 years (mean 41 months). PET with FDG was performed in all patients. A dose of 125 MBq of tracer was injected intravenously, and the measurements were started 30 min later. Multiple data sets were acquired during a total measuring time of 20 min. The data sets were then added and reconstructed to one set of images representing the activity distribution over the whole measurement time. A Scanditronix PCB2048-15B scanner was used for most of the studies, yielding 15 images with a slice thickness of 6.5 mm (full width at half-maximum FWHM). More recently, a Siemens Exact PET system has been used (47 slices, 3.5 mm slice thickness). No effort was made to generate metabolic maps showing such kinetic parameters of the tracer as metabolic rate. In 10 cases, the PET scans were repeated. A third PET scan was performed in 4 patients. The PET scans were visually evaluated by two neuroradiologists independently, and the uptake of FDG in the lesions was classified as increased, decreased or equal relative to that of normal white matter. A consensus was reached on the findings in a few cases otherwise the evaluators were unanimous. The analysis of the survival times was done by the Kaplan-Meier product-limit method.

Multiple computed tomography (CT) scans were performed during follow-up. An effort was made to estimate the volume of the lesion under study at the various CT examinations, simply by calculating the three maximum diameters and determining the volume of a sphere. This calculation was performed for comparison over time and not as an exact volume determination.

Verification of the diagnosis of the primary tumor was obtained in all patients. However, in 1 patient the diagnosis of lung cancer was later questioned, but no other primary cancer was found. Verification of the nature of the metastatic lesions was obtained in some patients with biopsy in connection with the radiosurgery procedure. In the remaining patients, the presence of multiple intracranial metastatic lesions in a patient with known malignant disease was considered sufficient evidence of the diagnosis. Verification of the PET findings was obtained in 4 patients at autopsy and in a further 16 at surgery. In some of the remaining patients, it was considered unethical for various reasons to obtain verification. The final diagnosis in these cases had to be based on probability.

Results

An increased accumulation of FDG in the lesions studied as compared to presumably normal white brain matter was found in 13 patients (group 1). Reduced accumulation was found in 17 patients (group 2). Two patients with a reduced FDG accumulation at a first PET scan showed an increased accumulation at a second scan, and they were included in group 1. Increased FDG uptake was first found at 14 weeks after Gamma Knife treatment. The latest observation was 1.6 years after treatment. Low uptake was first found 21 weeks after treatment. The age distribution was similar in both groups. The mean age in group 1 was 56 years (range 37–79 years), in group 2, 58 years (range 23–77 years). Patients in group 1 had 1–9 intracranial metastases at the time of treatment (mean, 2.9, median 2); patients in group 2 had 1–4 (mean, 2.2, median, 1).

All patients but 1 in group 1 were dead at the time limit of the follow-up. They had a mean survival after PET of 6.7 months (range 5 days to 15.8 months). The mean survival time after radiosurgery was 16.2 months (range 7.2 months to 2.4 years). One patient is still alive 1.7 years after PET and 2.5 years after radiosurgery. However, he was operated after PET and demonstrated a recurrent lung metastasis. The median survival for patients in group 1 was 53 weeks.

In group 2, the mean survival time was 3.4 years (range 8 months to 11.4 years). The median survival was 19.9 months. Six of the 17 patients were still alive at the time of evaluation. The mean survival time after PET was 1.5 years (range 2.6 months to 3.8 years). The Kaplan-Meier (fig. 1) plot revealed a significant difference in survival time between the two groups ($p < 0.05$).

In group 1, the PET findings were verified at autopsy (2 patients) and at open surgery (8 patients). Presence of viable metastatic tumor tissue was found in 9 of these 10 patients. The tenth patient was retreated in the Gamma Knife after PET showed increased accumulation of FDG in a previously treated lesion. Autopsy 2 months after the second treatment did not disclose the presence of any viable tumor cells. Histological verification was not obtained in 4 patients who died from recurrent cerebral metastases or widespread pulmonary metastases. Histological verification was obtained in 7 patients in group 2. Findings consistent with radiation necrosis were found in 5 of these patients and viable tumor tissue in 2. Histological verification was not obtained in the remaining patients, 5 of whom are still alive.

Three patients in group 2 died of cerebral disease. One patient died of postoperative infection and meningeal tumor spread. The second patient died of fulminant necrosis. The third died of a recurrent partially treated metastasis. One patient died of perforated peptic ulcer and one from ileus. The remaining patients died from manifestations of their malignant disease in locations outside the central nervous system. Four of the 13 patients in group 1 died of respiratory compli-

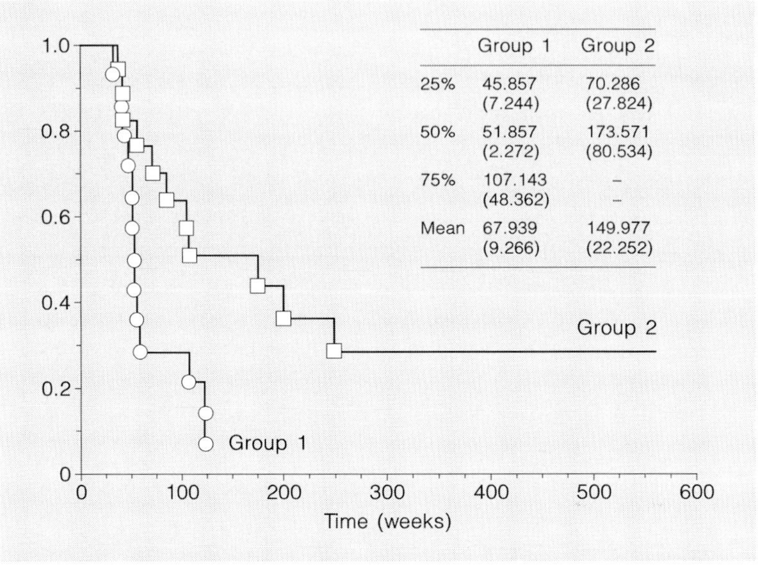

Fig. 1. Kaplan-Meier survival statistics (values in table, mean ± SE in parentheses) with positive (group 1; ○) and negative (group 2; □) FDG findings. One or more estimates of the mean are biased because the last observation in those strata/groups were censored.

cations or insufficiency. One died from uremia. One is still alive. The survival times in this series are summarized in table 1. The mean survival time in the total material treated with radiosurgery was 2.4 years (median 70 weeks).

The radiation dose differed slightly between the two groups, as shown in table 2.

Discussion

A volume increase in a radiosurgically treated metastasis may be due to continued growth of viable tumor, a reaction to radiation, or radiation-induced necrosis. Unfortunately, tumor recurrence and radiation necrosis have a very similar appearance on CT and magnetic resonance imaging (fig. 2, 3). Both lesions are characterized by increasing volume, surrounding edema and peripheral contrast enhancement [18–20]. Flickinger et al. [15] have suggested that tumor enlargement of more than 25% indicates recurrence rather than radiation injury. Others have claimed that delayed increase in tumor volume indicates a radiation reaction. It is, of course, very important to distinguish between recurrent tumor

Table 1. Survival after treatment

	1 year	2 years	3 years
Negative FDG	14/17 (82%)	10/17 (58%)	8/17 (47%)
Positive FDG	7/13 (54%)	4/13 (31%)	

Table 2. Radiation doses (Gy) in patients without and with increased FDG accumulation in the irradiated lesion

	Maximum	Minimum	Average	Integrated
Negative FDG	38–100 (63)	20–40 (29)	31–66 (45)	8–662 (242)
Positive FDG	43–83 (61)	18–30 (22)	28–54 (39)	35–835 (225)

Range given, with the mean in parentheses.

and radiation injury. Patronas et al. [3] and Di Chiro et al. [21] have used PET with FDG to distinguish between radiation necrosis and tumor recurrence in patients with primary brain tumors. They found an increased accumulation of tracer in tumor recurrence and a decreased uptake in radiation necrosis. Similar findings have been reported in patients with brain metastasis [22–24], but there is no unanimity in the literature. In a previous study, FDG-PET had a predictive value in patients with metastasis with failure of local control after radiosurgery: patients with an increased FDG uptake had a median survival of 40 weeks, while those with a reduced FDG uptake had a median survival of 168 weeks [24].

'Lost local control' is a term often used about the radiosurgical treatment of intracranial metastases. It may be defined as tumor growth regardless of treatment or tumor growth after an initially favorable response. Enlargement of an irradiated lesion with surrounding edema and peripheral contrast enhancement on magnetic resonance or CT may indicate tumor growth or radiation reaction. Differentiation is impossible in the individual case [18–20], but PET and FDG may help. It is believed that malignant tumors have an increased accumulation of FDG compared with normal white matter, but this is not necessarily true. It is conceivable that slowly growing tumors, even if malignant, may exhibit an FDG accumulation which does not differ markedly from that of normal cerebral white matter [23]. Thus, it is not surprising that a total correspondence between PET findings and histological findings is not found.

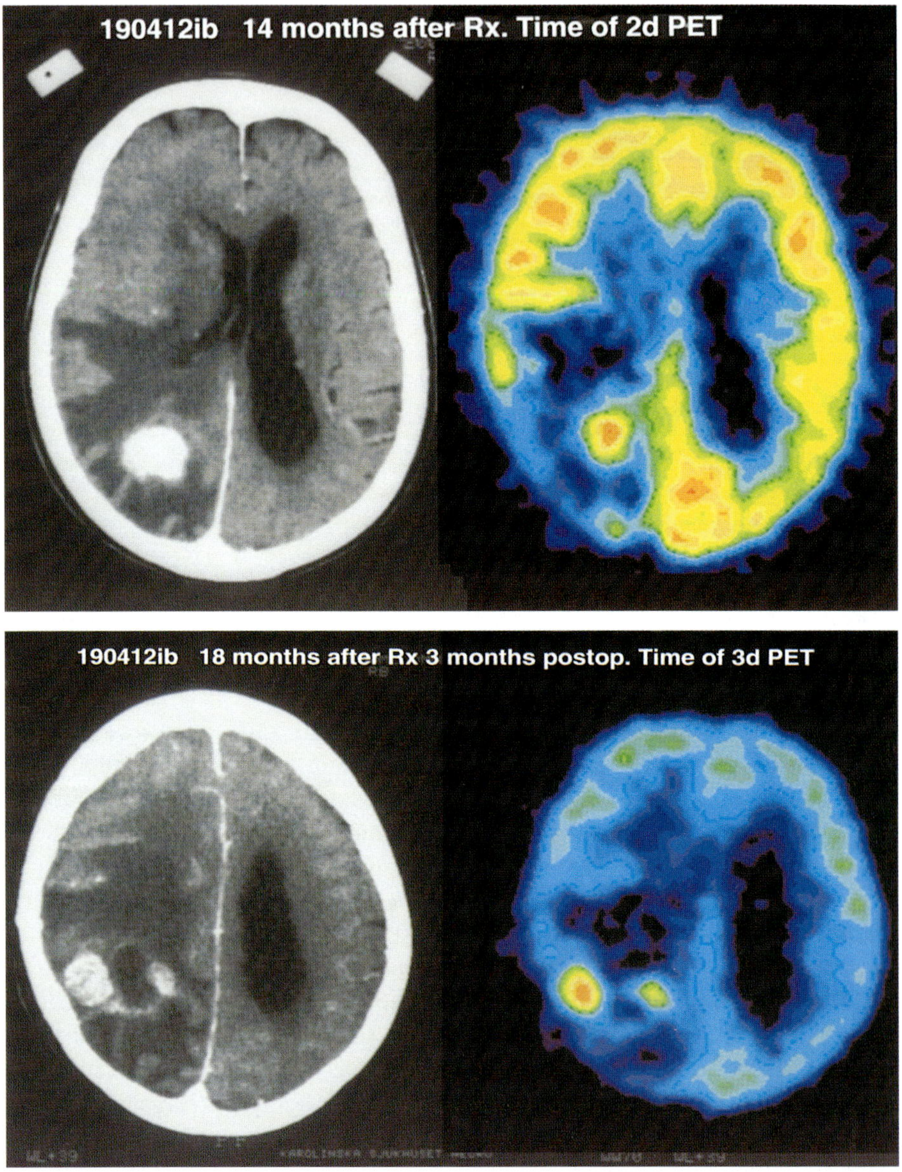

a

b

Fig. 2. **a** Moderately increased FDG accumulation at PET in a lesion with considerable contrast enhancement at CT. **b** Increased FDG accumulation in remaining parts of the tumor after open surgery verified malignant recurrent tumor and marked accumulation of new metastatic tumor.

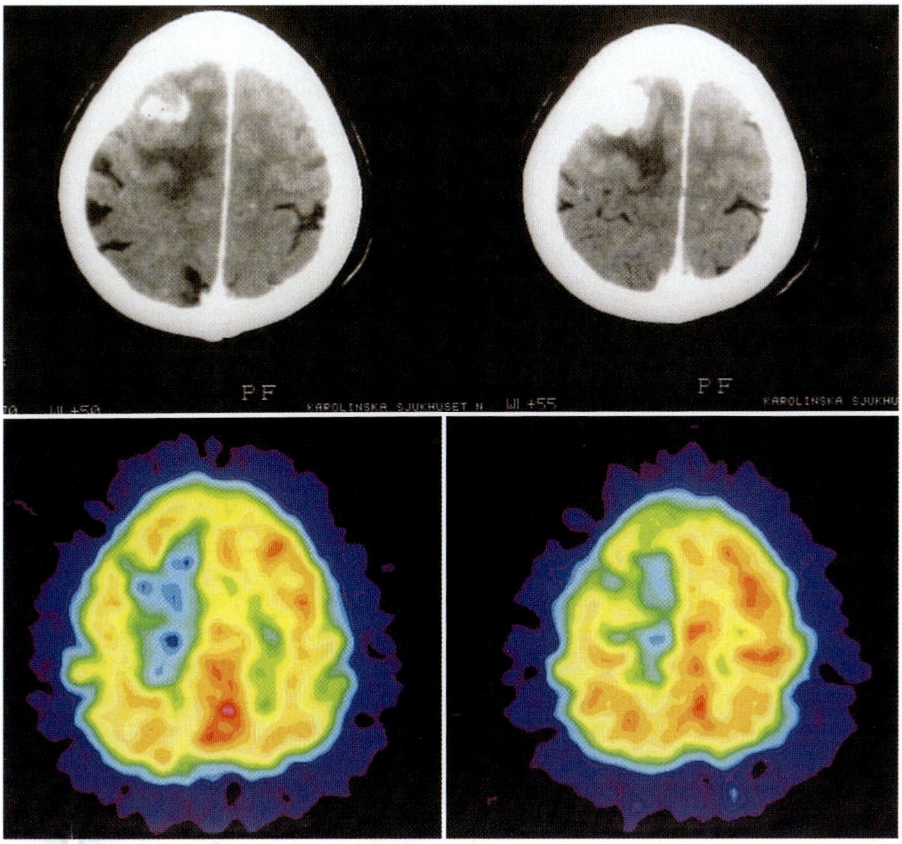

Fig. 3. Decreased accumulation of FDG in a lesion with marked, rather solid contrast enhancement in a recurrent lesion with surrounding edema. Stereotactic biopsy verified necrosis.

In the present series, the finding of a clearly increased FDG accumulation in a previously treated lesion prompted repeated radiosurgical treatment. The patient died 2 months later because of multiple lung metastases. At autopsy there were no viable tumor cells in the irradiated region of the brain, which may be explained by the repeated treatment. Two patients with reduced FDG uptake in irradiated cerebral lesions showed viable tumor cells at open surgery. In 1 patient, the recurrent tumor had a very thin contrast-enhancing capsule. Since the spatial resolution of the PET camera system used during the early part of this study was only 6–7 mm (FWHM), a partial volume artifact may well explain the negative PET study in this case. The newer PET system has a slightly higher resolution of

4–5 mm. In the other patient, viable tumor was found at open surgery, 9 months after the PET study. During this period, considerable growth of the irradiated tumor was seen on CT. It is quite conceivable that significant viable tumor was not present at the time of the PET study. Such a recurrence may be more likely to occur if the tumor was not initially treated optimally or not entirely covered. Another explanation may of course be that a new metastasis had developed. Moreover, 2 patients had an initial PET scan showing reduced FDG uptake at 8 and 5 months after surgery. A new PET scan after a further 5 and 2 months, respectively, showed a distinctly increased accumulation of tracer in combination with clinical deterioration. In these cases there may have been a temporary radiation reaction depressing the metabolic activity of the tumor tissue or masking it. In 6 patients, the repeat PET showed unchanged reduced accumulation of FDG. One patient initially had reduced FDG uptake which normalized completely at a second PET examination 10 months after radiosurgery and 5 months after the first PET.

The tumors in group 1 were slightly larger at the time of treatment compared with group 2 (mean 7.6 versus 5.8 cm^3). The mean time from radiosurgery to PET was 9.3 months in group 1 and 22 months in group 2. Thus, the tumors that were shown to be recurrences were growing much faster than those explained by radiation reactions. Differences like this may be easily seen in a series of patients, but will not be easily appreciated in the individual patient. Patients in group 2 had solitary metastases more often than those in group 1, which may explain the difference in survival between the two groups.

Between June 1991 and May 1994, 207 patients were treated with radiosurgery for intracranial metastases at this institution. The patients in the present series represent almost all patients with lost local control during this period and the percentage of these cases can then be determined to be about 10% [16]. In about half of the cases the lost control was due to tumor recurrence and in the remainder due to radiation reaction or radiation necrosis. Loss of local tumor control was defined by Flickinger et al. [15] as a significant sustained increase in tumor volume ($\geq 25\%$) on follow-up CT and/or MRI scans. With this definition, 4 of 13 patients in our series with tumor recurrence and high uptake of FDG could not be considered out of control, since the volume increase did not exceed 25%. On the other hand, 8 lesions with radiation reaction/necrosis did show a volume increase of more than 25% and may have been candidates for further therapy. Thus it seems important in the individual case to differentiate between radiation reaction/necrosis and recurrence, and this cannot be reliably done with CT/MR.

The time factor is of some importance since no recurrent tumor was encountered at or later than 19 months after radiosurgery.

A recent report on the use of MR in creating maps of the cerebral blood volume indicates that this is a sensitive method in the differentiation between radiation necrosis and tumor progress [25]. However, the experience with this technique is still limited.

In conclusion, PET is of definite help in the differential diagnosis between tumor progression and radiation reaction, while CT and MR are usually not.

References

1 Black P: Brain metastasis: Current status and recommended guidelines for management. Neurosurgery 1979;5:617–631.

2 Cairncross J, Posner J: The management of brain metastases; in Walker AE (ed): Oncology of the Nervous System. Boston, Nijhoff, 1983, pp 341–377.

3 Patronas N, Di Chiro G, Brooks R, DeLaPaz R, Kornblith P, Smith B, Rizzoli H, Kessler R, Manning R, Channing M, Wolf A, O'Connor C: Work in progress: 18-F Fluorodeoxyglucose and positron emission tomography in the evaluation of radiation necrosis of the brain. Radiology 1982;144: 885–889.

4 Lang E, Slater J: Metastatic brain tumors: Results of surgical and nonsurgical treatment. Surg Clin North Am 1964;44:865–872.

5 Pladdet I, Boven E, Nauten J, Pinedo HM: Palliative care for brain metastases of solid tumour types. Neth J Med 1989;34:10–21.

6 Byrne TN, Cascino TL, Posner JB: Brain metastasis from melanoma. J Neurooncol 1983;1:313–317.

7 Gay PC, Litchy WJ, Cascino TL: Brain metastasis in hypernephroma. J Neurooncol 1987;5:51–56.

8 Patchell R, Tibbs P, Walsh J, Dempsey R, Maruyama Y, Kryscio R, Markesbery W, Macdonald J, Young B: A randomized trial of surgery in the treatment of single metastases to the brain. N Engl J Med 1990;322:494–500.

9 Buatti J, Friedman W, Bova F, Mendenhall W: Treatment selection factors for stereotactic radiosurgery of intracranial metastases. Int J Radiat Oncol Biol Phys 1995;32:1161–1166.

10 Coffey R, Lunsford DL, Flickinger JC: The role of radiosurgery in the treatment of malignant brain tumors. Neurosurg Clin North Am 1992;23:231–244.

11 Davey P, O'Brien P, Schwartz M, Cooper P: A phase I/II study of salvage radiosurgery in the treatment of recurrent brain metastases. Br J Neurosurg 1994;8:717–723.

12 Jokura H, Takahashi K, Kayama T, Yoshimoto T: Gamma Knife radiosurgery of a series of only minimally selected metastatic brain tumours. Acta Neurochir Suppl (Wien) 1994;62:77–82.

13 Kihlström L, Karlsson B, Lindquist C: Gamma Knife surgery for cerebral metastases: Implications for survival based on 16 years experience. Stereotact Funct Neurosurg 1993;62(suppl 1):45–50.

14 Somaza S, Kondziolka D, Lunsford DL, Kirkwood J, Flickinger JC: Stereotactic radiosurgery for cerebral metastatic melanoma. J Neurosurg 1993;79:661–666.

15 Flickinger JC, Kondziolka D, Lunsford DL, Coffey R, Goodman M, Shaw W, Hudgins W, Weiner R, Harsh GT, Sneed P, Larson D: A multi-institutional experience with stereotactic radiosurgery for solitary brain metastasis. Int J Radiat Oncol Biol Phys 1994;28:797–802.

16 Karlsson B, Kihlström L, Lindquist C: Medical controversy: Is Gamma Knife surgery the treatment of choice for cerebral metastases? Forum 1994;4:396–402.

17 Kihlström L, Karlsson B, Lindquist C, Norén G, Rähn T: Gamma knife surgery for cerebral metastasis. Acta Neurochir Suppl (Wien) 1991;52:87–89.

18 Dooms G, Hecht S, Brant-Zawadzki M, Berthiaume Y, Norman D, Newton T: Brain radiation lesions: MR imaging. Radiology 1986;158:149–155.

19 Graeb D, Steinbok P, Robertson W: Transient early computed tomographic changes mimicking tumour progression after brain tumour irradiation. Radiology 1982;144:813–817.

20 Mikhael M: Radiation Necrosis of the brain: Correlation between computed tomography, pathology and dose distribution. J Comput Assist Tomogr 1978;2:71–80.

21 Di Chiro G, Oldfield E, Wright D, De Michele D, Katz D, Patronas N, Doppman J, Larson S, Ito M, Kufta C: Cerebral necrosis after radiotherapy and/or intra-arterial chemotherapy for brain tumors: PET and neuropathologic studies. Am J Roentgenol 1988;150:189–197.

22 Kim E, Chung S, Haynie T, Kim C, Cho B, Podolff D, Tilbury R, Yang D, Yung W, Moser RJ: Differentiation of residual or recurrent tumors from posttreatment changes with F-18 FDG PET. Radiographics 1992;12:269–279.

23 Landis K, Rich K, Dehdashti F, Simpson J, Fusselman M, McGuire A, Siegel B: Brain metastases from non-central nervous system tumors: Evaluation with PET. Radiology 1993;186:37–44.

24 Mogard J, Kihlström L, Ericson K, Karlsson B, Guo WY, Stone-Elander S: Recurrent tumor vs. radiation effects after Gamma Knife radiosurgery of intracerebral metastases: Diagnosis with PET–FDG. J Comput Assist Tomogr 1994;18:177–181.

25 DeLaPaz R, Ott I, Tulipano P: Recurrent brain tumor vs. radiation necrosis: Comparison of MR rCBV maps and FDG-PET. Proc Soc Magnetic Resonance and Eur Soc for Magnetic Resonance in Med and Biol, Nice, 1995. Berkeley, Society of Magnetic Resonance, 1995.

Proc 7th Int Meeting Leksell Gamma Knife® Society,
Island of Lana'i, Hawaii, November 1995
Stereotact Funct Neurosurg 1996;66(suppl 1):225–230

Stereotactic and Functional Neurosurgery

Gamma Knife Radiosurgery for Brain Stem Metastases: Two Autopsy Cases

M. Tago[a], *Y. Aoki*[a], *A. Terahara*[a], *K. Nakagawa*[a], *Y. Sasaki*[a], *H. Kurita*[b], *S. Kawamoto*[b], *S. Murayama*[c]

Departments of [a] Radiology, [b] Neurosurgery, and [c] Neurology, Faculty of Medicine, University of Tokyo, Japan

Key Words

Gamma Knife · Radiosurgery · Metastatic brain tumor · Autopsy · Neuropathology

Abstract

Early neuropathological findings were obtained at autopsy in two cases of brain stem metastasis treated with the Gamma Knife. In both cases, light microscopy radiation changes were strictly localized. Residual tumor tissue in the irradiation field showed marked degenerative changes including multinuclear cells, atypical nuclei and vacuolar degeneration. A characteristic finding in the irradiation field was fibrosis associated with hyalinized and thickened vessels. In more peripheral regions, demyelination and vacuolar degeneration were seen. This is the first report demonstrating extravascular fibrosis in the irradiated field following radiosurgery.

Introduction

Radiosurgery with the Leksell Gamma Knife is widely used for arteriovenous malformations [1–6], acoustic neurinomas [7, 8], meningiomas [9, 10] and metastatic brain tumors [11, 12]. However, very few neuropathological reports are available. We report early neuropathological changes in two autopsy cases treated with the Gamma Knife.

KARGER

E-Mail karger@karger.ch
Fax + 41 61 306 12 34
http://www.karger.ch

1011–6125/96/0665–0225$10.00/0

M. Tago, MD
7-3-1, Hongo, Bunkyo-ku
Tokyo 113 (Japan)

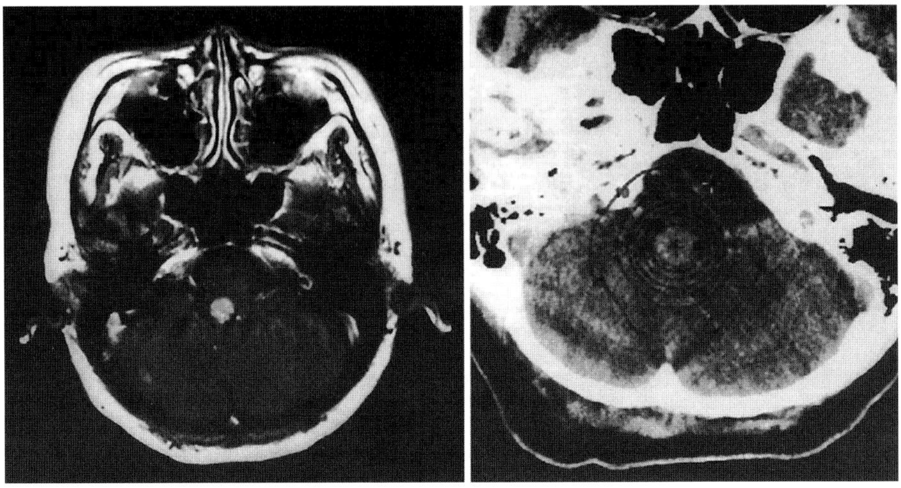

a b

Fig. 1. Case 1. **a** Medulla oblongata breast cancer metastasis shown on MRI. **b** Same lesion demonstrated on computed tomography with superimposed dose plan.

Case Reports

Case 1

A 58-year-old woman had multiple brain metastases from breast cancer, demonstrated on magnetic resonance imaging (MRI). One of these lesions in the medulla oblongata was irradiated with the Gamma Knife, using a maximum dose of 33.3 Gy and a peripheral dose of 20 Gy (fig. 1). Eleven days after treatment, the irradiated tumor showed a decrease in central contrast enhancement on MRI. One month later, it was smaller. However, 2 months after treatment, the patient died from heart failure. At autopsy, light microscopy histology revealed strictly localized radiation changes (fig. 2a). Residual tumor tissue in the irradiation field showed marked degenerative change, with multinucleated cells, atypical nuclei and vacuolar degeneration. There were almost no viable cells (fig. 2b). Prominent fibrosis was observed in the field, associated with hyalinized and thickened small vessels (fig. 2c). In more peripheral regions, myelin was not preserved, while axons were relatively well preserved, suggesting demyelination (fig. 2d, e). Vacuolar degeneration was also recognized in these peripheral regions.

Case 2

A 69-year-old man was shown on MRI to have multiple brain metastases from small-cell lung cancer. One of these lesions in the pons was irradiated with the Gamma Knife, using a maximum dose of 28.6 Gy and a peripheral dose of 20 Gy (fig. 3). Twenty-four days after treatment, the patient died of acute renal failure associated with a hepatorenal syndrome. Neuropathological findings were almost identical with those in case 1. Light microscopy radiation changes were again strictly localized, and residual tumor tissue in the irra-

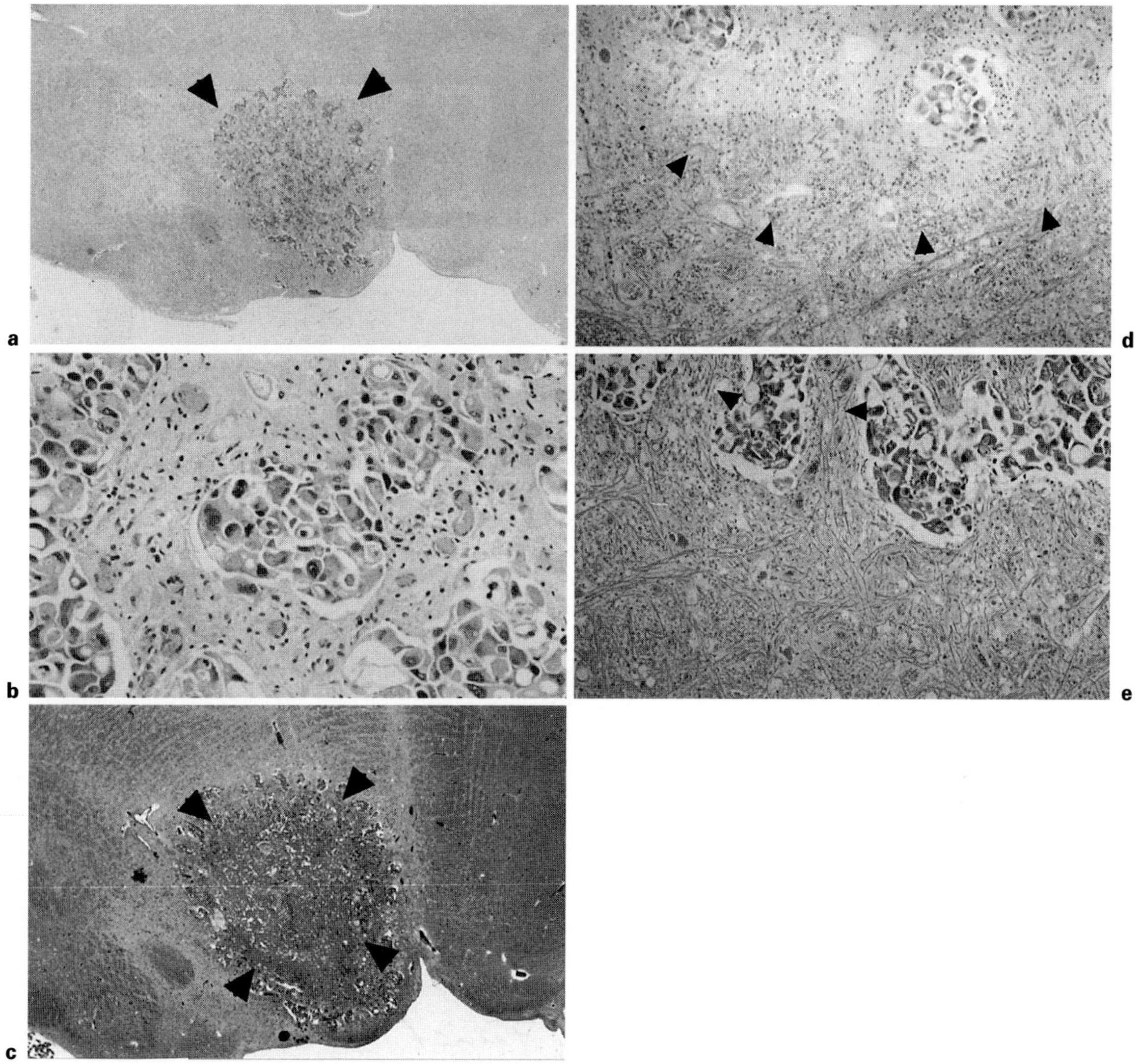

Fig. 2. Case 1. Light microscopy of the tumor shown in figure 1, obtained from the patient at autopsy after death due to heart failure. **a** Localized changes (arrowheads). HE. ×2.5. **b** Marked degenerative changes in the irradiated cells. HE. ×25. **c** Prominent fibrosis (arrowheads). Azan-Mallory. ×3.12. **d** Myelin is not preserved (arrowheads). Klüver-Barrera. ×25. **e** Axons relatively preserved (arrowheads), as in **d** suggesting demyelination. Bodian. ×25.

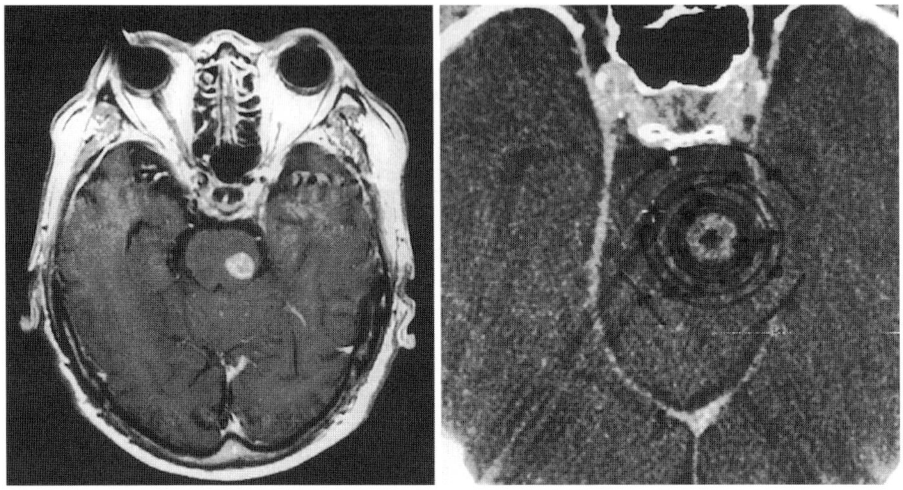

Fig. 3. Case 2. **a** Pons lung cancer metastasis shown on MRI. **b** Same lesion demonstrated on computed tomography with superimposed dose plan.

diated field revealed marked degenerative change. Fibrosis was also observed, although it was not prominent. In the peripheral regions, although vacuolar degeneration was observed, definite demyelination was not seen (fig. 4). Marginal hemorrhage was also observed.

Discussion

There are few reports of autopsy cases following radiosurgery. Koike et al. [13] reported an autopsy case 22 days after irradiation with the Gamma Knife for two metastatic brain tumors, finding almost complete loss of active tumor cells, reactive gliosis, and infiltration of macrophages. Yamamoto et al. [14] reported an autopsy case 26 months after treatment with the Gamma Knife for arteriovenous malformation, and found obstructed blood vessels due to intimal hypertrophy. However, they also found that some of the vessels had patent lumina. Necrosis, demyelination and gliosis were recognized surrounding the nidus. Coffey et al. [11] reported two autopsy cases treated with whole-brain fractionated radiotherapy followed by Gamma Knife radiosurgery. No tumor necrosis was found in one case 7 days after Gamma Knife treatment. In the other case examined 17 days after Gamma Knife radiation, extensive tumor necrosis was found. Thompson et al. [15] also reported an autopsy case treated with the same procedure, finding extensive tumor necrosis 14 days after radiosurgery.

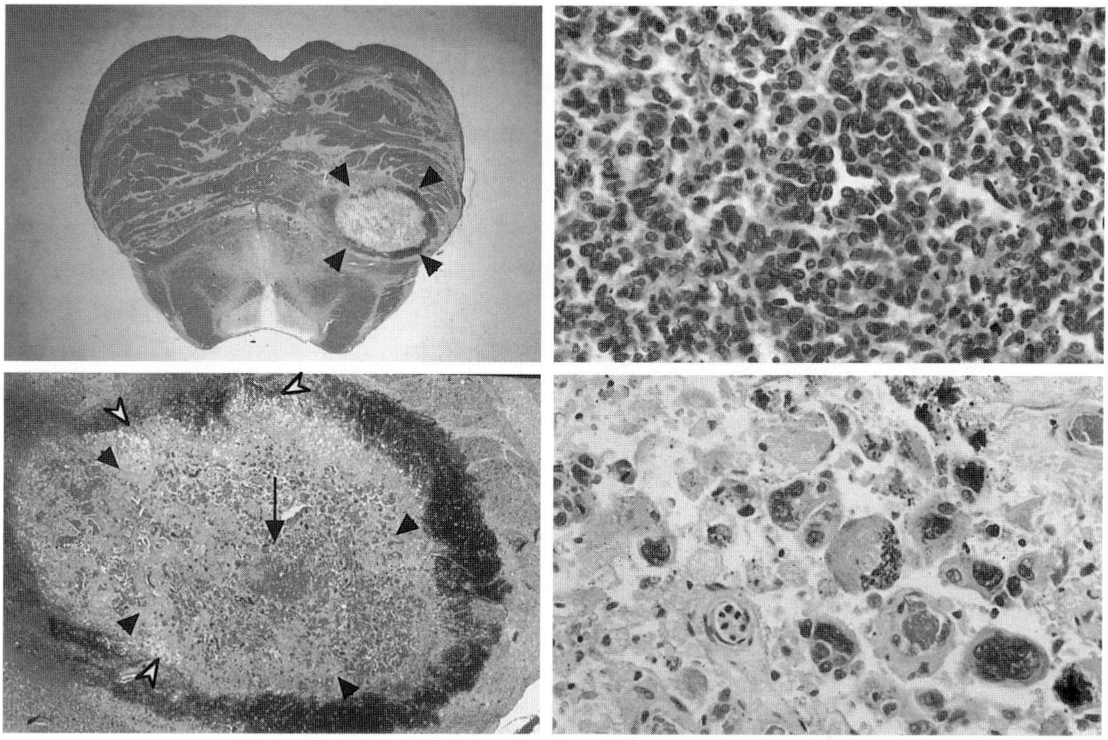

a b c d

Fig. 4. Case 2. Light microscopy of the tumor shown in figure 3, obtained from the patient at autopsy after death due to renal failure. **a** Strictly localized radiation changes (arrowheads). Klüver-Barrera. **b** Note coagulation necrosis (arrow), fibrosis (black arrowheads) and vacuolar degeneration (white arrowhead). Azan-Mallory. × 5. **c** Nonirradiated tumor cells. There are no degenerative changes. HE. × 100. **d** Irradiated tumor cells, revealing marked degenerative changes. HE. × 100.

Our two cases of metastatic brain tumors irradiated with the Gamma Knife alone revealed marked degenerative changes of the irradiated tumor cells. It is suggested that tumor necrosis or tumor cell degeneration occur between 1 and 2 weeks after radiosurgery. Demyelination was found in case 1, but was not definite in case 2. No gliosis was found in either case. Koike et al. [13], found gliosis and Yamamoto et al. [14] found demyelination and gliosis. The discrepancies may be due to the different intervals between irradiation and postmortem observation or to different dosage. However, further investigation is needed.

Yamamoto et al. [14] reported that irradiated blood vessels were strongly positive for collagen type III. Nonetheless, this is the first report demonstrating fibrosis in the radiosurgically irradiated field, associated with hyalinized and thickened vessels. Whether this fibrosis follows normal brain injury or tumor necrosis is not as yet clear. Thus, further investigation is needed, perhaps using an animal model.

References

1 Steiner L, Linquist C: Radiosurgery in cerebral arteriovenous malformations; in Tasker RR (ed): Neurosurgery: State of the Art Reviews. Philadelphia, Hanley and Belfus, 1987, pp 329–336.

2 Lindquist C, Steiner L: Stereotactic radiosurgical treatment of arteriovenous malformations; in Lunsford LD (ed): Modern Stereotactic Neurosurgery. Boston, Nijhoff, 1988, pp 491–505.

3 Lunsford LD, Kondziolka D, Flickinger JC, Bissonette DJ, Jungreis CA, Maitz AH, Horton JA, Coffey RJ: Stereotactic radiosurgery for arteriovenous malformations of the brain. J Neurosurg 1991;75:512–524.

4 Colombo F, Benedetti A, Pozza F, Marchetti C, Chierego G: Linear accelerator radiosurgery of cerebral arteriovenous malformations. Neurosurgery 1989;24:833–840.

5 Betti OO, Munari C, Rosler R: Stereotactic radiosurgery with the linear accelerator: Treatment of arteriovenous malformations. Neurosurgery 1989;24:311–321.

6 Loeffler JS, Alexander E 3rd, Siddon RL, Saunders WM, Coleman CN, Winston KR: Stereotactic radiosurgery for intracranial arteriovenous malformations using a standard linear accelerator. Int J Radiat Oncol Biol Phys 1989;17:673–677.

7 Norén G, Greitz D, Hirsch A, Lax I: Gamma Knife radiosurgery in acoustic neurinoma; in Steiner L, Lindquist C, Forster D, Backlund EO (eds): Radiosurgery: Baseline and Trends. New York, Raven Press, 1992, pp 141–148.

8 Flickinger JC, Lunsford LD, Linskey ME, Duma CM, Kondziolka D: Gamma knife radiosurgery for acoustic tumors: Multivariate analysis of four year results. Radiother Oncol 1993;27:91–98.

9 Lunsford LD, Kondziolka D, Flickinger JC: Stereotactic radiosurgery: Current spectrum and results. Clin Neurosurg 1992;38:405–444.

10 Engenhart R, Kimmig BN, Hover KH, Wowra B, Sturm V, van Kaick G, Wannemacher M: Stereotactic single high dose radiation therapy of benign intracranial meningiomas. Int J Radiat Oncol Biol Phys 1990;19:1021–1026.

11 Coffey RJ, Flickinger JC, Bissonette DJ, Lunsford LD: Radiosurgery for solitary brain metastases using the cobalt-60 gamma unit: Methods and results in 24 patients. Int J Radiat Oncol Biol Phys 1991;20:1287–1295.

12 Flickinger JC, Kondziolka D, Lunsford LD, Coffey R, Goodman M, Shaw E, Hudgins W, Weiner R, Harsh GT, Sneed P, Larson D: A multi-institutional experience with stereotactic radiosurgery for solitary brain metastasis. Int J Radiat Oncol Biol Phys 1994;28:797–802.

13 Koike Y, Hosoda H, Ishiwata Y, Sakata K, Hidaka K: Effect of radiosurgery using Leksell Gamma unit on metastatic brain tumor: Autopsy case report. Neurol Med Chir 1994;34:534–537.

14 Yamamoto M, Jimbo M, Kobayashi M, Toyoda C, Ide M, Tanaka N, Lindquist C, Steiner L: Long-term results of radiosurgery for arteriovenous malformation: Neuro-diagnostic imaging and histological studies of angiographically confirmed nidus obliteration. Surg Neurol 1992;37:219–230.

15 Thompson BG, Coffey RJ, Flickinger JC, Lunsford LD: Stereotactic radiosurgery of small intracranial tumors: Neuropathological correlation in three patients. Surg Neurol 1990;33:96–104.

Proc 7th Int Meeting Leksell Gamma Knife® Society,
Island of Lana'i, Hawaii, November 1995
Stereotact Funct Neurosurg 1996;66(suppl 1):231–239

Stereotactic and Functional Neurosurgery

Is Unchanged Tumor Volume after Radiosurgery a Measure of Outcome?

M. Yamamoto, M. Jimbo, M. Ide, Y. Umebara, S. Hagiwara, K. Takakura, T. Hirai

Departments of Neurosurgery, Dai-ni Hospital and Neurological Institute, Tokyo Women's Medical College, Tokyo, and Heisei Memorial Hospital, Fujieda, Japan

Key Words

Brain tumor · Neurinoma · Meningioma · Hemangioblastoma · Radiosurgery · Gamma Knife · Tumor doubling time

Abstract

We report three patients who underwent Gamma Knife radiosurgery for benign tumors (meningioma, neurinoma and hemangioblastoma), in whom an 'unchanged tumor volume' demonstrated by postirradiation follow-up neuroimaging could be regarded as a successful treatment results, as compared with preradiosurgery tumor growth. It is our view that unless significant tumor growth has been observed before radiosurgery, 'unchanged in size' after radiosurgery cannot be regarded as a successful treatment result. Because relatively few hemangioblastoma patients have been treated radiosurgically, this report emphasizes the course of one case with hemangioblastoma.

Introduction

Stereotactic radiosurgery has become increasingly important as an alternative to initial or repeated surgical resection of brain tumors, particularly in neurinomas and meningiomas [1–16]. The effects of radiosurgery on benign brain tumors are considered to be twofold: (1) a direct cytotoxic effect on the tumor cells and (2) delayed intratumoral vascular obliteration which leads to coagula-

KARGER

E-Mail karger@karger.ch
Fax + 41 61 306 12 34
http://www.karger.ch

1011–6125/96/0665–0231$10.00/0

Masaaki Yamamoto, MD
Department of Neurosurgery
Tokyo Women's Medical College Dai-ni Hospital
2-1-10 Nishiogu, Arakawa-ku
Tokyo 116 (Japan)

tion necrosis of the tumor [12, 13]. Gradual, and eventually permanent, tumor regression is regarded as the ideal treatment result in radiosurgery for brain tumors. Nevertheless, all reported series describing radiosurgery for benign brain tumors, such as neurinomas, meningiomas and pituitary tumors, include 40–50% of cases in which the sizes of the treated tumors remain unchanged for many years [2, 4–11, 13–16]. The notion that 'unchanged in size' after radiosurgery indicates successful treatment is based on the idea that the vast majority of untreated brain tumors, even if benign, show gradual growth. However, recent analyses of the natural courses of neurinomas and meningiomas using neuroimaging techniques have disclosed that some of these tumors do not grow for many years. On the other hand, spontaneous shrinkage is very rare [17–34]. Olivero et al. [28] reported recently that 35 (58%) of 60 meningiomas had shown no growth, with an average follow-up of 29 months (range 3–72 months). Therefore, it is our view that unless significant tumor growth has been observed before radiosurgery, 'unchanged in size' after radiosurgery cannot be regarded as a successful treatment result [35, 36]. Surprisingly, however, there have been no reports analyzing treatment results in radiosurgically treated brain tumors in relation to preradiosurgical growth patterns.

We report three patients who underwent Gamma Knife radiosurgery, in whom an 'unchanged tumor volume' demonstrated by postirradiation follow-up neuroimaging *can* be regarded as showing successful treatment results compared with preradiosurgical tumor growth. Furthermore, because relatively few hemangioblastoma patients have been treated radiosurgically [37, 38], this report also provides details of a hemangioblastoma patient who underwent Gamma Knife radiosurgery. In this patient, growth of the residual tumor, which had grown remarkably over the 6 years following surgical excision, has been well controlled for 3 postradiosurgical years. Tumor shrinkage has, however, been minimal.

Material and Methods

From our personal series of 30 patients who have been treated by Gamma Knife radiosurgery for various brain tumors since 1991, 14 patients were selected for evaluation of treatment results defined by postradiosurgical volume changes in relation to the tumor doubling time before irradiation. In all 14 patients, the preradiosurgical observation period using neuroimaging techniques was sufficiently long. Furthermore, the quality of all images obtained both before and after radiosurgery was adequate for the determination of tumor volume. In the 3 patients reported here, postirradiation volume changes have thus far been minimal.

Determination of Tumor Volume and Tumor Doubling (Half) Time

Tumor volume was determined by one of the authors (S.H.), who had been blinded to clinical data and the day of the examination. Gadolinium-enhanced magnetic resonance

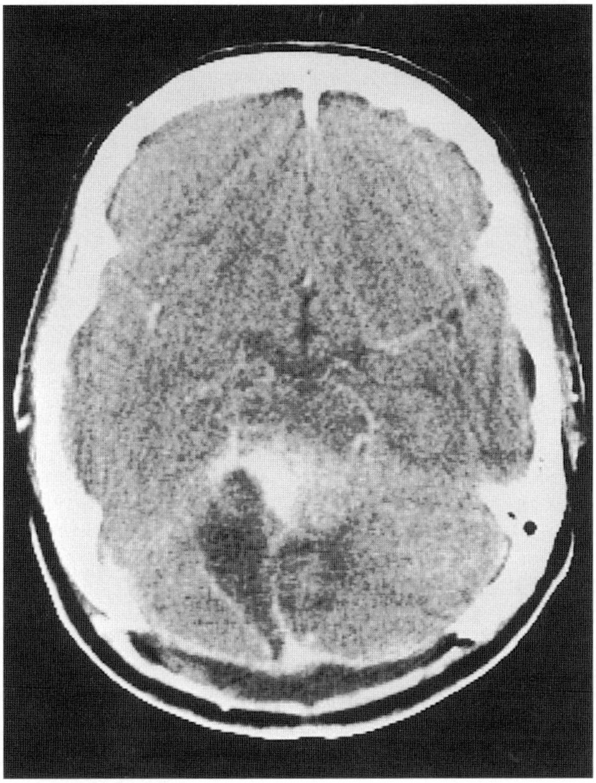

Fig. 1. Case 1. Post-contrast CT scan on June 25, 1986, showing a residual tumor.

imaging (MRI) or contrast-enhanced computed tomography (CT) scans with a 5-mm slice thickness were used. In two of the three cases where MR imaging was not available, tumor areas on the CT scans were measured in square centimeters using an image-analyzing program. Tumor volume was calculated as the total area multiplied by the slice thickness (0.5 cm). In the remaining case, volume was determined from MRI scans by the method reported by Nedzelski et al. [25]. Three diameters were used. Two were determined on an axial slice including a maximum diameter. The other was determined on a coronal slice. The diameters were measured in centimeters using the same image-analyzing program. Tumor volume was calculated by multiplication of the tree diameters by 0.52, as reported by Pasqualin et al. [39].

Tumor doubling time was calculated as $T \times \log2/(\log V_1 - \log V_0)$, where V_0 was the initial tumor volume, V_1 was the last tumor volume before radiosurgery and T was the period in days between two examinations. Similarly, the postradiosurgical tumor half time was calculated using the same function, in which V_0 was the most recent tumor volume and V_1 was the preradiosurgical tumor volume.

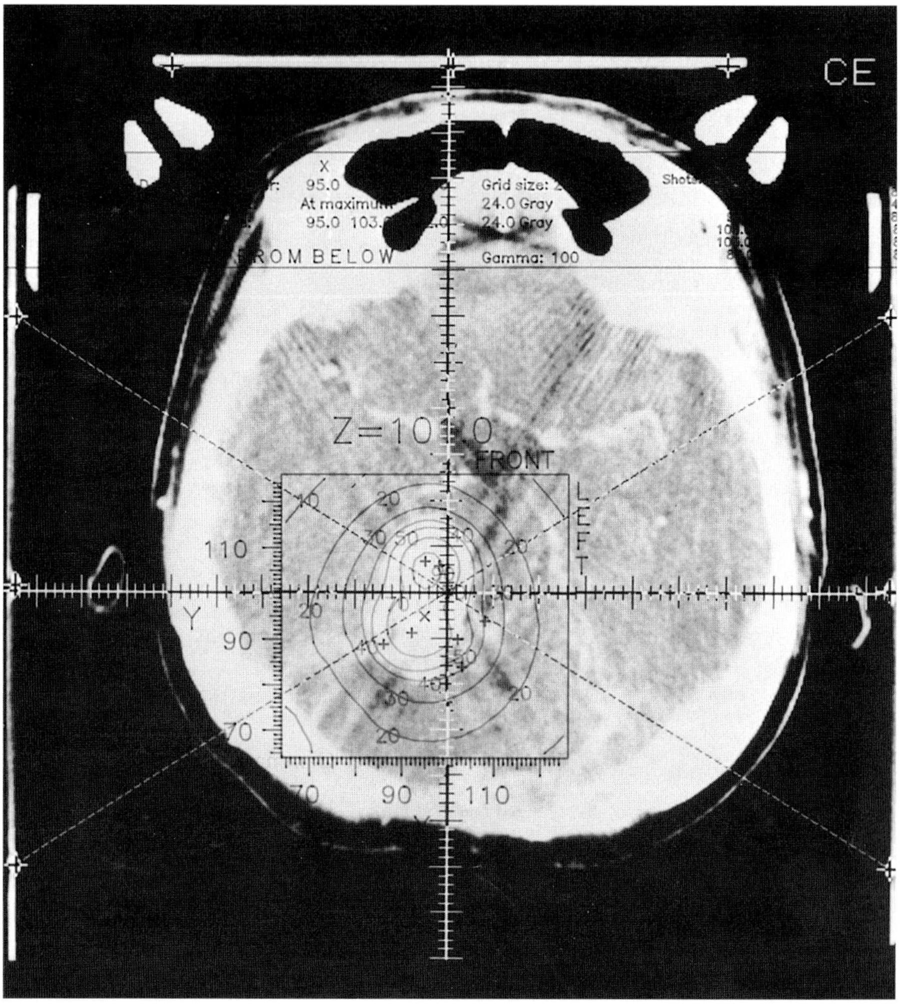

Fig. 2. Case 1. Post-contrast CT scan obtained during Gamma Knife radiosurgery showing remarkable regrowth of the tumor. Percent isodose gradient is superimposed.

Case Studies

Case 1 – Hemangioblastoma

Before Radiosurgery. This 34-year-old woman, who had shown no signs of von Hippel-Lindau syndrome, underwent partial resection of a cerebellar hemangioblastoma on June 10, 1986 (fig. 1). This procedure was followed by insertion of a ventriculoperitoneal shunt a week later. As the presurgical tumor growth had been relatively rapid radiation ther-

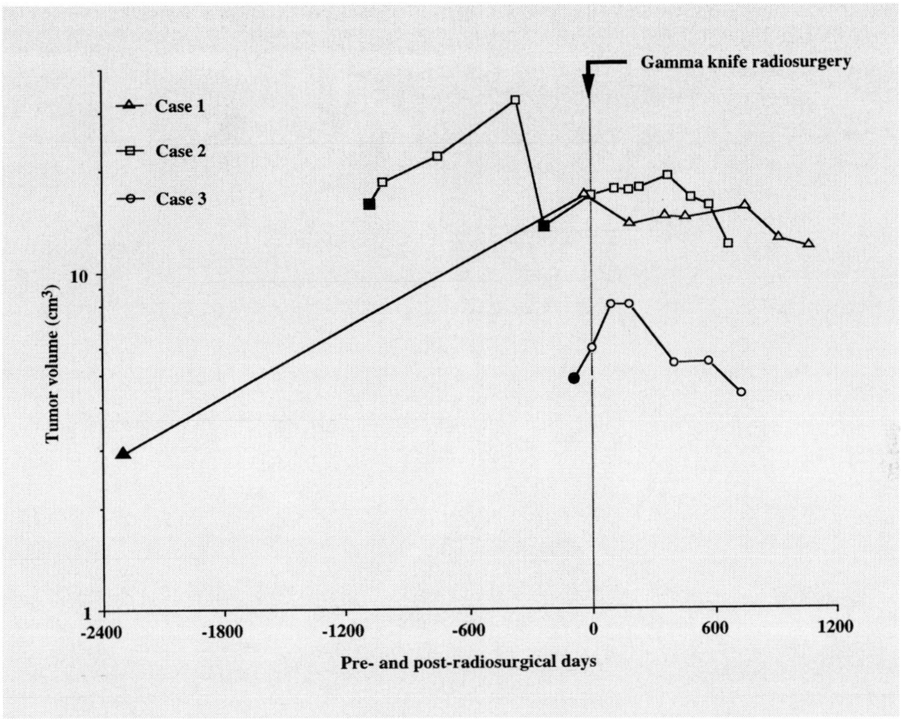

Fig. 3. Changes in tumor volume before and after Gamma Knife radiosurgery. The closed symbols indicate surgical removal.

apy was given to the residual tumor. A linear accelerator was used and the total dose was 56 Gy, delivered in 2.0 Gy fractions. Although this patient had mild truncal ataxia, right cerebellar hemispheric signs and a right hearing disturbance, her posttreatment course was uneventful through June 1992. At that time, the 40-year-old patient was again seen at our facility with the new symptom of diplopia. Neurodiagnostic imaging demonstrated remarkable regrowth of the cerebellar tumor with a volume of 15.5 cm^3. Tumor doubling time was determined to be 895 days.

Radiosurgery. As the patient refused reoperation, Gamma Knife radiosurgery was carried out on October 8, 1992 (fig. 2). The tumor was covered with a 50% isodose volume. A central dose of 24 Gy was used to obtain a marginal dose of 12 Gy.

After Radiosurgery. Serial postradiosurgical neuroimaging follow-up demonstrated the transient appearance of central nonenhanced areas, and no tumor growth has been observed as of September 16, 1995 (fig. 3, 4). The volume reduction rate and the tumor half time, which were determined using the most recent imaging examinations obtained on postradiosurgical day 1,073, were 86.1% and 2,101 days, respectively.

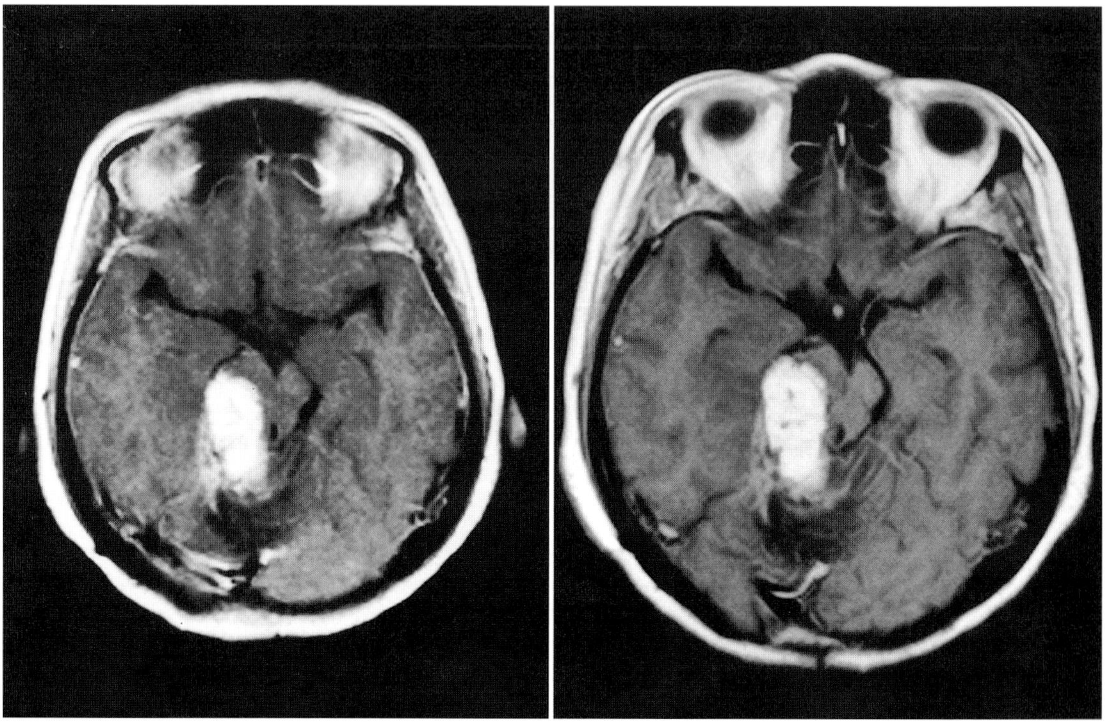

a b

Fig. 4. Case 1. Serial MRI obtained 1.5 (**a**) and 3 (**b**) years after radiosurgery showing no change in the tumor volume.

Case 2 – Meningioma

This 71-year-old woman underwent partial resection of a cerebellopontine angle meningioma on November 27, 1990. Serial CT scans obtained after surgery demonstrated gradual growth of the residual tumor. Therefore, this patient underwent reoperation on March 2, 1993. Neurodiagnostic imaging performed after the second operation demonstrated remarkable regrowth of the tumor with a volume of 16.8 cm^3. Tumor doubling time was determined to be 771 days (fig. 3). Gamma Knife radiosurgery was carried out on November 5, 1993. The tumor was covered with a 50% isodose volume. A central dose of 30 Gy was used to obtain a marginal dose of 15 Gy. Serial postradiosurgical neuroimaging follow-up demonstrated transient growth with almost the same tumor doubling time as that demonstrated prior to radiosurgery. This continued until the 400th postradiosurgical day, at which time the start of volume reduction was observed. The volume reduction rate and the tumor half time, which were determined using the most recent imaging examinations obtained on postradiosurgical day 670, were 71.5% and 1,380 days, respectively (fig. 3).

Case 3 – Acoustic Neurinoma

This 68-year-old man underwent partial resection of an acoustic neurinoma on January 26, 1993. Neurodiagnostic imaging performed after the operation demonstrated remarkable regrowth of the tumor with a volume of 5.9 cm^3. Tumor doubling time was determined to be 296 days (fig. 3). Gamma Knife radiosurgery was carried out on May 14, 1993. The tumor was covered with a 50% isodose volume. A central dose of 24 Gy was used to obtain a marginal dose of 12 Gy. Serial postradiosurgical neuroimaging follow-up demonstrated transient growth with almost the same tumor doubling time as that demonstrated prior to radiosurgery until the 90th postradiosurgical day, at which time the tumor was observed to be shrinking. The volume reduction rate and the tumor half time, determined using the most recent imaging examinations obtained on postradiosurgical day 732, were 73.4% and 1,604 days, respectively (fig. 3).

Discussion

Although many reports have focused on radiosurgical treatment for benign tumors, in particular acoustic neurinomas and meningiomas [1–16], relatively few hemangioblastoma patients have been treated radiosurgically [37, 38]. Therefore, we will briefly discuss radiosurgical treatment for a hemangioblastoma only. Chandler et al. [37] reported a patient who underwent stereotactic radiosurgery using a linear accelerator system for a small hemangioblastoma in the fourth ventricle. The tumor was covered with a 50% isodose volume using a 16-mm collimator and the selected dose was 15 Gy at the tumor periphery. Two-year neuroimaging follow-up studies demonstrated no enlargement of the treated tumor. However, the 'unchanged tumor volume' shown in this case could not be regarded as an outcome of radiosurgery because preradiosurgical tumor growth was not demonstrated.

Lunsford [38] reporting on eight hemangioblastoma patients treated with Gamma Knife radiosurgery was only cautiously optimistic about the potential role of radiosurgery. According to his results of six patients with follow-up ranging from 7 to 33 months, the tumor seemed to be adequately controlled in only three patients. The case reported here demonstrates that Gamma Knife radiosurgery can genuinely reduce the growth of a hemangioblastoma. Nevertheless, further studies involving larger series of patients must be designed to resolve the debate as to whether a hemangioblastoma patient is a good candidate for radiosurgery.

In conclusion, we consider these types of analyses to be essential for confirmation that, as reported by several authors, an 'unchanged tumor volume' demonstrated by postirradiation follow-up neuroimaging can be regarded as an outcome of radiosurgery [2, 6, 8–13, 15, 16]. Further studies involving larger series of patients should be designed to resolve the debate as to whether 'unchanged in volume' following radiosurgery for benign brain tumors constitutes a good treatment result.

Acknowledgment

The authors are very grateful to Bierta E. Barfod, MD, University of Washington School of Medicine, for her assistance in preparing the English manuscript.

References

1 Backlund EO: Stereotactic radiosurgery in intracranial tumours and vascular malformations; in Krayenbühl H, Brihaye J, Loew F, Logue V, Mingrino S, Pertuiset B, Symon L, Troupp H, Yasargil MG (eds): Advances and Technical Standards in Neurosurgery. Berlin, Springer, 1979, vol 6, pp 3–37.
2 Flickinger JC, Lunsford LD, Coffey RJ, Linskey ME, Bissonette DJ, Maitz AH, Kondziolka D: Radiosurgery of acoustic neurinomas. Cancer 1991;67:345–353.
3 Ganz JC: Gamma Knife Radiosurgery. Berlin, Springer, 1993.
4 Hirato M, Inoue HK, Nakamura M, Ohye C, Shibazaki T, Andou Y: Gamma Knife radiosurgery in acoustic neurinoma: Early effects and the preservation of hearing. Acta Neurochir (Wien) 1993; 122:165.
5 Hirsh A, Norén G: Audiological findings after stereotactic radiosurgery in acoustic neurinomas. Acta Otolaryngol (Stockh) 1988;106:244–251.
6 Hitchcock E, Kitchen G, Dalton E, Pope B: Stereotactic LINAC radiosurgery. Br J Neurosurg 1989; 3:305–312.
7 Kamerer DB, Lunsford LD, Møller M: Gamma Knife: An alternative treatment for acoustic neurinomas. Ann Otol Rhinol Laryngol 1988;97:631–635.
8 Kondziolka D, Lunsford LD: Radiosurgery of meningiomas. Neurosurg Clin North Am 1992;3: 219–230.
9 Linskey ME, Lunsford LD, Flickinger JC: Neuroimaging of acoustic nerve sheath tumors after stereotactic radiosurgery. AJNR Am J Neuroradiol 1991;12:1165–1175.
10 Linskey ME, Lunsford LD, Flickinger JC: Tumor control after stereotactic radiosurgery in neurofibromatosis patients with bilateral acoustic tumors. Neurosurgery 1992;31:829–839.
11 Linskey ME, Lunsford LD, Flickinger JC, Kondziolka D: Stereotactic radiosurgery for acoustic tumors. Neurosurg Clin North Am 1992;3:191–205.
12 Lunsford LD, Kamerer DB, Flickinger JC: Stereotactic radiosurgery for acoustic neuromas. Arch Otolaryngol Head Neck Surg 1990;116:907–909.
13 Norén G, Arndt J, Hindmarsh T, Hirsh A: Stereotactic radiosurgical treatment of acoustic neurinomas; in Lunsford LD (ed): Modern Stereotactic Neurosurgery. Boston, Nijhoff, 1988, pp 481–489.
14 Stephanian E, Lunsford LD, Coffey RJ, Bissonette DJ, Flickinger JC: Gamma Knife surgery for sellar and suprasellar tumors. Neurosurg Clin North Am 1992;3:207–218.
15 Steiner L, Lindquist C, Steiner M: Radiosurgery; in Symon L, Calliauw L, Cohadon F, Lobo J, Loew F, Nornes H, Pásztor E, Pickard JD, Strong AJ, Yasargil MG (eds): Advances and Technical Standards in Neurosurgery. Berlin, Springer, 1992, vol 19, pp 19–102.
16 Yamamoto M, Norén G: Stereotactic radiosurgery in acoustic neurinomas (in Japanese, English abstract). No-Shinkei-Geka 1990;18:1101–1106.
17 Bederson JB, von Ammon K, Wichmann WW, Yasargil MG: Conservative treatment of patients with acoustic tumors. Neurosurgery 1991;28:646–651.
18 Clark WC, Moretz WH Jr, Acker JD, Gardner LG, Eggers F, Robertson JH: Nonsurgical management of small and intracanalicular acoustic tumors. Neurosurgery 1985;16:801–803.
19 Firsching RP, Fischer A, Peters R, Thun F, Klug N: Growth rate of incidental meningiomas. J Neurosurg 1990;73:545–547.
20 Ide M, Hagiwara S, Umebara Y, Yamamoto M, Jimbo M, Kubo O: Peritumoral brain edema with meningiomas (abstract). 54th Annu Meet Jpn Neurosurg Soc, Oct 1995, p 256.
21 Ide M, Jimbo M, Yamamoto M, Umebara Y, Hagiwara S, Kubo O: Growth rate of intracranial meningioma: Tumor doubling time and proliferating cell nuclear antigen staining index. Neurol Med Chir (Tokyo) 1995;35:289–293.

22 Kusakari J, Kobayashi T, Inamura N, Shibuya M, Ohdaira H, Kawase T, Takeyama M, Kikuchi T, Takasaka T, Kawamoto K: Studies on the growth rate of acoustic tumor (in Japanese, English abstract). J Otolaryngol Jpn 1987;90:324–328.
23 Lassonen EM, Troupp H: Volume growth rate of acoustic neurinomas. Neuroradiology 1986;28: 203–207.
24 Nagar GT: Acoustic neurinomas: Pathology and differential diagnosis. Arch Otolaryngol 1969;89: 252–279.
25 Nedzelski JM, Canter RJ, Kassel EE, Rowed DW, Tator CH: Is no treatment good treatment in the management of acoustic neuromas in the elderly? Laryngosocope 1989;96:825–829.
26 Nedzelksi JM, Schessel DA, Pfeiderer A, Kassel EE, Rowed DW: Conservative management of acoustic neuromas. Otolaryngol Clin North Am 1992;25:691–705.
27 Ogawa K, Kanzaki J, Ogawa S, Yamamoto M, Ikeda S, Shiobara R: The growth rate of acoustic neuromas. Acta Otolaryngol Suppl (Stockh) 1991;487:157–163.
28 Olivero WC, Lister JR, Elwood PW: The natural history and growth rate of asymptomatic meningiomas: A review of 60 patients. J Neurosurg 1995;83:222–224.
29 Silverstein H, McDaniel A, Norrell H, Wazen J: Conservative management of acoustic neuroma in the elderly patient. Laryngoscope 1985;95:766–770.
30 Thomsen J, Tos M: Acoustic neuroma: Clinical aspects, audiovestibular assessment, diagnostic delay, and growth rate. Am J Otol 1990;11:12–19.
31 Valvassori GE, Guzman M: Growth rate of acoustic neuromas. Am J Otol 1989;10:174–176.
32 Wazen J, Silverstein H, Norrell H, Besse B: Preoperative and postoperative growth rates in acoustic neuromas documented with CT scanning. Otolaryngol Head Neck Surg 1985;93:151–155.
33 Wennerberg J, Mercke U: Growth potential of acoustic neuromas. Am J Otol 1989;10:293–296.
34 Zöllner C, Bockenheimer S: The growth rate of acoustic neuromas: A report of three cases. Arch Otorhinolayngol 1985;241:259–264.
35 Yamamoto M, Hagiwara S, Ide M, Jimbo M, Hirai T, Nakamura Y: Radiosurgery for acoustic neurinoma with rapid growth and relatively high staining indexes for PCNA and MIB-1: A case report. Neurol Med Chir (Tokyo) 1996;36:241–245.
36 Yamamoto M, Ide, Umebara Y, Hagiwara S, Takakura K: Gamma knife radiosurgery in brain tumors: Post-irradiation volume changes compared with pre-radiosurgical growth fractions. Neurol Med Chir (Tokyo) 1996;36:358–363.
37 Chandler HC Jr, Friedman WA: Radiosurgical treatment of a hemangioblastma: Case report. Neurosurgery 1994;34:353–355.
38 Lunsford LD: Radiosurgery for hemangioblastoma. Neurosurgery 1994;34:355.
39 Pasqualin A, Barone G, Cioffi F, Rosta R, Scienza R, Pian RD: The relevance of anatomic and hemodynamic factors to a classification of cerebral arteriovenous malformations. Neurosurgery 1991;28:370–379.

Proc 7th Int Meeting Leksell Gamma Knife® Society,
Island of Lana'i, Hawaii, November 1995
Stereotact Funct Neurosurg 1996;66(suppl 1):240–259

Stereotactic and Functional Neurosurgery

Irradiation Effects on the Metabolism of Metastatic Brain Tumors: Analysis by Positron Emission Tomography and ^{1}H-Magnetic Resonance Spectroscopy

E. Yoshino[a], *Y. Ohmori*[a], *Y. Imahori*[a], *T. Higuchi*[a], *S. Furuya*[b], *S. Naruse*[a,b], *T. Mori*[c], *K. Suzuki*[c], *T. Yamaki*[a], *S. Ueda*[a], *T. Tsuzuki*[d], *S. Takai*[d]

Departments of [a] Neurosurgery and [b] Radiology,
Kyoto Prefectural University of Medicine,
[c] Department of Neurosurgery, Matsushita Memorial Hospital, and
[d] Gamma Knife Department, Takai Hospital, Kyoto, Japan

Key Words

Stereotactic radiosurgery · Metastastic brain tumor · Radiation necrosis · Tumor regrowth · Positron emission tomography · Proton magnetic resonance spectroscopy

Abstract

To evaluate irradiation effects on the metabolism of metastatic brain tumors treated by Gamma Knife radiosurgery, positron emission tomography (PET) and ^{1}H-magnetic resonance spectroscopy (MRS) studies were performed on five patients. The tumor origins were lung cancer in three patients and breast cancer in two. Treatment volume was 0.4–10.1 cm^3 (mean: 5.5 cm^3). The marginal dose to the tumor was 24–30 Gy (mean: 26.2 Gy). The follow-up period was 5–19 months (mean: 13.4 months). No patients had conventional whole-brain radiation therapy. ^{18}F-fluoroboronophenylalanine (^{18}FBPA) or ^{18}F-fluorodeoxyglucose (^{18}FDG) were used as tracers for the PET study. Using ^{1}H-MRS, several metabolites were simultaneously measured in metastatic brain tumor and adjacent brain. In the PET study of the representative case, the uptake rate of ^{18}FBPA that is actively transported to the tumor decreased markedly 15 days after radiosurgery and continued to decrease thereafter. In the ^{1}H-MRS study, choline, which is characteristically high in metastatic brain tumors, also decreased over time. In two cases with suspected radiation injury, the enhanced region, which was decreased in size in early follow-up, enlarged progressively and was accompanied by edema. However, ^{18}FBPA and ^{18}FDG were not transported to the enhanced region. The peak of free lipid, which might show destruction of the cell membrane, was recognized in the enhanced region and adjacent brain in these cases. This study revealed that radiation effects on the metabolism of metastatic brain tumors occur at an early stage after radiosurgery and continue over several months. In particular, in the case of radiation injury, PET and ^{1}H-MRS studies made it possible to distinguish between regrowth of the tumor and radiation injury.

KARGER

E-Mail karger@karger.ch
Fax + 41 61 306 12 34
http://www.karger.ch

1011–6125/96/0665–0240$10.00/0

Eiji Yoshino, MD, PhD
Department of Neurosurgery
Shakaihoken Kobe Central Hospital
2-1-1 Sohyamacho Kita-Ku
Kobe 651-11 (Japan)

Introduction

Surgical resection followed by whole-brain radiation therapy (WBRT) significantly prolongs the survival of patients with metastatic brain tumors when compared with WBRT alone [1]. It has become increasingly accepted that stereotactic radiosurgery is also effective therapy for metastatic brain tumors, achieving tumor control with a low morbidity [2, 3]. A local control rate equal or superior to surgical resection and WBRT has been recorded [3]. Radiosurgery effectively controls the growth of tumors considered 'resistant' to conventional radiotherapy [4]. A majority of tumors treated with radiosurgery shrink or stop growing within 1 month. During this time, peritumoral edema usually declines. In a few cases, peritumoral edema may progress again, and the irradiated tumor (enhanced region) may then increase in size. In such cases, it is difficult to differentiate between tumor progression and radiation injury with conventional computed tomography (CT) or magnetic resonance imaging (MRI), which makes it difficult to decide whether to repeat the treatment or not.

The metabolic alteration of metastatic brain tumors after stereotactic radiosurgery has not been well understood. Positron emission tomography (PET) and magnetic resonance spectroscopy (MRS) have both been used to study the in vivo metabolism of various pathological conditions, such as brain tumor [5, 6], cerebral infarction [7, 8] and head injury [9, 10]. However, data in the field of radiosurgery are limited.

The present study was performed for two purposes: (1) to evaluate radiation effects on the metabolism of metastatic brain tumors and normal brain adjacent to a tumor after Gamma Knife radiosurgery, using PET and proton (^{1}H-)MRS; (2) to examine the usefulness of these modalities in differentiating regrowth of the tumor from radiation necrosis.

Materials and Methods

PET

^{18}Fluoroboronophenylalanine (^{18}FBPA) and ^{18}F-fluorodeoxyglucose (^{18}FDG) were used as radioactive tracers. The PET images were obtained with a Headtome PET scanner (Shimazu, Japan). The spatial resolution was 8.6 mm in full width at half maximum in plane resolution, while the average axial resolution was 13.6 mm.

^{18}FBPA-PET. After intravenous injection of 185 MBq (5 mCi) of ^{18}FBPA, a dynamic study (lasting for 60 min) and arterial blood sampling were performed. PET data were collected continuously 15 times with a 4-min collection time. To analyze the ^{18}FBPA data, mean values (cps) for the tumor were compared with those for the contralateral normal cortex. The ratio of radioactivity in the tumor and the normal cortex (T/N ratio) was then obtained. The ^{18}FBPA-PET scan was performed on two patients before and after radiosurgery and on three patients after the treatment.

Table 1. Patient characteristics

No.	Age years	Sex	Tumor origin	Tumor volume cm^3	Max. dose Gy	Marginal dose Gy	Internal dose mJ	PET before radio-surgery	PET after radio-surgery	^{1}H-MRS before radio-surgery	^{1}H-MRS after radio-surgery	Outcome
1	60	F	breast	6.1	50	25	202.5	^{18}FBPA	^{18}FBPA	yes	yes	alive (18 months)
2	53	F	lung	(1) 0.4 (2) 4.6	(1) 30 (2) 60	(1) 27 (2) 30	(1) 11.3 (2) 210.5	^{18}FBPA	^{18}FBPA ^{18}FDG	no	yes	alive (19 months); radiation necrosis histologically verified
3	63	F	lung	1.6	60	30	74.5	no	^{18}FBPA ^{18}FDG	no	yes	alive (17 months); radiation necrosis suspected
4	69	M	lung	(1) 10.1 (2) 1.4* 0.4**	(1) 50 (2) 50* 30**	(1) 25 (2) 25* 27**	(1) 350.0 (2) 44.7* 10.0**	no	^{18}FBPA	no	no	dead 9 months after radiosurgery (pneumonia)
5	58	F	breast	9.3	60	24	349.9	no	^{18}FBPA	no	yes	dead 5 months after radiosurgery (CSF dissemination)

(1) = First Gamma Knife radiosurgery; (2) = second Gamma Knife radiosurgery; * = regrowth; ** = new metastatic tumor.

^{18}FDG-PET. Prior to scanning, 3.7 MBq/kg of ^{18}FDG were administered intravenously. The actual images were obtained from 40 to 60 min after the ^{18}FDG injection. The regional metabolic rate of glucose (rCMRglc) was estimated by the formula of Hutchins et al. [11] using the lumped constant and rate constants described by Phelps et al. [12]. The ^{18}FDG-PET scan was performed on two patients with suspected radiation necrosis.

^{1}H-MRS

The system used was a Magnetom H15 (Siemens, Germany) with a 1.5-Tesla magnet. ^{1}H-MRS was measured by three-dimensional chemical shift imaging (CSI) methods [13]. The CSI was obtained by applying 2-directional 16 × 16 phase encoding on an 18 × 18 cm field of view (FOV). In the FOV, an 8 × 8 × 2 cm volume of interest was selected by the spin echo method with water and fat suppression. Consequently 256 voxels, 1 × 1 × 2 cm in size, were obtained simultaneously. Repetition time/echo time was 3000/135 ms and accumulation was performed three times. After applying two-dimensional Fourier transformation of acquired data, the baseline and the phase were corrected automatically in all voxels. The ^{1}H-MRS study was performed on four patients.

Patients and Gamma Knife Radiosurgery

Patient characteristics are summarized in table 1. No patient had conventional WBRT either before or after radiosurgery. Tumor volume varied from 0.4 to 10.3 cm^3 (mean:

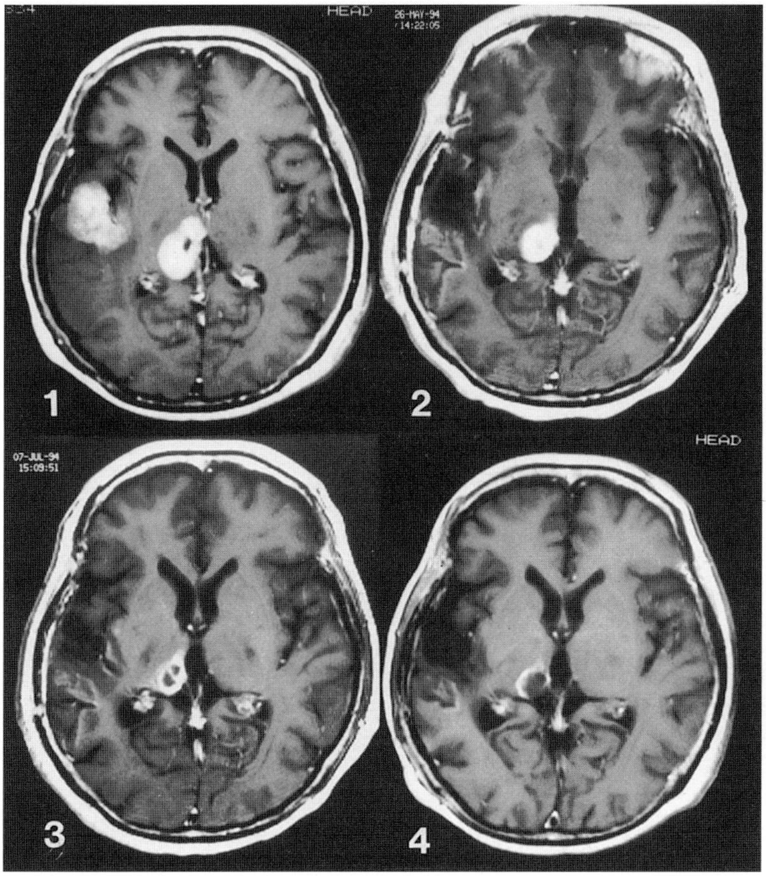

1a

(For fig. 1b, 1c see pp. 244 and 245.)

Fig. 1. Patient 1. **a** MR images before and after radiosurgery. (1) Before radiosurgery. Right temporal tumor was surgically removed. (2) 31 days after radiosurgery. (3) 73 days after radiosurgery. (4) 18 months after radiosurgery. **b** ^{18}FBPA-PET images before and after radiosurgery. A distinct focus of high ^{18}FBPA accumulation is seen corresponding to the tumor. The T/N ratio reduced over time. (1) Before radiosurgery (T/N ratio: 2.3). (2) 15 days after radiosurgery (T/N ratio: 1.7). (3) 43 days after radiosurgery (T/N ratio: 1.4). (4) 15 months after radiosurgery (T/N ratio: 0.3). **c** ^{1}H-MRS before and after radiosurgery. The choline signal which was extremely high before radiosurgery was chronologically reduced. (1) Before radiosurgery. CSI of each metabolite is also shown: Spectrum from normal brain (A) and tumor (B). (2) 5 days after radiosurgery. (3) 31 days after radiosurgery. (4) 73 days after radiosurgery (arrow = lactate). (2)–(4) Upper spectrum from the tumor, lower spectrum from normal brain adjacent to the tumor.

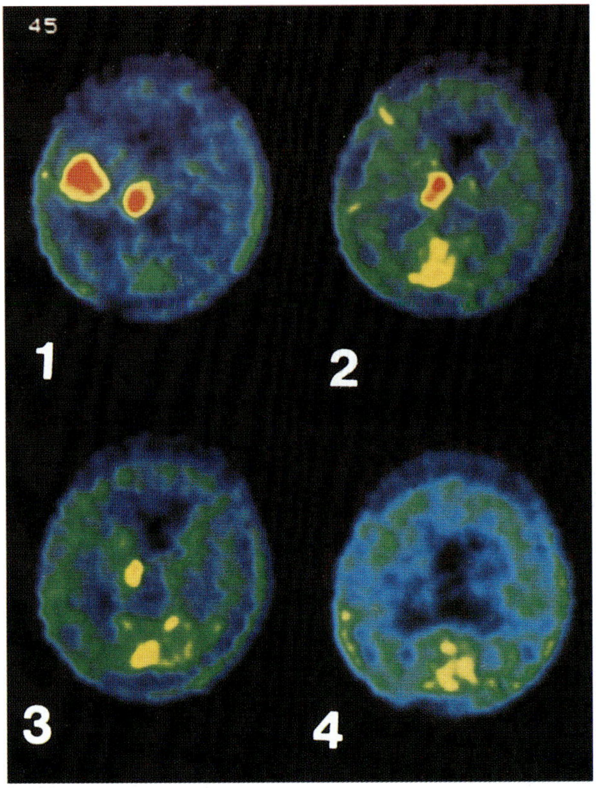

1b

(For legend see p. 243.)

5.5 cm^3) and the marginal tumor dose was 24–30 Gy (mean: 26.2 Gy). The follow-up period was 5–19 months (mean: 13.4 months).

Radiosurgery was performed with the Leksell Gamma Knife type B (Elekta, Sweden). MR images were obtained before Gamma Knife radiosurgery with gadolinium enhancement using 4-mm axial and coronal T_1-weighted images without a gap. At the time of treatment, dose planning was performed using the KULA dose planning system. Subsequently, tumor volume and tumor dose distributions were obtained using GammaPlan.

Results

Patient 1 (fig. 1)

This 60-year-old woman had cerebral metastases in the right temporal lobe and right thalamus, originating from an adenocarcinoma of the breast. After total removal of the temporal tumor, the thalamic tumor was treated with radiosurgery

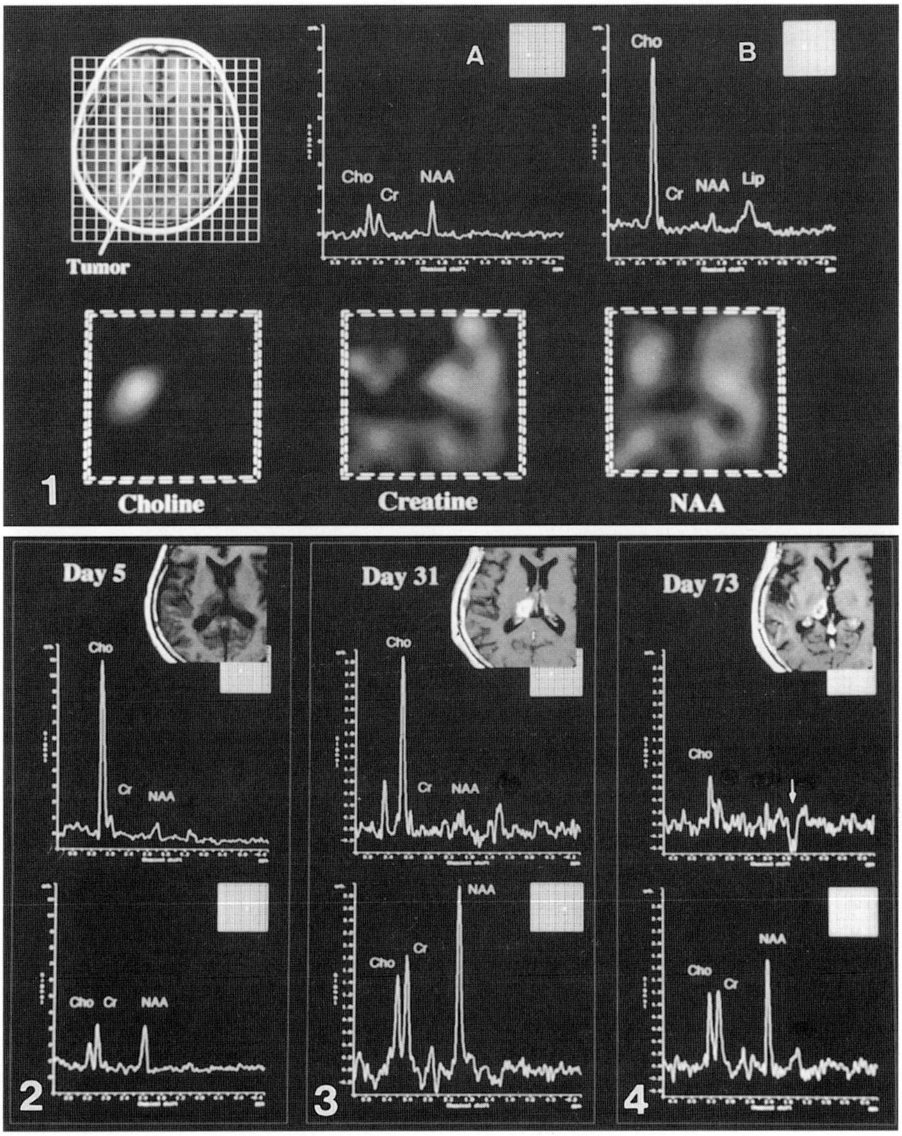

1c

(For legend see p. 243.)

with a marginal dose of 25 Gy. The tumor decreased in size and remained unchanged as a small cystic mass. High uptake of ^{18}FBPA (T/N ratio: 2.3) was noted before radiosurgery. The T/N ratio was reduced to 1.7, 15 days after radiosurgery and continued to decrease over time. There was no ^{18}FBPA uptake 15 months after the treatment. In the ^{1}H-MRS study, the peak of N-acetylaspartate

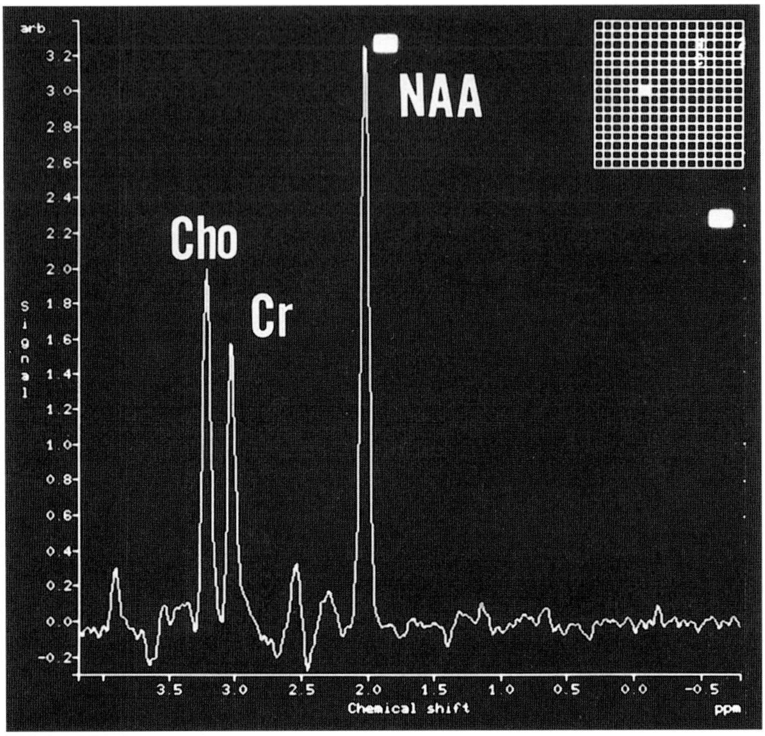

Fig. 2. The spectrum of ^{1}H-MRS in normal brain. Choline (Cho), creatine (Cr) and N-acetyl aspartate (NAA) are clearly detected.

(NAA), creatine and choline were consistently observed in normal brain (fig. 2). The NAA peak was as about twice as high as the choline and creatine peaks. In this patient, a remarkably high choline signal was obtained before radiosurgery. It decreased gradually over time. Seventy-three days later, only low peaks of choline and lactate were observed. She had no neurological deficits 18 months after the treatment, and remains well.

Patient 2 (fig. 3)

This 53-year-old woman had adenocarcinoma of the lung with a left frontal metastasis. Both tumors were totally removed 6 years ago. A new metastasis in the right deep white matter was noted 1 year later and slowly increased in size. At ^{18}FBPA-PET before radiosurgery, the uptake of ^{18}FBPA to the tumor was slightly lower than that of normal cortex (T/N ratio: 0.9) and higher than that of white matter (tumor and white matter ratio: 1.3). She underwent radiosurgery with a marginal dose of 27 Gy. The irradiated tumor enlarged with surrounding edema 5 months after treatment. At this time, ^{18}FBPA was not transported to the enhanced mass. However, 3 months later, ^{18}FBPA uptake was noted again. With ^{1}H-MRS, a marked elevation of the free lipid peak was observed. NAA and choline peaks of the enhanced mass and adjacent white matter were lower than those of white matter distant from the lesion. Treatment was repeated with 30 Gy to the tumor margin. After the second treatment, the enhanced mass increased in size while the gadolinium enhancement became less pronounced. Surrounding edema was not reduced except when steroid and glycerol were used. At ^{18}FDG-PET after the second treatment, the rCMRglc of the enhanced mass and the contralateral white matter were 4.5 and 5.0 mg/100 g per minute, respectively. At ^{1}H-MRS, the peak of free lipid remained high. The NAA and choline signals of the mass and adjacent white matter were lower compared with the previous ^{1}H-MRS study. The mass was stereotactically removed 9 months after the second radiosurgical procedure. Histology disclosed radiation necrosis. At present, she is troubled by a mild left hemiparesis.

Patient 3 (fig. 4)

This 63-year-old woman was operated for lung cancer (adenocarcinoma) 5 years ago. A left thalamic metastasis was discovered 4 years later. She underwent radiosurgery with 30 Gy to the tumor margin. The irradiated tumor decreased in size during the early follow-up period but enlarged progressively thereafter until 8 months after treatment. The enlargement was accompanied by edema. The enhanced mass has remained unchanged since then. At ^{18}FBPA-PET, the ^{18}FBPA accumulation of the mass was lower than that of the contralateral thalamus. At ^{18}FDG-PET, the rCMRglc of the mass and the contralateral thalamus were 4.6 and 5.9 mg/100 g per minute, respectively. The rCMRglc of normal white matter was 4.8 mg/100 g per minute. At ^{1}H-MRS, all visible signals of the enhanced mass were lower than those of the contralateral thalamus. Twelve months after radiosurgery, a peak of free lipid was noted in the enhanced mass and the region of surrounding edema. At present, the patient suffers from a mild right hemiparesis and hemihypesthesia.

Patient 4 (fig. 5)

This patient was a 69-year-old man. A cerebellar metastasis originating from an adenocarcinoma of the lung was treated with a marginal dose of 25 Gy. The irradiated tumor decreased in size but enlarged again and a new metastatic lesion appeared in the left frontal lobe 8 months after the treatment. There was a high uptake of ^{18}FBPA in both lesions (T/N ratio: 1.7 and 1.9). Gamma Knife radiosurgery was repeated. Nevertheless, the patient died of pneumonia due to the progression of lung cancer, 1 month after the second radiosurgical procedure.

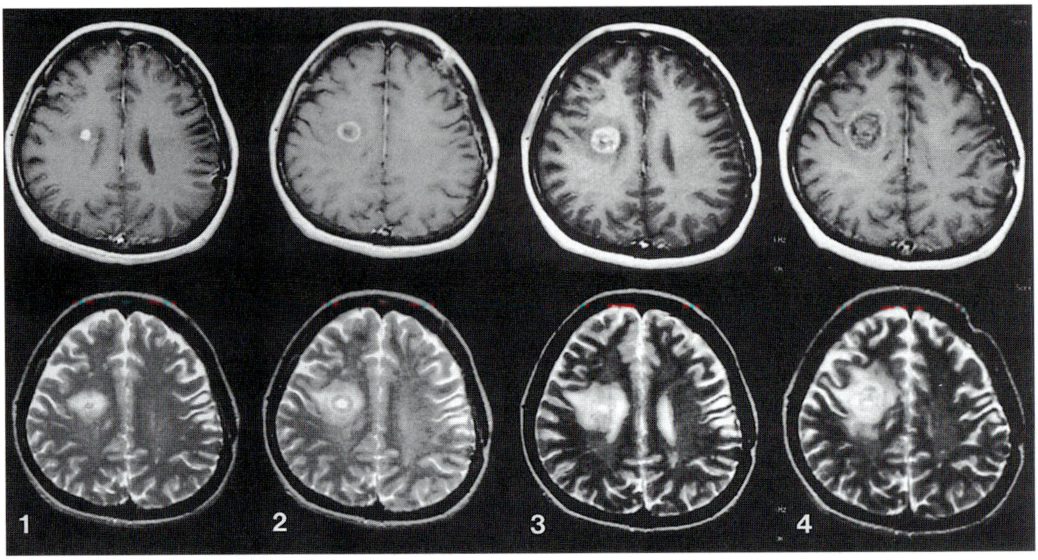

3a

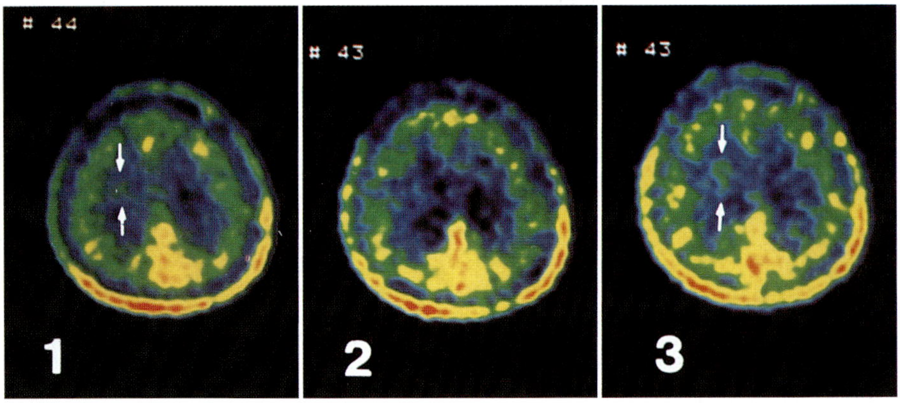

3b

Fig. 3. Patient 2. **a** MR images before and after radiosurgery. The second radiosurgery was performed 9 months after the first radiosurgery. (1) Before radiosurgery. (2) 5 months after radiosurgery. (3) 8 months after radiosurgery. (4) 8 months after the second radiosurgery. **b** ^{18}FBPA-PET images before and after radiosurgery. The uptake of ^{18}FBPA (arrows) was noted again 8 months after the first radiosurgery. (1) Before radiosurgery. (2) 5 months after radiosurgery. (3) 8 months after radiosurgery. **c** ^{18}FDG-PET image 74 days after the second radiosurgery. Low uptake of ^{18}FDG is noted in the enhanced mass. (rCMRglc of the lesion and contralateral white matter: 4.5 and 5.5 mg/100 per minute, respectively.) **d** ^{1}H-MRS before and after the second radiosurgery. Elevation of the free lipid signal is conspicuous. Decrease of NAA is observed, especially after the second radiosurgery. A = Spectrum from the mass lesion; B = spectrum from the surrounding edema; C = spectrum from the white matter distant from the lesion. (1) 8 months after the first radiosurgery. (2) 4 months after the second radiosurgery.

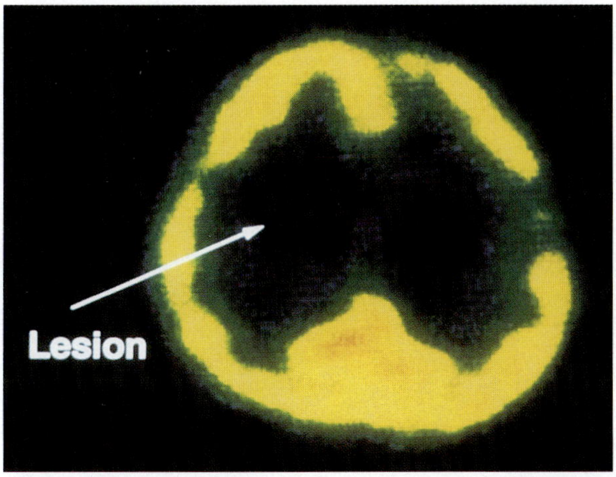

3c

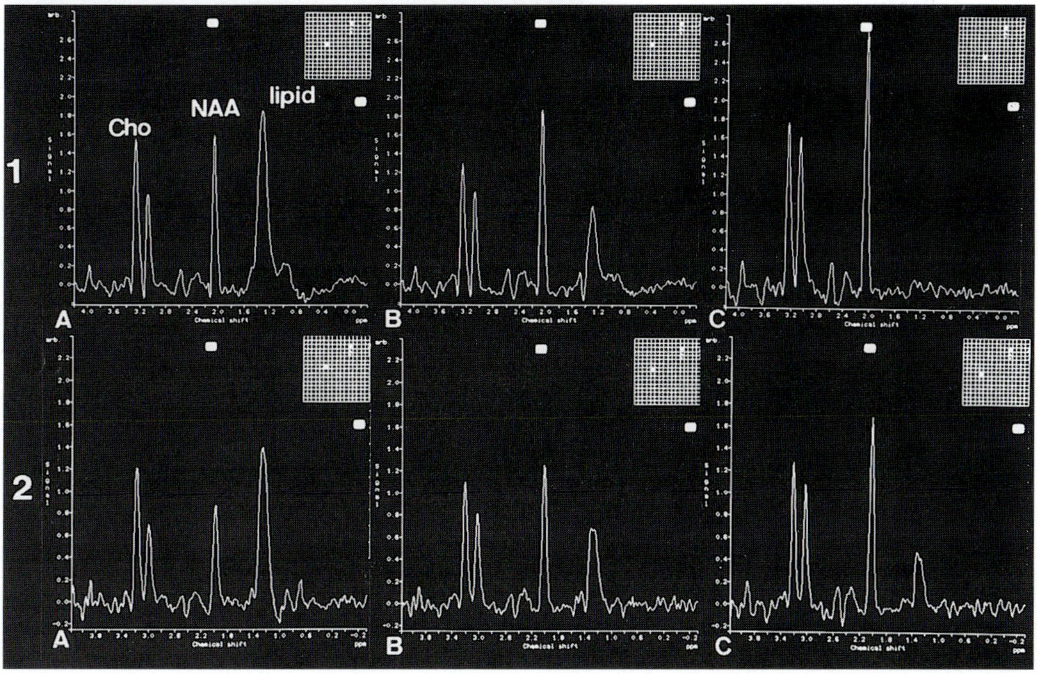

3d

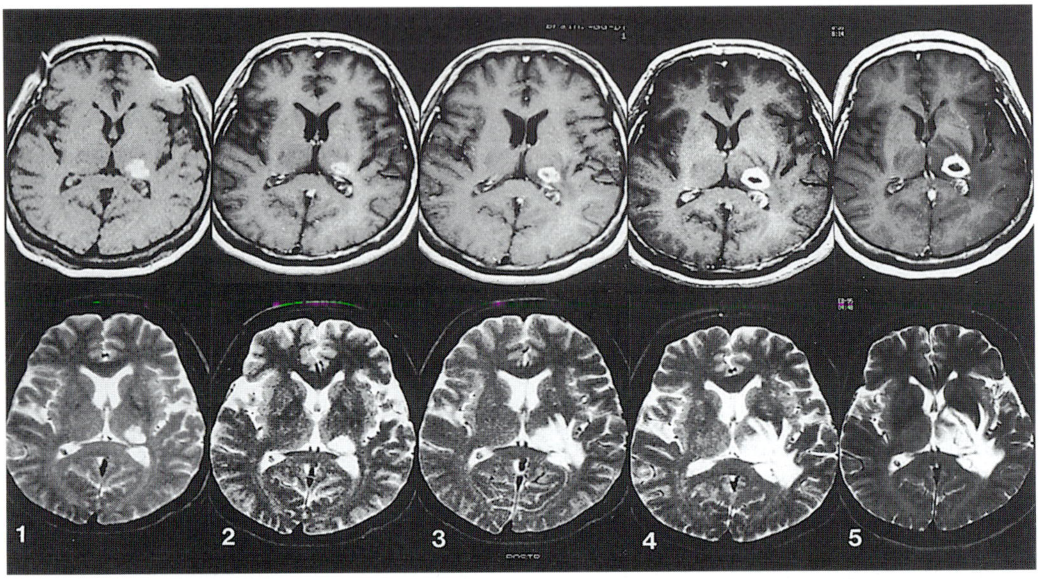

4a

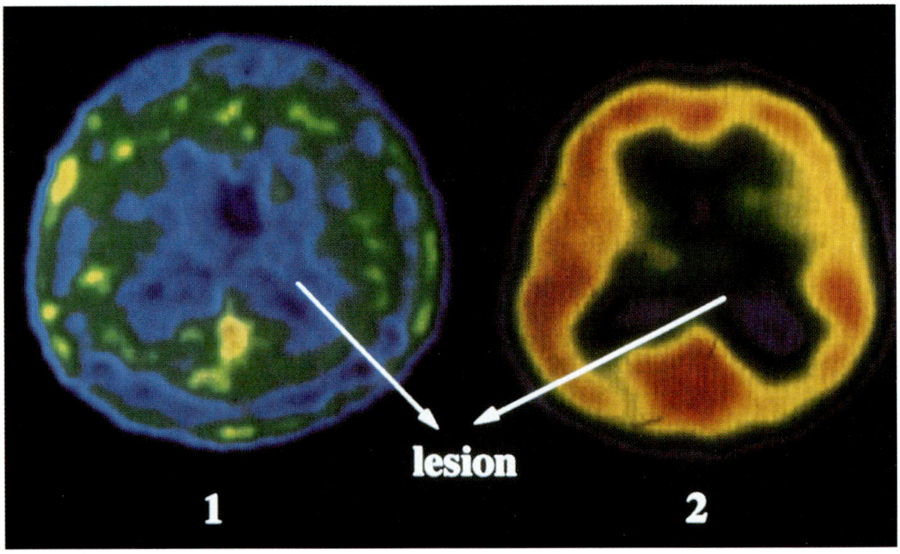

4b

Fig. 4. Patient 3. **a** MR images before and after radiosurgery. (1) Before radiosurgery. (2) 57 days after radiosurgery. (3) Four months after radiosurgery. (4) Eight months after radiosurgery. (5) 13 months after radiosurgery. **b** ^{18}FBPA- (1) and ^{18}FDG-PET (2) images. Uptake of both tracers into the lesion is lower than that of the contralateral thalamus. **c** ^{1}H-MRS 4 (1) and 12 (2) months after radiosurgery. All visible signals of the lesion (1-A) are lower than those of the contralateral thalamus (1-B). Free lipid was observed 12 months after radiosurgery.

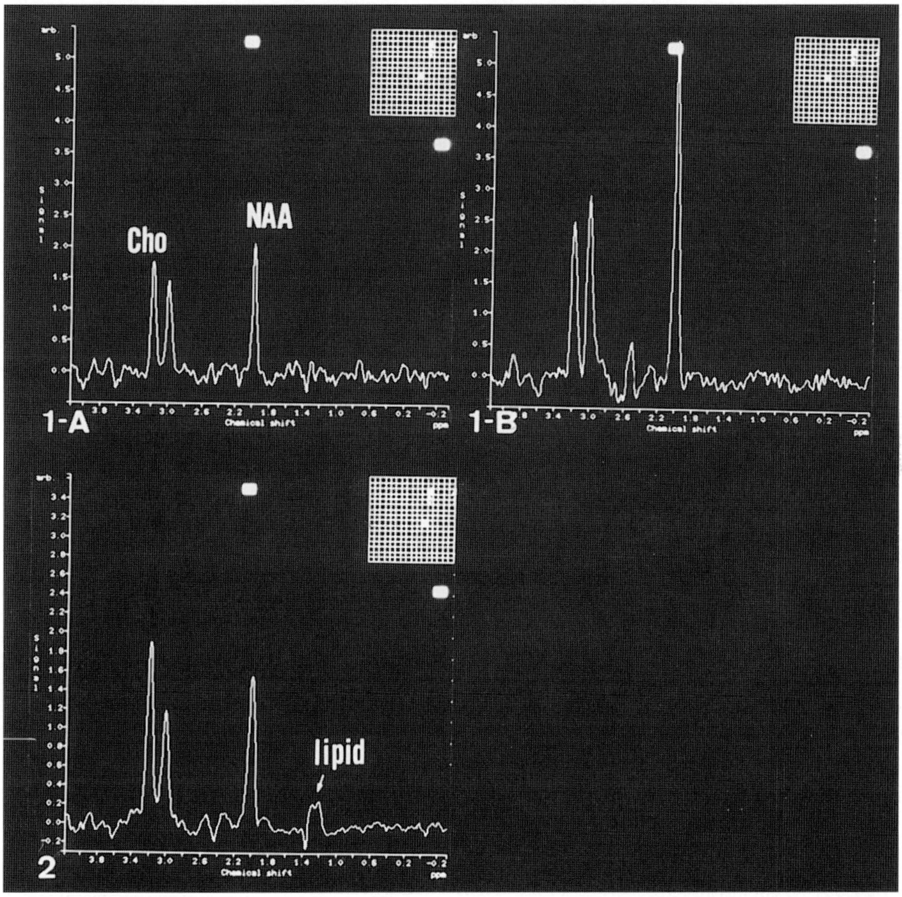

4c

(For fig. 5 and 6 see pp. 252 and 253.)

Fig. 5. Patient 4. **a** MR images before and after radiosurgery. Regrowth of the tumor and new metastatic tumor were noted 8 months after radiosurgery. (1) Before radiosurgery. (2) Four months after radiosurgery. (3) Eight months after radiosurgery. **b** ^{18}FBPA-PET images 8 months after radiosurgery. High uptake of ^{18}FBPA is noted in the regrowing tumor and new metastatic tumor.

Fig. 6. Patient 5. **a** MR images before (1) and 30 days after (2) radiosurgery. **b** ^{1}H-MRS 54 days after radiosurgery, showing a peak of free lipid.

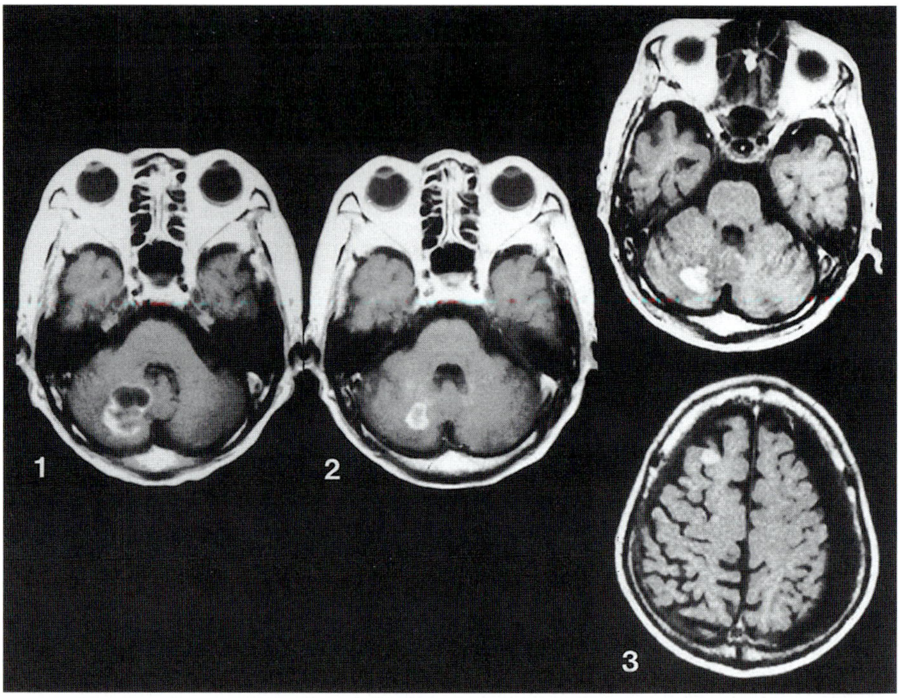

5a

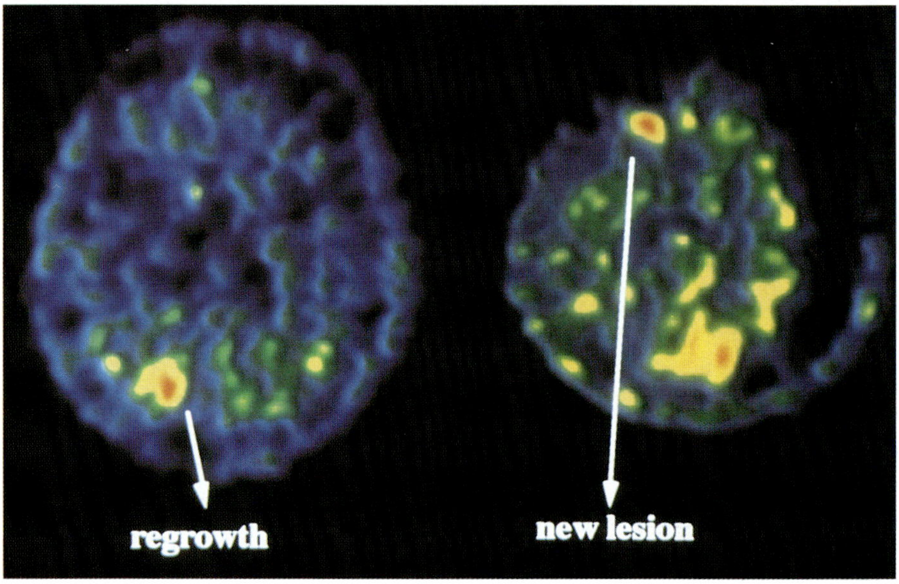

5b

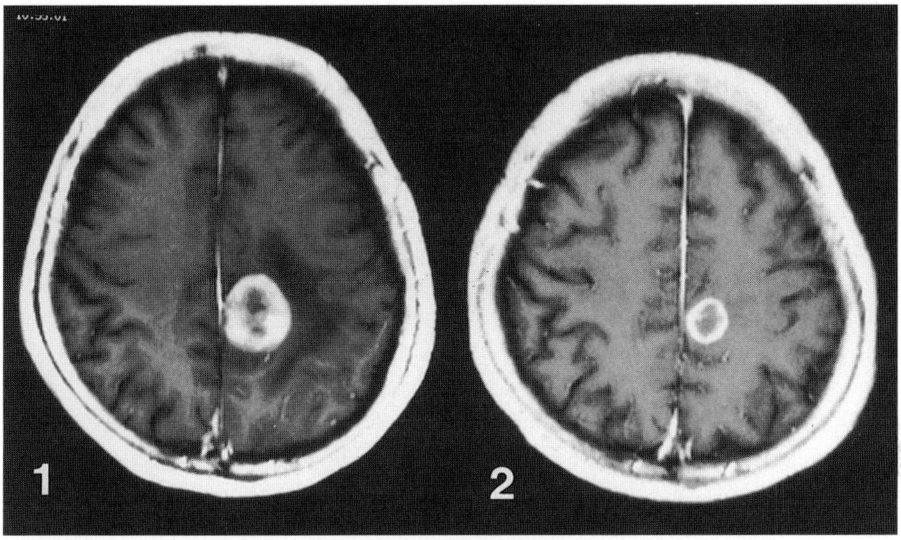
1
2

6a

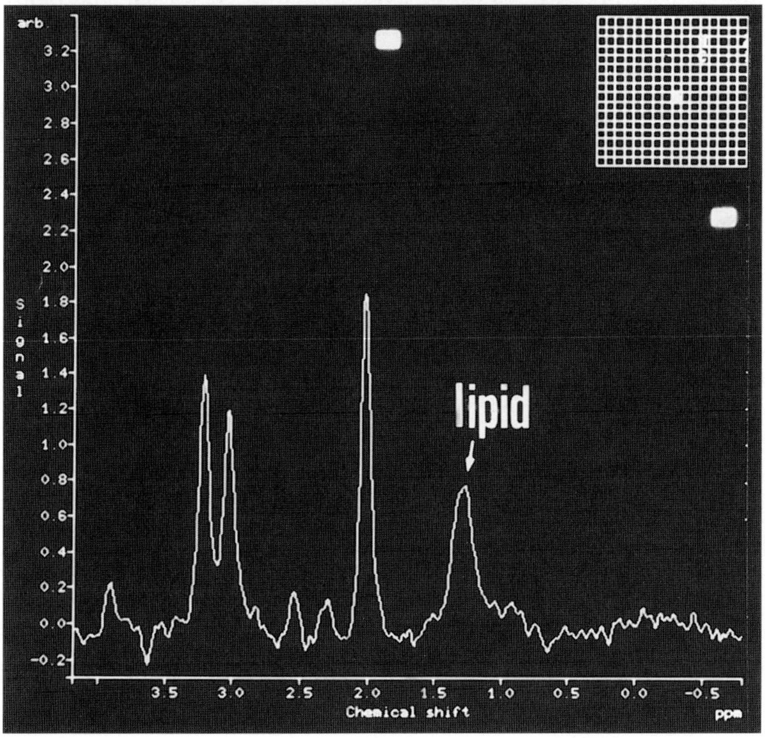
arb.
3.2
3.0
2.8
2.6
2.4
2.2
2.0
1.8
1.6
1.4
1.2
1.0
0.8
0.6
0.4
0.2
0.0
-0.2
Signal
lipid
3.5
3.0
2.5
2.0
1.5
1.0
0.5
0.0
-0.5
Chemical shift
ppm

6b

Patient 5 (fig. 6)

This 58-year-old woman presented with headache and a mild right hemiparesis due to a metastasis from an adenocarcinoma of the breast. She underwent radiosurgery with a margin dose of 24 Gy. ^{18}FBPA-PET studies were performed 34 and 94 days after the treatment. The T/N ratio was reduced from 1.7 to 1.3. At ^{1}H-MRS 54 days after the treatment, a free lipid signal was observed in the tumor. The patient died of cerebrospinal fluid dissemination 5 months after radiosurgery.

Discussion

Metastastic brain tumors are a manifestation of systemic malignant diseases, and life expectancy is limited in many patients. The aim of stereotactic radiosurgery is to improve or maintain the quality of life [14]. If the irradiated tumors are completely controlled, recent improvements in the treatment for the primary lesion may provide patients with a longer useful life. However, severe complications such as radiation necrosis undermine the useful effects of radiosurgery. Radiation necrosis after radiosurgery for metastatic brain tumors has been thought to be a rare complication [3]. We suspect that the longer radiosurgery improves survival, the more often radiation necrosis will be seen. Careful follow-up of all patients having radiosurgery is important to determine the true incidence of radiation necrosis [15]. To avoid radiation injury, radiation effects on the metabolism of metastatic brain tumor and normal brain adjacent to the tumor should be clarified. In this study, PET and ^{1}H-MRS were used to investigate the metabolic alteration.

^{18}FDG-PET and ^{18}FBPA-PET

For PET, ^{18}FDG is conventionally employed to monitor glucose utilization. Lesion uptake of ^{18}FDG is equal to or greater than that of gray matter in the majority of malignant gliomas [16] and more than white matter in metastatic brain tumors [17]. In the case of glioma, it has been widely accepted that it is possible with ^{18}FDG-PET to differentiate between tumor progression and radiation necrosis [18]. Mograd et al. [19] also stated that their differentiation after Gamma Knife radiosurgery could be made more confidently with ^{18}FDG-PET than with CT or MRI. In this study, ^{18}FDG-PET was applied to two patients suspected of suffering from radiation necrosis. In patient 2 with histologically verified radiation necrosis, the rCMRglc of the lesion including the surrounding edema showed lower values than did normal white matter. In patient 3, the rCMRglc of the thalamic lesion was lower than that of the contralateral thalamus. The enhanced region with its surrounding edema did not increase in size between

8 and 13 months after Gamma Knife radiosurgery. These findings would indicate that the enhanced region was a radiation necrosis. However, recent studies have reported that ^{18}FDG-PET results could not be correlated accurately with tumor progression and radiation necrosis [17, 20]. Valk et al. [21] evaluated patients undergoing ^{18}FDG-PET after interstitial brachytherapy. Histological examination of biopsied tissue after ^{18}FDG-PET was performed on 18 patients (9 with positive and 9 with negative uptake). There were viable cells as well as necrosis in all cases. They stated that some cells in ^{18}FDG-negative cases might be morphologically intact, but had little or no metabolic activity.

The current study used both ^{18}FDG and ^{18}FBPA. BPA has been used as a tumor-selective boron carrier for boron neutron capture therapy (BNCT) in malignant melanoma [22]. In the same way, it is thought to be a potential boron carrier for BNCT of malignant glioma, due to its high rate of incorporation into malignant glioma cells [23]. ^{11}C-Methionine and ^{11}C-tyrosine have been previously used as amino acid tracers [24, 25]. ^{11}C-Tyrosine has a higher rate of transport across the blood-brain barrier and may be used in protein synthesis [26], although nonselective transport of ^{11}C-methionine has been reported [27]. In an ^{18}FBPA study in gliomas, time-activity curves demonstrated the accumulation pattern. This supports the evidence for its intracellular capture and its use in protein synthesis [23]. A chronological ^{18}FBPA-PET study was performed on patients 1 and 2. In patient 1, the decrease in ^{18}FBPA transport to tumor cells was observed 15 days after Gamma Knife radiosurgery, and this continued for a long time. There was finally no ^{18}FBPA transport to the irradiated tumor.

Considering the results of ^{1}H-MRS, irradiation effects on amino acid metabolism appeared in the early stage after radiosurgery. This might indicate that indirect ionizing reactions with free radicals directly affecting cellular organelles [28] occurred in some parts of the tumor. In the remaining part of the tumor, there was probably DNA damage leading slowly to cell death. Such early effects on the tumor were histologically verified in the autopsy cases 14–22 days after radiosurgery [4, 29, 30]. In patient 2, the enhanced region increasing in size over time together with surrounding edema was strongly indicative of radiation necrosis. Nonetheless, we consider that tumor regrowth occurred, since ^{18}FBPA uptake was noted again. At present, we believe that this enhanced region represented a combination of tumor regrowth and radiation necrosis. In patient 4, the irradiated tumor certainly regrew, because there was a similar uptake of ^{18}FBPA in both the irradiated tumor and the new metastasis. In patient 5, the T/N ratio was reduced from 1.7 to 1.3 within 60 days, consistent with MRI findings.

^{1}H-MRS

Four main peaks, namely choline, creatine, NAA and free lipid, were obtained in the present ^{1}H-MRS study. Choline is a cell membrane constituent and a major phospholipid in brain [31]. NAA is a brain metabolite with high concentrations normally found only in neurons. The role of NAA is not well understood, but it is considered to be an indicator of neuronal function [31]. In many brain tumors including metastases, an increase of choline and a decrease or loss of NAA have been observed [6, 32]. The increase in the choline level may be related to enhanced phospholipid turnover in the cell membrane of proliferating tumor cells [33]. The response to conventional radiation therapy has been studied using ^{1}H-MRS. A reduction of choline accompanied by tumor shrinkage was observed in gliomas [34, 35]. The reduction of choline possibly reflects attenuation of tumor cell proliferation and cell membrane production [34]. In patient 1, the slight decrease of choline began in 5 days and there was a remarkable decrease within 31 days after Gamma Knife radiosurgery. In 73 days, only small choline and lactate peaks were observed. This result was consistent with that of the ^{18}FBPA study. Considering both results, this tumor would appear to have been undergoing complete necrosis.

After Gamma Knife radiosurgery, the peak of free lipid was noted in the tumor itself and/or the brain adjacent to the tumor in this study. In patient 1, preirradiated tumor showed the peak of free lipid. Some tumors originally have free lipid signals [6, 36]. In patient 2, who showed typical radiation necrosis, free lipid was markedly elevated in the enhanced mass and adjacent brain 8 months after the first radiosurgery. At this time, the enhanced mass was thought to be a combination of tumor regrowth and radiation necrosis because of the presence of ^{18}FBPA uptake. The increase in the free lipid value most likely reflects radiation necrosis and it could be due to the increase of products of destroyed cell membrane. Free lipid signals were also obtained in the brain of patients with cerebral infarction [37] and multiple sclerosis [38]. After the second treatment with the Gamma Knife, lower NAA was observed in the adjacent brain accompanied by surrounding edema, which might indicate severe damage of the brain after the second radiosurgery treatment. Histological findings of radiation necrosis are as follows: vascular changes (thickened vessel walls, endothelial proliferation, fibrinoid necrosis, hyaline and amyloid deposition, perivascular lymphocytic infiltration and intraluminal thrombosis) and parenchymal changes (coagulative necrosis, cystic cavitation with gliosis and patchy demyelination) [15]. The decrease in NAA and choline, and the presence of free lipid might partially reflect the histological findings. If the necrosis is complete, the spectra showed a decrease in all peaks beneath the noise level [39]. In patients 3 and 5, the free lipid signal was also observed in the enhanced mass. We suspect that the former was due to radiation injury and the latter to the destruction of the tumor.

Finally, irradiation effects on the metabolism of the metastatic brain tumor occurred within 15 days. Radiation necrosis occurred several months after Gamma Knife radiosurgery. Low or absent uptake of ^{18}FBPA and ^{18}FDG, and the decrease in NAA and increase in free lipid in ^{1}H-MRS, were useful indicators of radiation necrosis. PET and ^{1}H-MRS together were useful to differentiate between tumor progression and radiation necrosis. However, there are cases where radiation necrosis combines with tumor regrowth. The pattern of metabolic alteration and the incidence of radiation necrosis seem to depend, e.g., on tumor size, location, histology and volume dose. Further studies are needed to make these modalities really useful.

Acknowledgment

We thank Mrs. Maki Oyake for her secretarial assistance.

References

1 Patchell RA, Tibbs PA, Walsh JW, Dempsey RJ, Maruyama Y, Kryscio RJ, Markesbery WR, Macdonald JS, Young B: A randomized trial of surgery in the treatment of single metastases to the brain. N Engl J Med 1990;322:494–500.

2 Kihlström L, Karlsson B, Lindquist C: Gamma Knife surgery for cerebral metastases: Implications for survival based on 16 years experience. Stereotact Funct Neurosurg 1993;61:45–50.

3 Flickinger JC, Kondziolka D, Lunsford LD, Coffey RJ, Goodman ML, Shaw EG, Hudgins WR, Weiner R, Harsh GR, Sneed PK, Larson DA: A multi-institutional experience with stereotactic radiosurgery for solitary brain metastasis. Int J Radiat Oncol Biol Phys 1994;28:797–802.

4 Coffey RJ, Flickinger JC, Bissonette DJ, Lunsford LD: Radiosurgery for solitary brain metastases using the cobalt-60 gamma unit: Methods and results in 24 patients. Int J Radiat Oncol Biol Phys 1991;20:1287–1295.

5 Di Chiro G, DeLaPaz RL, Brooks RA, Sokoloff L, Kornblith PL, Smith BH, Patronas NJ, Kufta CV, Kessler RM, Johnston GS, Manning RG, Wolf AP: Glucose utilization of cerebral gliomas measured by [^{18}F]fluorodeoxyglucose and positron emission tomography. Neurology 1982;32: 1323–1329.

6 Bruhn H, Frahm J, Gyngell ML, Merboldt KD, Hanicke W, Sauter R, Hamburger C: Noninvasive differentiation of tumors with use of localized H-1 MR spectrosocpy in vivo: Initial experience in patients with cerebral tumors. Radiology 1989;172:541–548.

7 Wise RJS, Bernardi S, Frackowiak RSJ, Legg NJ, Jones T: Serial observations on the pathophysiology of acute stroke. Brain 1983;106:197–222.

8 Bruhn H, Frahm J, Gyngell ML, Merboldt KD, Hanicke W, Sauter R: Cerebral metabolism in man after acute stroke: New observations using localized proton NMR spectroscopy. Magn Res Med 1989;9:126–131.

9 Langfitt TW, Obrist WD, Alavi A, Grossman RI, Zimmerman R, Jaggi J, Uzzell B, Reivich M, Patton DR: Computerized tomography, magnetic resonance imaging, and positron emission tomography in the study of brain trauma. J Neurosurg 1986;64:760–767.

10 Furuya S, Naruse S, Yamaki T, Horikawa Y, Ebisu T, Ueda S, Tanaka C, Higuchi T, Umeda M: Neuroimaging of cerebral metabolism in severe diffuse brain injury in chronic stage. Part 2: MR spectroscopy and spectroscopic imaging; in Nakamura N, Hashimoto T, Yasue M (eds): Recent Advances in Neurosurgery. Tokyo, Springer, 1993, pp 196–199.

11 Hutchins GD, Holden JE, Koeppe RA, Halama JR, Gatley SJ, Nickles RJ: Alternative approach to single-scan estimation of cerebral glucose metabolic rate using glucose analogs, with particular application to ischemia. J Cereb Blood Flow Metab 1984;4:35–40.

12 Phelps ME, Huang SC, Hoffman EJ, Selin C, Sokoloff L, Kuhl DE: Tomographic measurement of local cerebral glucose metabolite rate in humans with (F-18) 2-fluoro-2-deoxy-*D*-glucose: Validation of method. Ann Neurol 1979;6:371–388.
13 Naruse S, Furuya S, Ide M, Murakami K, Tanaka C, Umeda M, Horikawa Y, Ebisu T, Ueda S, Miyazaki T, Yamamoto T: Clinical application of ^{1}H-chemical-shift imaging (CSI) to brain disease. Prog CI 1992;14:161–171.
14 Jokura H, Takahashi K, Kayama T, Yoshimoto T: Gamma Knife radiosurgery of a series of only minimally selected metastatic brain tumours. Acta Neurochir 1994;62:77–82.
15 Statham P, Macpherson P, Johnston R, Forster DM, Adams JH, Todd NV: Cerebral radiation necrosis complicating stereotactic radiosurgery for arteriovenous malformation. J Neurol Neurosurg Psychiatry 1990;53:476–479.
16 Coleman RE, Hoffman JM, Hanson MW, Sostman HD, Schold SC: Clinical application of PET for the evaluation of brain tumors. J Nucl Med 1991;32:616–622.
17 Davis WK, Boyko OB, Hoffman JM, Hanson MW, Schold SC, Burger PC, Friedman AH, Coleman RE: [^{18}F]2-Fluoro-2-deoxyglucose-positron emission tomography correlation of gadolinium-enhanced MR imaging of central nervous system neoplasia. Am J Neuroradiol 1993;14:515–523.
18 Patronas NJ, Di Chiro G, Brooks RA, DeLaPaz RL, Kornblith PL, Smith BH, Rizzoli HV, Kessler RM, Manning RG, Channing M, Wolf AP, O'Connor CM: Work in progress: [^{18}F]fluorodeoxyglucose and positron emission tomography in the evaluation of radiation necrosis of the brain. Radiology 1982;144:885–889.
19 Mograd J, Kihlström L, Ericson K, Karlsson B, Guo WY, StoneElander S: Recurrent tumor vs. radiation effects after Gamma Knife radiosurgery of intracerebral metastases: Diagnosis with PET-FDG. J Comput Assist Tomogr 1994;18:177–181.
20 Janus TJ, Kim EE, Tilbury R, Bruner JM, Yung WKA: Use of [^{18}F]fluorodeoxyglucose positron emission tomography in patients with primary malignant brain tumors. Ann Neurol 1993;33:540–548.
21 Valk PE, Budinger TF, Levin VA, Silver P, Gutin PH, Doyle WK: PET of malignant cerebral tumors after interstitial brachytherapy. J Neurosurg 1988;69:830–838.
22 Mishima Y, Honda C, Ichihashi M, Obara H, Hiratsuka J, Fukuda H, Karashima H, Kobayashi T, Kanda K, Yoshino Y: Treatment of malignant melanoma by single neutron capture treatment with melanoma-seeking 10B-compound. Lancet 1989;ii:388–389.
23 Imahori Y, Ueda S, Ohmori Y, Yoshino E, Ono K, Kobayashi T, Ido T, Mishima Y: A basic concept for PET-BNCT system; in Mishima Y (ed): Cancer Neutron Capture Therapy. New York, Plenum, in press.
24 Derlon JM, Bourdet C, Bustany P, Chatel M, Theron J, Darcel F, Syrota A: [^{11}C]*L*-Methionine uptake in gliomas. Neurosurgery 1989;25:720–728.
25 Go KG, Keuter EJW, Kamman RL, Pruim J, Metzemaekers JDM, Staal MJ, Paans AMJ, Vaalburg W: Contribution of magnetic resonance spectroscopic imaging and *L*-[1-^{11}C]tyrosine positron emission tomography to localization of cerebral gliomas for biopsy. Neurosurgery 1994;34:994–1002.
26 Paans AMJ, Elsinga PH, Vaalburg W: Carbon-11 labeled tyrosine as a probe for modeling the protein synthesis rate; in Mazoyer BM, Heiss WD, Comar D (eds): PET Studies on Amino Acid Metabolism and Protein Synthesis. Boston, Kluwer, 1993, pp 161–174.
27 Schober O, Duden C, Meyer GJ, Mueller JA, Hundeshagen H: Non-selective transport of [^{11}C-methyl]-*L*- and *D*-methionine into a malignant glioma. Eur J Nucl Med 1987;13:103–105.
28 Ganz JC: Biologic effects of ionising radiation; in Ganz JC (ed): Gamma Knife Surgery: A Guide for Referring Physicians. Berlin, Springer, 1993, pp 35–49.
29 Koike Y, Hosoda H, Ishiwata Y, Sakata K, Hidaka K: Effect of radiosurgery using Leksell gamma unit on metastatic brain tumor: Autopsy case report. Neurol Med Chir 1994;34:534–537.
30 Thompson BG, Coffey RJ, Flickinger JC, Lunsford LD: Stereotactic radiosurgery of small intracranial tumors: Neuropathological correlation in three patients. Surg Neurol 1990;33:96–104.
31 Miller BL: A review of chemical issues in ^{1}H NMR spectroscopy. N-acetyl l-aspartate, creatine and choline. NMR Biomed 1991;4:47–52.
32 Ott D, Hennig J, Ernst T: Human brain tumors: Assessment with in vivo proton MR spectroscopy. Radiology 1993;186:745–752.

33 Luyten PR, Marien AJH, Heindel W, van Gerwen PHJ, Herholz K, den Hollander JA, Friedmann G, Heiss WD: Metabolic imaging of patients with intracranial tumors: H-1 MR spectroscopic imaging and PET. Radiology 1990;176:791–799.
34 Heesters MAAM, Kamman RL, Mooyaart EL, Go KG: Localized proton spectroscopy of inoperable brain gliomas: Response to radiation therapy. J Neurooncol 1993;17:27–35.
35 Fulham MJ, Bizzi A, Dietz MJ, Shih HH, Raman R, Sobering GS, Frank JA, Dwyer AJ, Alger JR, Di Chiro G: Mapping of brain tumor metabolites with proton MR spectroscopic imaging: Clinical relevance. Radiology 1992;185:675–686.
36 Bizzi A, Movsas B, Tedeschi G, Phillips CL, Okunieff P, Alger JR, Di CG: Response of non-Hodgkin lymphoma to radiation therapy: Early and long-term assessment with H-1 MR spectroscopic imaging. Radiology 1995;194:271–276.
37 Berkelbach van der Sprenkel JW, Luyten PR, van Rijen PC, Tulleken CAF, den Hollander JA: Cerebral lactate detected by regional proton magnetic resonance spectroscopy in a patient with cerebral infarction. Stroke 1988;19:1556–1560.
38 Larsson HB, Christiansen P, Jensen M, Frederiksen J, Heltberg A, Olesen J, Henriksen O: Localized in vivo proton spectroscopy in the brain of patients with multiple sclerosis. Magn Reson Med 1991;22:23–31.
39 Nakakoshi T, Matsuzawa H, Houkin K, Miyasaka K, Arimoto T: Two cases of proton MR spectroscopy of the brain after irradiation. Radiat Med 1994;12:139–142.

Proc 7th Int Meeting Leksell Gamma Knife® Society,
Island of Lana'i, Hawaii, November 1995
Stereotact Funct Neurosurg 1996;66(suppl 1):260–268

Stereotactic and Functional Neurosurgery

Prediction of Results following Gamma Knife Surgery for Brain Stem and Other Centrally Located Arteriovenous Malformations: Relation to Natural Course

B. Karlsson[a], *I. Lax*[b], *M. Söderman*[c], *L. Kihlström*[a], *C. Lindquist*[a]

Departments of [a] Neurosurgery, [b] Hospital Physics, and [c] Neuroradiology, Karolinska Hospital, Stockholm, Sweden

Key Words

Brain · Arteriovenous malformation · Risk · Gamma Knife · Radiosurgery

Abstract

Two models for predicting the results of Gamma Knife surgery for brain stem and other centrally located arteriovenous malformations (AVMs) are presented. By using these models, the probability of total obliteration and the risk of complications can be predicted. The model to predict the probability for obliteration is based on the following two observations. First, there is a positive relationship between the minimum dose given to the AVM nidus and the incidence of obliteration. Second, there is a negative relationship between the AVM nidus volume and the minimum dose given in the obliterated cases. The risk estimation model is also based on two observations. First, centrally located AVMs carry a higher risk of complications than those located peripherally. Second, the average dose to volumes which are large for radiosurgery is related to the incidence of complications. The findings of this study may be used to estimate the consequences of Gamma Knife treatment for every individual case prior to the treatment. This makes a comparison between different treatment options and no treatment possible. The risk of hemorrhage without any treatment is also quantified.

KARGER

E-Mail karger@karger.ch
Fax + 41 61 306 12 34
http://www.karger.ch

1011–6125/96/0665–0260$10.00/0

Bengt Karlsson, MD, PhD
Department of Neurosurgery
Karolinska Hospital
S–171 76 Stockholm (Sweden)

Introduction

The management of brain stem arteriovenous malformations (AVMs) is controversial. If the AVM nidus is intraparenchymal, microsurgery as well as embolization are considered to be either excluded or at best extremely dangerous. Drake [1] reported five operated brain stem AVMs, where three were 'operated upon inadvertently in the mistaken view that they lay on or only shallowly in the brainstem'. Attempts at resection of two small mesencephalic-pontine AVMs ended fatally. Some years later, he and colleagues reported their experience with 15 brain stem AVMs [2]. Two were excised safely, 4 patients died as a result of surgery, and 9 were explored unsuccessfully. On the other hand, Lawton et al. [3] reported 8 brain stem AVMs which were cured. Four were embolized and all were operated. Only one deteriorated after surgery.

It is obvious that the dangers of microsurgery differ significantly from center to center, even among the most prestigious institutions in the world. Gamma Knife surgery has a significant advantage for this group of patients because the treatment results should be similar and reproducible in all centers, if the treatment plans and doses are similar, a most important prerequisite for designing models that can predict the results of treatment, including the degree of success and the complication rate. The aims of this report are threefold. It should assist Gamma Knife users to quantify the expected results of a proposed AVM treatment before it is undertaken. It should enable an assessment of the relative risks of Gamma Knife surgery, microsurgery and embolization, in order to recommend the best treatment option in each individual case. It should allow the expected results following Gamma Knife surgery to be compared with the natural course of the disease.

Materials and Methods

Risk for Hemorrhage without Treatment

The assessment of the risk for an untreated AVM in this report is based on a novel method of defining the natural course of the disease [4, 5]. This analysis is based on the observation that in a large patient group there is a defined relation between the risk of hemorrhage and the age distribution at the initial AVM rupture. The conclusions in the studies cited above were based on 1,479 patients with a known date for the initial AVM rupture.

Using only the age at the initial hemorrhage as input, it could be shown that the risk for hemorrhage increases with AVM size and patient age [4, 5]. Furthermore, it was found that the risk for AVM rupture after Gamma Knife treatment is independent of the presence or absence of prior hemorrhage [6]. This would indicate that the number of previous hemorrhages is of limited or no importance when the risk of future hemorrhage is estimated.

Risk of Radiation-Induced Complications following Gamma Knife Treatment

A complication was defined as a radiation-induced new or aggravated neurological deficit. This can be transitory or permanent, and occurs together with radiological evidence of edema or radionecrosis.

Starting in 1988, we have used the predicted risk of complications to compare different treatment alternatives, in order to design an optimal dose plan. Additionally, the prescription dose was decided after taking the calculated risk of complications into consideration. Thus, from the point of view of estimating risk, the patient material after 1988 can be considered prospective. To this end, we compared the predicted number of complications with the observed number in all patients not previously treated with radiotherapy who received Gamma Knife surgery for the first time between January 1, 1988 and September 1, 1993.

Probability of Total Obliteration following Gamma Knife Surgery

It has been shown that the higher the lowest dose to the AVM nidus (lowest peripheral dose = margin dose = minimum dose), the higher the incidence of obliteration [7]. In the same paper, it was also shown that there was an inverse relationship between AVM size and the minimum dose effective in obliterating malformations. Thus, the larger the AVM, the lower the peripheral dose needed to obliterate it. One possible explanation for this is based on the assumption that it is sufficient to obliterate every vessel in the AVM once to obtain total obliteration. It is known that radiation induces sublethal damage in the vessel wall, which triggers a repair process resulting either in a progressive increase in the vessel wall thickness leading finally to obliteration or to restoration of the vessel. For stochastic reasons, the longer the vessel, the higher the likelihood that the repair process will end in total constriction of the vessel at one point. The total vessel length is related to (AVM volume)$^{1/3}$ which has the dimension (cm).

It seems reasonable to combine these two findings. This prompted us to relate the obliteration rate to the product of the minimum dose and (AVM volume)$^{1/3}$. This is expressed as the K index and is calculated as follows:

$$\text{K index} = \text{minimum dose} \times (\text{AVM volume})^{1/3}.$$

The AVM volume was defined as the volume included in the prescription isodose. This calculation was performed for all 945 AVMs with adequate follow-up treated at the Karolinska Hospital and the University of Virginia from 1970 to 1990 inclusive.

Results

Risk of Hemorrhage without Treatment

A graph can be constructed to estimate the risk of future hemorrhage, using the natural course assessment described above. In figure 1, the cumulative risk of hemorrhage is plotted against the number of years at risk. The different curves represent different patient ages at the time of the risk assessment, combined in 5-year steps from 10 to 50 years of age. For instance, a 25-year-old patient has about a 43% risk for hemorrhage in 10 years and a 70% risk in 20 years. Using this graph, the risk without treatment can be estimated for every individual patient and compared to the risk following different treatment options.

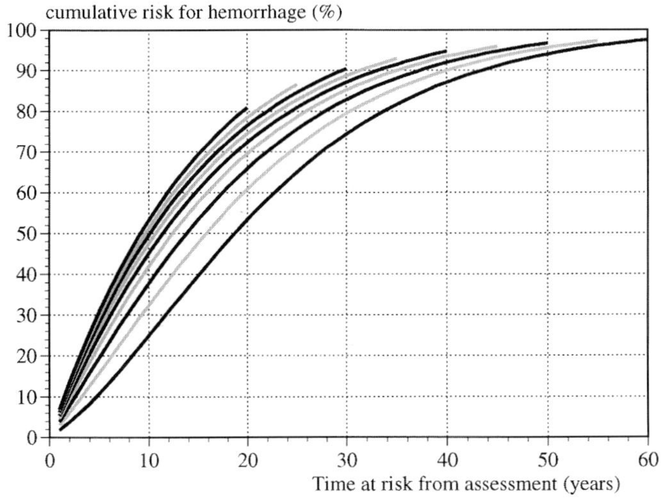

Fig. 1. Graph illustrating the cumulative risk of hemorrhage for different age groups from the time of assessment. The lowest line is for a patient of 10 years, the next for a 15-year-old patient and so on in 5-year steps up to 50 years of age.

Risk of Radiation-Induced Complications following Gamma Knife Treatment

In the prospective material of 444 patients, the number of complications was lower than predicted when the target was peripheral and higher when it was central. In this context, a central location was defined as situated in the mesencephalon, thalamus, corpus callosum or basal ganglia. For the 176 central AVMs that could be analyzed prospectively, 13 complications were observed and 8.7 predicted. Thus, it would seem that centrally located AVMs have higher risk of complications than those situated more peripherally.

The risk estimation in this report is based on the notion that a relationship exists between the average dose in the 20 cm^3 of tissue receiving the most radiation and the incidence of complications [8]. Figure 2 illustrates this relationship for the 491 centrally located AVMs treated at the Karolinska Hospital from 1970 to September 1, 1993 inclusive.

Probability of Total Obliteration following Gamma Knife Surgery

The obliteration rate increased linearly with the K index up to a value of around 27. For higher K values, the obliteration rate was a constant 80% suggesting that a maximum probability of obliteration can be achieved when the K index

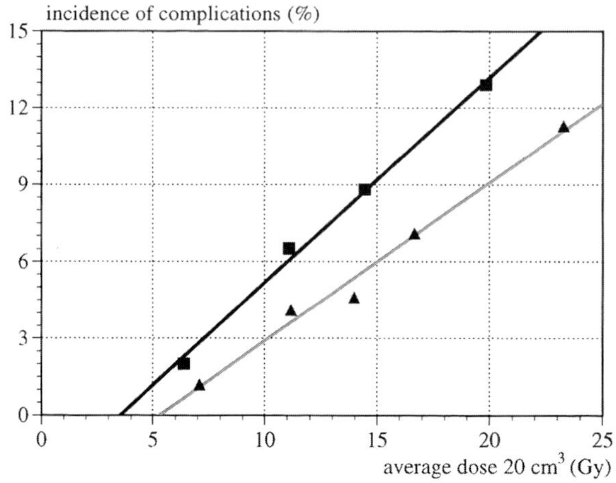

Fig. 2. The relationship between the incidence of complications and the average dose to the 20 cm^3 receiving the most radiation for central lesions (■). For comparison, the same relation is also illustrated for the whole material (▲). This graph can be used to give a rough estimate of the risk of complications for centrally located AVMs prior to treatment.

is around 27. A higher K index value would appear to increase the risk of complications without any additional benefit for the patient.

The probability of obliteration does not seem to be location dependent [9], making it possible to use the K index to predict the probability of obliteration for any AVM. In figure 3, the K index is plotted against the incidence of obliteration. The equation for the linear regression of the first part of the curve is:

$$f(x) = 3.073x - 3.3385.$$

Thus, if the K index is 17, the probability of total obliteration is 50%. If it is 21, the probability is 60%. If it is 24, the probability is 70%. If it is 27, the probability is 80%.

Case Report

A small intraaxial brain stem AVM in a 15-year-old boy is illustrated in figure 4 [10]. The AVM volume was estimated to be 0.77 cm^3. It could be covered using three 8-mm shots. From figures 2 and 3, it can be calculated that the minimum dose needed to obtain a 50% chance for total obliteration is 19 Gy, associated with a 2.5% risk of complications.

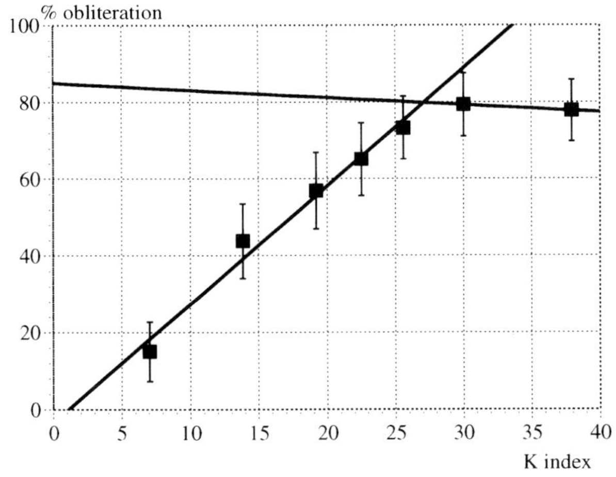

Fig. 3. K index plotted against the incidence of obliteration. The index may be used to estimate the probability of total obliteration before treatment. In the absence of prospective verification of the accuracy of the predicted value of the index, the findings must be interpreted with caution.

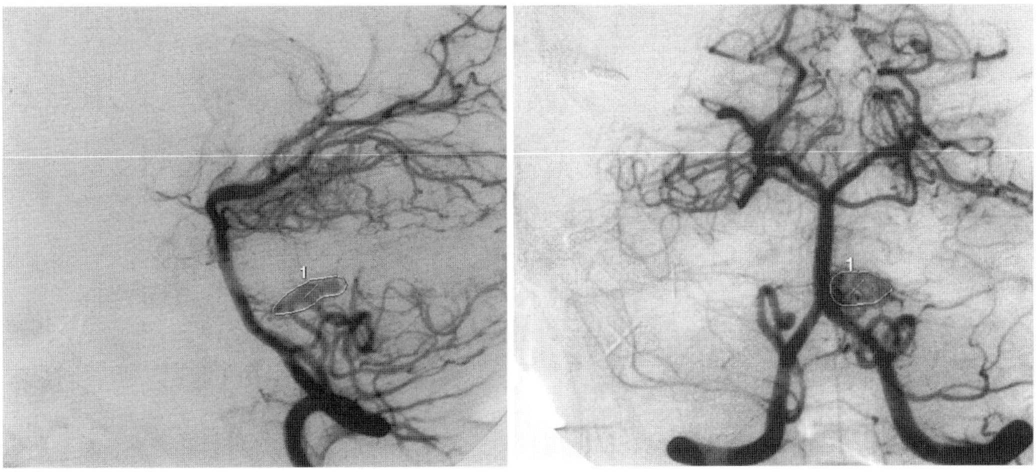

Fig. 4. Lateral and posteroanterior view of the AVM on distortion-corrected digital subtraction angiography images [10].

Table 1. Risk/benefit relations for different dose levels in one case

Probability of total obliteration, %	Minimum dose Gy	Risk of complications, %
50	19	2.5
60	23	2.9
70	26	3.4
80	29	3.8

The risk/benefit relations in this case are illustrated in table 1. Thus, for this patient, if 27 Gy is given as the lowest or peripheral dose, there would be an expected 3.8% risk for complications and an 80% chance of total obliteration.

Discussion

Risk of Hemorrhage without Treatment

The magnitude of the annual risk of hemorrhage from AVMs is controversial. There is a considerable range in the reported annual incidence of hemorrhage, from less than 1% to 5% [11–18]. The incidence of hemorrhage has usually been related to the size of the AVM, and most investigators have found that small AVMs are more prone to spontaneous rupture [19–21]. However, the contrary finding that larger AVMs carry the highest risk of hemorrhage has also been reported [22]. It has been suggested that a correlation exists between age and the risk of rupture [23]. However, to our knowledge, this has previously been neither substantiated nor quantified.

In this study we have used our own assessment of the natural course of the disease. The resulting risk does not differ dramatically from that obtained if the 4% constant risk reported by Ondra et al. [18] is used. It is therefore reasonable to assume that the magnitude of the risk of hemorrhage, illustrated in figure 1, is accurate. This should hold true even if the risk of hemorrhage is frighteningly high over a longer observation time.

Risk for Radiation-Induced Complications following Gamma Knife Treatment

A risk prediction model has been used at the Karolinska Hospital since 1988. The model was initially based on the first 611 AVM cases treated with the Gamma Knife. This analysis showed that the incidence of complications was independent of the AVM location [8]. This finding can be interpreted in two ways. One possibility is that there is no difference in radioresponsiveness between central and peripheral structures. The other possibility is that the dose to the more central structures was deliberately kept lower in this series, in order to minimize the risk of complications. This report shows that the latter interpretation is the correct one. Only patients treated more than 2 years ago have been included in this study because of the observation that more than 90% of the complications occur within 18 months following treatment [24].

It has previously been shown that the average dose in a large volume correlates with the incidence of complications [8]. This finding can be used together with figure 2 to give a rough estimate of the risk of complications for a centrally located AVM, prior to treatment. Nonetheless, the good fit of the linear regression ($R^2 = 0.99$) can give a false impression of accuracy. It should be kept in mind that the confidence intervals for the points are large, due to the fact that only 481 patients are included in the analysis. Therefore, the error limits of the predicted risk are large. However, the value does give an estimate of the magnitude of the risk for complications prior to treatment. It would, of course, be more accurate to use a biological model for the risk estimation. This requires that the parameters of the model be defined, which was done recently [25].

Probability of Total Obliteration following Gamma Knife Surgery

A number of theories can be postulated to explain the relation between the K index and the incidence of obliteration. One is described above (see Materials and Methods). Another theory is based on the fact that the larger the malformation, the larger the volume of normal brain tissue that will be included in the target volume, defined from angiography films in two projections only. Therefore, the larger the malformation, the higher the probability that the estimated minimum dose is lower than the true minimum dose.

Once more, it must be kept in mind that the K index is based on a retrospective study only. Although appealing, the predictive value of the K index still needs to be validated in a prospective study. Moreover, we need to uncover the radiobiological explanation underlying the relationship. Until this is achieved, the index must be used with caution. For instance, it is probable that there are AVM volume and dose limitations for the validity of the index. The best guess at present is that an index between 17 and 27 can be used, and that the limit of the AVM nidus volume may be around 10 cm^3. Nonetheless, it seems reasonable to suggest that using the index is better than making no assessment at all of the probability of AVM obliteration.

References

1 Drake CG: Cerebral arteriovenous malformations: Considerations for and experience with surgical treatment in 166 cases. Clin Neurosurg 1979;26:145–208.
2 Drake CG, Friedman H, Peerless SJ: Posterior fossa arteriovenous malformations. J Neurosurg 1986;64:1–10.
3 Lawton MT, Hamilton MG, Spetzler RF: Multimodality treatment of deep arteriovenous malformations: Thalamus, basal ganglia and brain-stem. Neurosurgery 1995;37:29–36.
4 Karlsson B, Lindquist C, Johansson A, Steiner L: Risk of initial hemorrhage from untreated cerebral AVM. Fourth Int Workshop Cerebrovasc Surgery, Chicago, 1995, p 71.
5 Karlsson B, Lindquist C, Johansson A, Steiner L: Annual risk of hemorrhage from untreated cerebral arteriovenous malformations. Minim Invasive Neurosurg, in press.
6 Karlsson B, Lindquist C, Steiner L: The effect of Gamma Knife surgery on the risk of rupture prior to AVM obliteration: Minimally Invasive Neurosurgery 1996;39:21–27.
7 Karlsson B, Lindquist C, Steiner L: Factors of importance for obliteration after Gamma Knife surgery for cerebral arteriovenous malformations. Neurosurgery, in press.
8 Lax I, Karlsson B: Prediction of complications in Gamma Knife radiosurgery of arteriovenous malformations. Acta Oncol 1996;35:49–55.
9 Duma CL, Lunsford LD, Kondziolka D, Bissonette DJ, Somaza S, Flickinger JC: Radiosurgery for vascular malformations of the brain-stem. Acta Neurochir Suppl 1993;58:92–97.
10 Söderman M, Picard C, Ericson K: An algorithm for correction of the distortion in stereotaxic digital subtraction angiography. Neuroradiology 1996, in press.
11 Brown RJ, Wiebers DO, Forbes GS: Unruptured intracranial aneurysms and arteriovenous malformations: Frequency of intracranial hemorrhage and relationship of lesions. J Neurosurg 1990;73:859–863.
12 Crawford PM, West CR, Chadwick DW, Shaw MD: Arteriovenous malformations of the brain: Natural history in unoperated patients. J Neurol Neurosurg Psychiatry 1986;49:1–10.
13 Davis C, Symon L: The management of cerebral arteriovenous malformations. Acta Neurochir (Wien) 1985;74:4–11.
14 Graf CJ, Perret GE, Torner JC: Bleeding from cerebral arteriovenous malformations as part of their natural history. J Neurosurg 1983;58:331–337.
15 Heros RC, Tu YK: Is surgical therapy needed for unruptured arteriovenous malformations? Neurology 1987;37:279–286.
16 Horton JC, Chambers WA, Lyons SL, Adams RD, Kjellberg RN: Pregnancy and the risk of hemorrhage from cerebral arteriovenous malformations. Neurosurgery 1990;27:867–871.
17 Luessenhop A: Cerebral arteriovenous malformations. Contemp Neurosurg 1989;11:1–5.
18 Ondra SL, Troupp H, George ED, Schwab K: The natural history of symptomatic arteriovenous malformations of the brain: A 24-year follow-up assessment. J Neurosurg 1990;73:387–391.
19 Graf CJ, Perret GE, Torner JC: Bleeding from cerebral arteriovenous malformations as part of their natural history. J Neurosurg 1983;58:331–337.
20 Itoyama Y, Uemura S, Ushio Y, Kuratsu J, Nonaka N, Wada H, Sano Y, Fukumura A, Yoshida K, Yano T: Natural course of unoperated intracranial arteriovenous malformations: Study of 50 cases. J Neurosurg 1989;71:805–809.
21 Spetzler RF, Hargraves R, McCormick P, Zabramski J, Flom R, Zimmerman R: Relationship of perfusion pressure and size to risk of hemorrhage from arteriovenous malformations. J Neurosurg 1992;76:918–923.
22 Jomin M, Lesoin F, Lozes G: Prognosis for arteriovenous malformations of the brain in adults based on 150 cases. Surg Neurol 1985;23:362–366.
23 Harbaugh K, Harbaugh R: Arteriovenous malformations in elderly patients. Neurosurgery 1994;35:579–584.
24 Guo WY: Radiological aspects of Gamma Knife radiosurgery for arteriovenous malformations and other non-tumoral disorders of the brain. Acta Radiol 1993;34:22.
25 Karlsson B: Gamma knife surgery of cerebral arteriovenous malformations; thesis, Karolinska Institute, Stockholm, 1996.

Proc 7th Int Meeting Leksell Gamma Knife® Society,
Island of Lana'i, Hawaii, November 1995
Stereotact Funct Neurosurg 1996;66(suppl 1):269–277

Stereotactic and Functional Neurosurgery

Dynamic and Static Scintigraphic Evaluation of Cerebral Arteriovenous Malformations to Evaluate Radiosurgical Treatment

K.A. Leber[a], *R. Aigner*[b], *R. Nicoletti*[b], *G.F. Fueger*[b], *G. Pendl*[a]

Departments of [a] Neurosurgery, and [b] Radiology (Division of Nuclear Medicine),
Karl Franzens University School of Medicine, Graz, Austria

Key Words

Arteriovenous malformation · Gamma Knife · Radiosurgery · Scintigraphy · Single photon emission computed tomography · Technetium-99m · Blood pool scintigraphy

Abstract

The radiobiologic changes induced by cobalt-60 gamma irradiation in cerebral arteriovenous malformations (AVMs) is a torpid process. Complete obliteration may take 1 or 2 years or even longer. Neuroradiological modalities like magnetic resonance imaging (MRI) and magnetic resonance angiography (MRA) do not provide sufficient information to comprehend this process. Digital subtraction angiography represents an invasive method and is therefore most often performed when complete obliteration is expected. The purpose of this study was to investigate the value of blood pool scintigraphy and functional imaging, such as single photon emission computed tomography (SPECT), to gain more knowledge about the volumetric changes of AVMs treated by radiosurgery. Twenty consecutive candidates for Gamma Knife treatment were selected for comparative MRI/MRA and scintigraphic studies. All lesions ranging from 0.6 to 18.6 cm^3 could be identified on blood pool and SPECT images. Seven patients had repetitive examinations at 3-month intervals to compare the relative volumetric change of the lesion. In 5 cases, a marked decrease in blood pooling was noticed after 3 months, and in 2 patients no significant change was evident. In contrast, MRI/MRA scans done at the same time did not similarly indicate progressive obliteration changes. This preliminary result indicates that scintigraphic evaluation using the blood pool technique is a very sensitive method to describe the relative volumetric change of radiosurgically treated AVMs.

KARGER

E-Mail karger@karger.ch
Fax + 41 61 306 12 34
http://www.karger.ch

1011–6125/96/0665–0269$10.00/0

Klaus A. Leber, MD
Department of Neurosurgery
Karl Franzens University
School of Medicine
A–8036 Graz (Austria)

Introduction

The obliteration of nidus vessels of cerebral arteriovenous malformations (AVMs) after cobalt-60 gamma irradiation is a slowly evolving radiobiological reaction that may take 1 or 2 years, depending on the volume of the lesion and the dose [1]. In some rare instances it may even take longer or be incomplete.

Little is known about the effect of ionizing radiation on biological tissues in general and blood vessels in particular [2–4]. Neuroradiological modalities do not provide sufficient information for understanding this process of progressive obliteration. Angiography is still the procedure of choice to demonstrate the actual state of angioarchitecture, but it is an invasive method, and most patients will not comply with frequent angiographic follow-ups. Most radiosurgery centers recommend it as a final documentation when complete obliteration has been indicated by other means.

Blood pool scintigraphy, using ^{99m}Tc autologous erythrocytes, has been known as a screening method for vascular malformations of abdominal organs, as well as for gastrointestinal bleeding [5–8]. It is suggested that cerebral AVMs pool these labeled blood cells, which may possibly indicate the actual volume of the lesion, enabling quantification of the lesion volume after gamma irradiation.

Material and Methods

The present study examined 20 consecutive patients harboring an intracerebral AVM, at different stages of treatment. All were candidates for endovascular and/or Leksell Gamma Knife treatment. Criteria for exclusion were multiple, clustered lesions and associated aneurysms. Diagnosis was made by magnetic resonance imaging (MRI) combined with magnetic resonance angiography (MRA) and confirmed by digital subtraction angiography (DSA). There were 5 male and 15 female patients with a mean age of 39 years (16–67). The volume of the AVM was calculated from the target volume defined by the dose plan, considering only the nidus. Draining veins were excluded. All patients had an MRI and a scintigraphic evaluation before the radiosurgical procedure to serve as a baseline for later comparison. Seven had follow-ups at 3-month intervals. The region of the nidus was measured in three different planes, and the change in average size was expressed as a percentage of the initial value.

Scintigraphic Techniques

^{99m}Tc-labeled autologous erythrocytes (15 mCi) were administered intravenously before the investigations (in vitro labeling technique). Dynamic radionuclide angiography (RNA) was first performed to gain insight into hypo- or hyperperfusion of the region of interest (ROI). Static imaging was performed in four planar projections (anterior, posterior, left lateral, right lateral) 10 min after the administration of the labeled erythrocytes. In addition, an extracorporeal equivalent blood sample was imaged to obtain reference values and to estimate the blood volume of the AVM. The count rate of the ROI was measured from these scans and expressed as a percent change compared to the baseline value. Single photon emission computed tomography (SPECT) was carried out immediately after the static planar scintigraphy to provide tomographic images and, if required, an optional three-dimensional reconstruction. RNA and the planar images were acquired from a dual-head scintillation camera (Elscint Helix). SPECT was obtained from a triple-headed scintillation camera (Picker PRISM 3000).

Results

According to the radiosurgical target volume, the size of the AVMs ranged from 0.5 to 3.3 cm maximum diameter, equivalent to a volume of 0.6–18.6 cm^3.

MRI revealed radiation-induced alterations such as moderate perinidal edema, gliosis and a decrease in the lumen of draining veins. It also showed the extent of signal void representing patent nidus vessels within the nidus itself. No radionecrosis was diagnosed by neuroimaging. One patient could not be exposed to a high magnetic field because of intracranial ferromagnetic clips from a prior attempt at surgical resection of the lesion.

In all 20 patients, the AVMs could be demonstrated in each of the three scintigraphic studies. The smallest was a spherical cerebellar lesion of 0.6 cm^3, in which the actual nidus was difficult to distinguish on MRI. However, SPECT unequivocally identified this AVM in the upper left hemisphere of the cerebellum as a spherical blood pool (fig. 1). The scintigraphic appearance seemed to be slightly larger than the target volume calculated from the angiogram, because the ectatic draining vein encircled the core of the lesion halfway so it could not be separated from the true nidus by this means.

Figure 2 demonstrates a nonbleeding right temporobasal AVM of 2.6 cm in maximal diameter (4.9 cm^3). An early filling vein drains into the vein of Galen. Fragments of this pathological vein are visible on three-dimensional SPECT. Another late filling vein across the right frontal cortex leading into the superior sagittal sinus was found as an anatomical variant.

Comparative follow-up studies were performed in 7 patients. Two could be examined at the time of radiosurgery. In 5 patients, the first data were obtained 2, 3, 6 or 12 months after treatment. Follow-up was carried out at 3-month intervals. There was a marked scintimetric decrease of local blood pool volume in all 5 cases, even if the MRI and MRA did not reveal any significant change in size. Only one AVM showed an increase in volume of 25% after 2 months. However, a decrease of 60% was found after 6 months. In two patients, the volume of the lesions did not change significantly within one follow-up interval. The percentage variation of the measured volumes is graphically summarized in figure 3.

1a

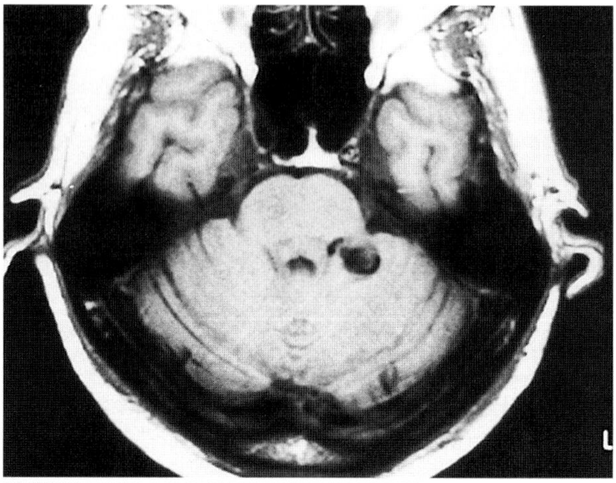

1b

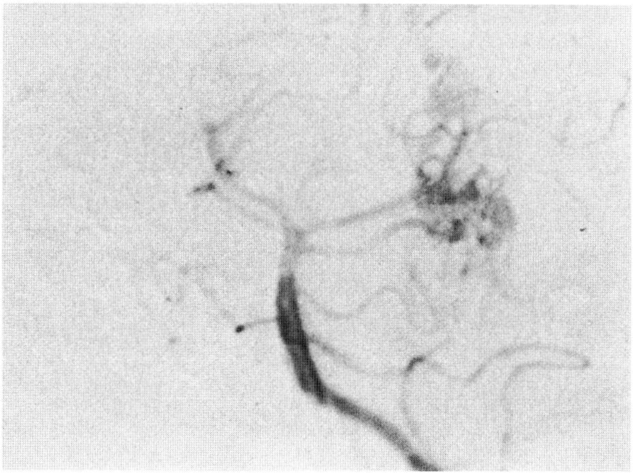

Fig. 1. Left cerebellar AVM 0.6 cm (0.6 cm^3), bleeding. **a** T_1-weighted MRI. **b** Left vertebral angiogram, posteroanterior. **c** Blood pool scintigram, left lateral skull. Region of increased tracer activity (arrow), normal extracranial tracer distribution (paranasal sinuses). **d** Three-dimensional SPECT and two-dimensional scans, AVM arrowed. SSS = Superior sagittal sinus; LLS = Left lateral sinus; RCS = right cavernous sinus.

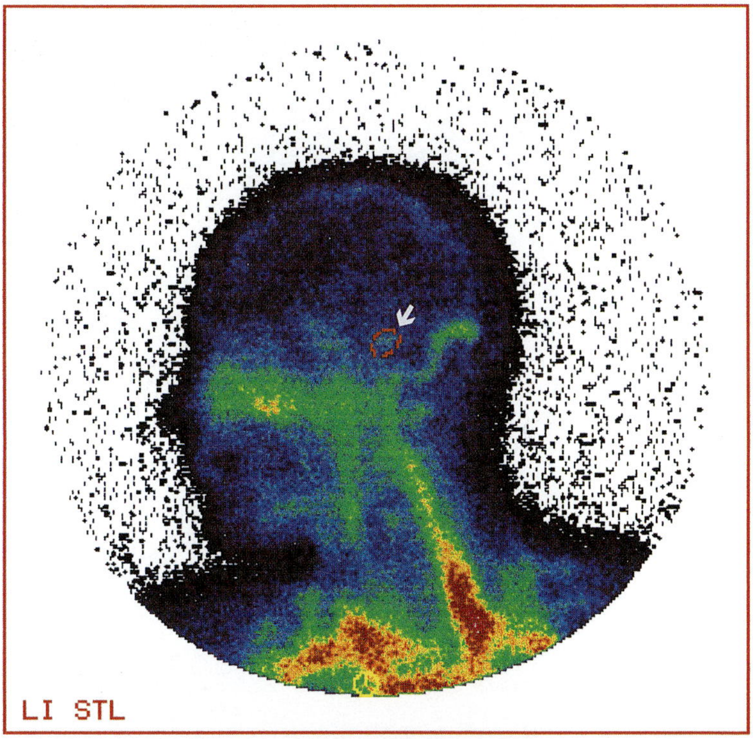

1c

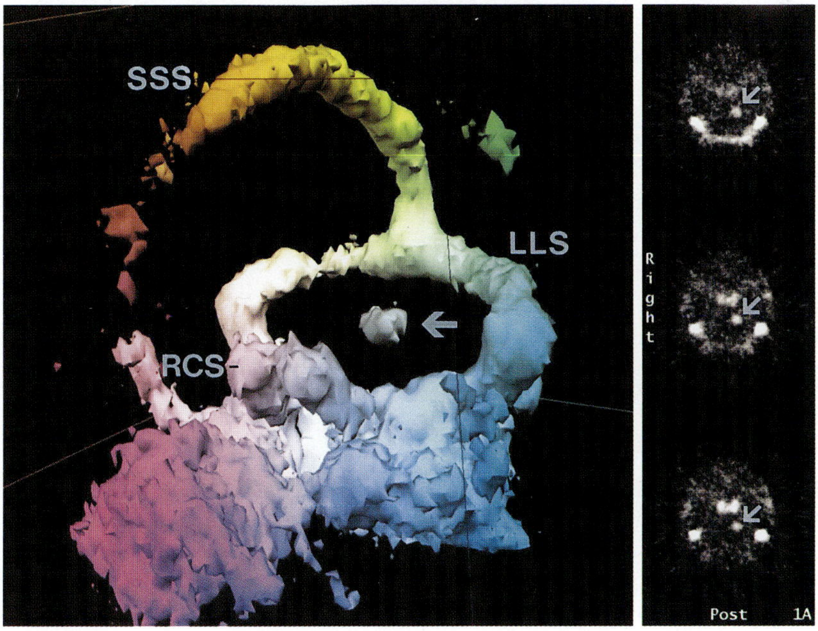

1d

2a

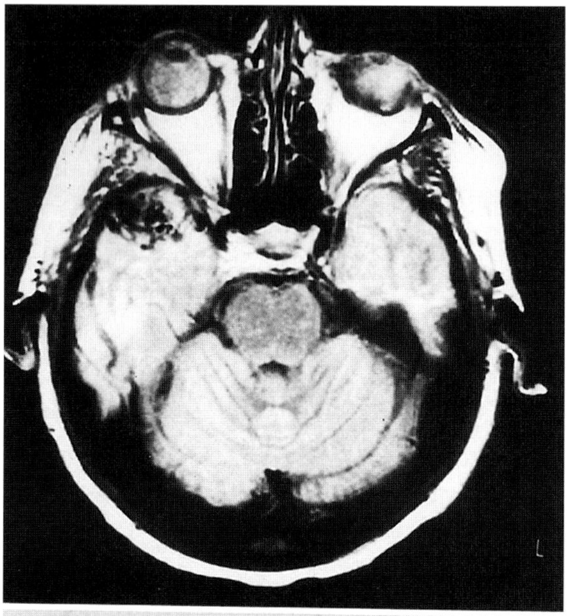

2b

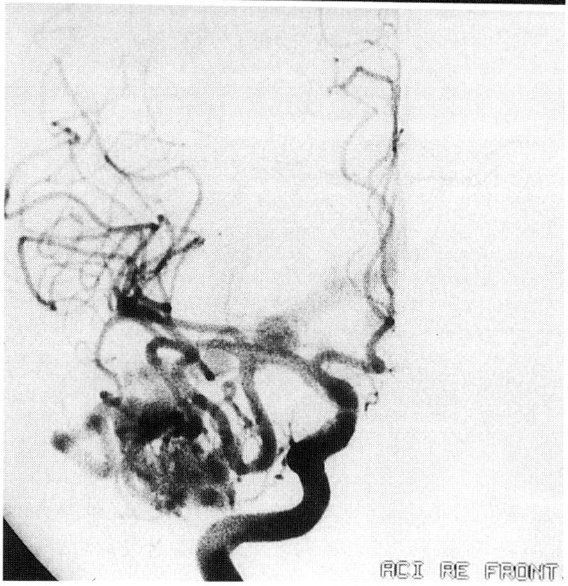

Fig. 2. Right temporobasal AVM 2.6 cm (4.9 cm^3), nonbleeding. **a** T_1-weighted MRI. **b** Right carotid angiogram, posteroanterior. **c** Blood pool scintigram, right lateral skull. Region of increased tracer activity (arrow). **d** Two-dimensional scans and three-dimensional SPECT. SSS = Superior sagittal sinus; LLS = left lateral sinus; LCS = left cavernous sinus; arrowheads = fragments of draining vein; arrow = normal superficial frontal vein leading into SSS.

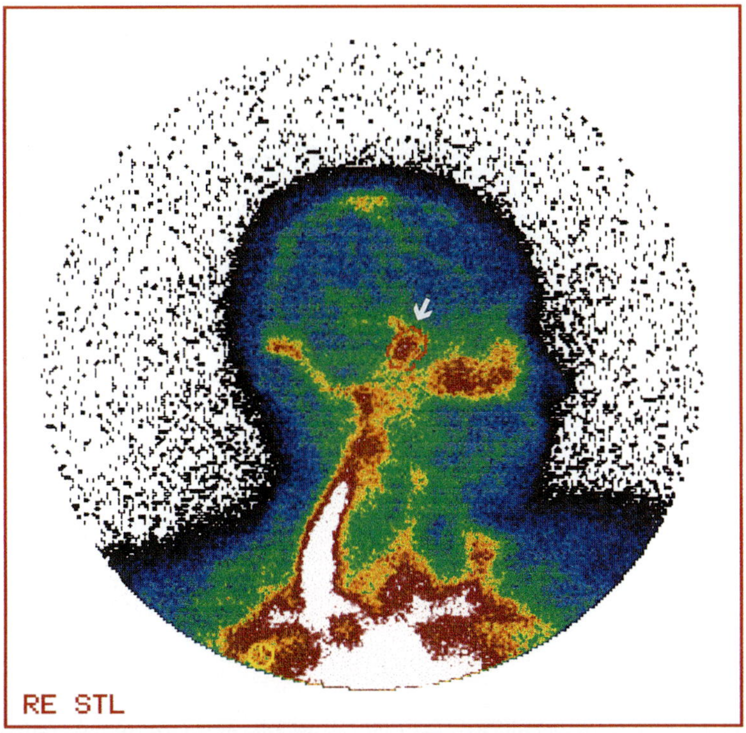

2c

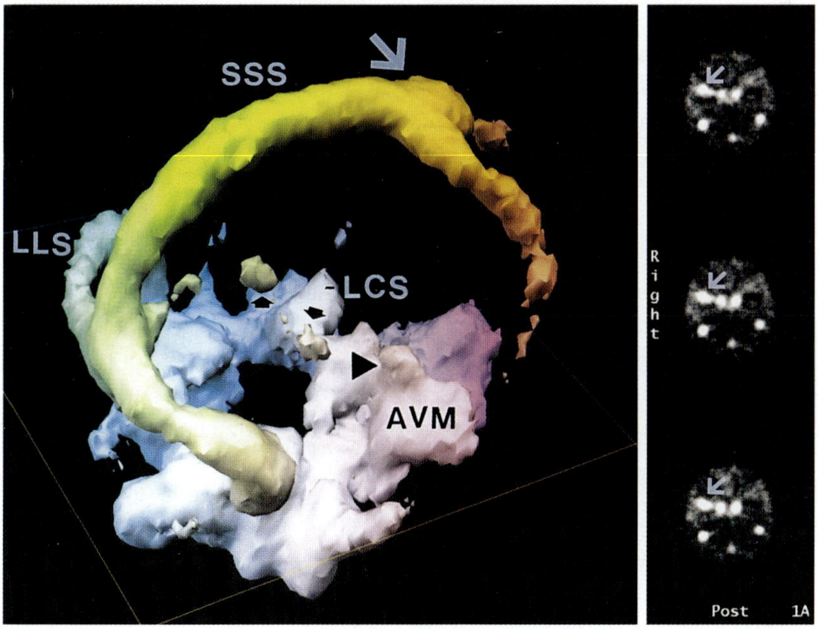

2d

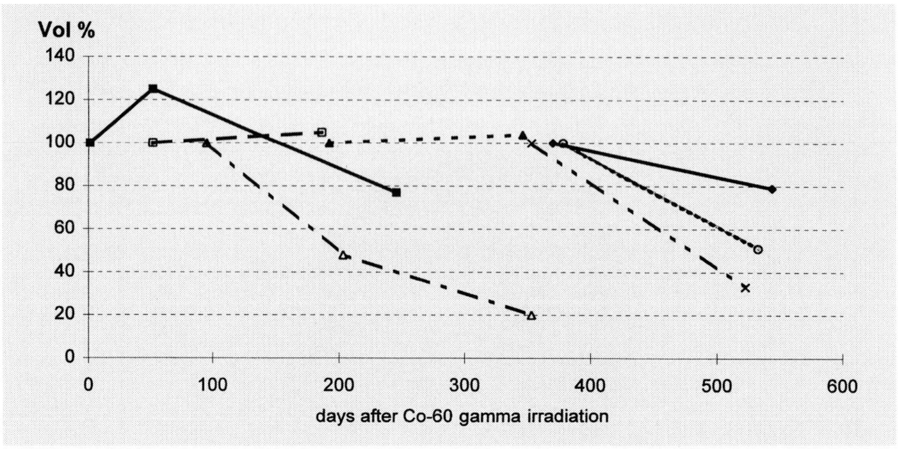

Fig. 3. Percent change of the AVM volume after radiosurgery in 7 patients. Note the marked decrease within a short observation time of 3–4 months, and the paradoxical increase in 1 patient after 2 months.

Discussion

Stereotactic radiosurgery has proved to be an effective treatment modality for carefully selected cerebral AVMs. However, the time-dependent hemodynamic changes within such vascular lesions still remain the subject of scientific debate. To date, neither a morphological nor a functional examination method can provide a quantitative or semiquantitative estimate of the AVM blood volume after radiosurgical treatment. A mathematical model has been suggested to simulate the compartmental hemodynamics of AVMs treated by stereotactic radiosurgery in terms of predictive calculations [9]. This model represents an important hypothesis, but these projections still need further confirmation by clinical data. Total obliteration of the entire lesion is presently claimed as the only secure way to prevent further bleeding. Total occlusion is defined as the disappearance of the nidus and the draining vein on angiography. There has been recent discussion that a remaining enlarged vein from the obliterated nidus might not be as dangerous as previously thought [10]. The latency period between radiosurgical treatment and final obliteration of the lesion certainly attracts clinical attention.

MRI gives some information about the volumetric changes of the nidus or the draining vein, but this information is more a subjective estimation than a true measurement. The signal alterations produced by hemosiderin after bleeding, progressive gliosis and different flow phenomena are sometimes difficult to distinguish, let alone quantify. The same applies to MRA, which illustrates the morphology of the lesion nicely but was disappointing when applied to comparative results in this series.

In contrast, the results of the present study have indicated that static scintigraphic examination is a simple and noninvasive semiquantitative method to follow the slow process of obliteration after gamma irradiation of cerebral AVMs. It has to be pointed out that this method is based on the intravascular pooling of labeled blood cells as can be demonstrated impressively by SPECT. From these preliminary data, it would appear that scintigraphic examinations can show lesions as small as 6 mm in diameter and enable reproducible measurements of relative nidus volume. However, it has not been possible to separate draining veins from the true nidus. Therefore, it is proposed that the origin of veins draining the nidus are included in these measurements. Once the end point of obliteration has been achieved, the size of these veins will return to normal and will no longer represent a pathological blood pool. However, exact knowledge of the topographic localization of the AVM is essential to delineate the ROI needed to quantify the volume of the lesion. An overlapping projection of the nidus and the venous sinuses or other heavily pooling structures like the paranasal sinuses will nullify any useful information. At present, an ongoing study is attempting to compare the volume measured in milliliters, at scintigraphy to the actual calculated target volume. In addition, an attempt is being made to quantify the results obtained by SPECT.

References

1 Lunsford LD, Kondziolka D, Bissonette DJ, Maitz AH, Flickinger JC: Stereotactic radiosurgery of brain vascular malformations. Neurosurg Clin North Am 1992;3:79–98.

2 Kihlström L, Lindquist C, Adler J, Collins P, Karlsson B: Histological studies of Gamma-Knife lesions in normal and hypercholesterinemic rabbits; in Steiner L (ed): Radiosurgery: Baseline and Trends. New York, Raven Press, 1992, pp 111–119.

3 Altschuler E, Lunsford LD, Kondziolka D, Wu A, Maitz A, Sclabassi R, Martinez AJ, Flickinger JC: Radiobiologic models for radiosurgery. Neurosurg Clin North Am 1992;3:61–77.

4 Lo EH, Frankel KA, De La Paz RL: Cerebrovascular and metabolic perturbations in delayed heavy charged particle radiation injury. Brain Res 1989;504:168–172.

5 Fueger GF, Schuschnigg C: Intestinale Blutungs-Szintigraphie mit 99m-Technetium markierten Erythrozyten. Wien Med Wochenschr 1986;17:431–435.

6 Markisz J, Front D, Royal HD, Sacks B, Parker JA, Kolodny GM: An evaluation of 99m-Tc-labeled blood-pool-scintigraphy for the detection and localisation of gastrointestinal bleeding sites. Gastroenterology 1982;83:394–398.

7 Winzelberg GG, Castronovo FP, Callahan JR, McKusick KA, Strauss HW: 111-In-Oxine labelled red cells for detection of simulated lower gastrointestinal bleeding in an animal model. Radiology 1980;135:455–461.

8 Lull RJ, Morris GL: Scintigraphic detection of gastrointestinal hemorrhage: Current status. J Nucl Med Technol 1986;14:79–88.

9 Lo EH, Fabrikant JI, Levy RP, Phillips MH, Frankel KA, Alpen EL: An experimental compartmental flow model for assessing the hemodynamic response of intracranial arteriovenous malformations to stereotactic radiosurgery. Neurosurgery 1991;28:251–259.

10 Pollock BE, Flickinger JC, Lunsford LD, Bissonette DJ, Kondziolka D: Hemorrhage risk after stereotactic radiosurgery of arteriovenous malformations (abstract). 2nd Congr Int Stereotact Radiosurg Soc Boston, Jun 1995, p 28.

Proc 7th Int Meeting Leksell Gamma Knife® Society,
Island of Lana'i, Hawaii, November 1995
Stereotact Funct Neurosurg 1996;66(suppl 1):278–287

Stereotactic and Functional Neurosurgery

Pathobiology of Cerebral Gliomas in Children and the Role of Radiosurgery

H.K. Inoue, H. Kohga, A. Zama, M. Hirato, T. Shibazaki, Y. Andou, C. Ohye

Department of Neurosurgery, Gunma University School of Medicine, Maebashi, and The Gamma Unit Center, Hidaka Hospital, Takasaki, Japan

Key Words

Cerebral hemisphere · Glioma · Children · Radiosurgery

Abstract

Twenty-five gliomas of the cerebral hemisphere in children were examined. Most hemispheric gliomas in children have relatively clear margins and less infiltrative potential. Radiosurgery has a role in the treatment of these tumors in addition to reducing the risk of radiation injuries developing later. Fifteen patients were alive 1–27 years (mean 8.4) following treatment and 10 patients died. Histologic examination demonstrated 10 differentiated gliomas, 10 poorly differentiated gliomas and 5 other gliomas. Most tumors had relatively clear margins on computed tomography and/or magnetic resonance images, and peritumoral edema was slight. In 9 autopsy cases, tumor dissemination and/or metastasis were seen in 7. However, tumor infiltration was not extensive, and clear tumor margins were found in some cases. Thus, cerebral gliomas in children have relatively clear margins and low infiltrative potential. Radiosurgery has a role in the treatment of these tumors.

Introduction

Gliomas in children have different pathobiologic features to those in adults. Tumor sites are predominantly in the cerebellum, brain stem and optic pathway, rather than the cerebral hemispheres, and many gliomas in adults arise in the cerebrum [1, 2]. Benign gliomas such as pilocytic astrocytoma and ependymoma

KARGER

E-Mail karger@karger.ch
Fax + 41 61 306 12 34
http://www.karger.ch

1011–6125/96/0665–0278$10.00/0

Hiroshi K. Inoue, MD, PhD
Department of Neurosurgery
Gunma University School of Medicine
3-39-15, Showa-machi
Maebashi, Gunma 371 (Japan)

are common, while malignant gliomas (glioblastoma) are relatively rare [3]. Moreover, malignant gliomas in children have a tendency to be undifferentiated and composed of small round tumor cells. Heterogeneity and polymorphism are found in small groups such as giant-cell glioblastomas and pleomorphic xanthoastrocytomas [4]. Determining the pathobiology of cerebral gliomas is important for current treatment modalities, including radiosurgery.

A standard treatment for cerebral gliomas in children is surgical removal followed by conventional irradiation. However, a recent report has shown that the routine use of radiotherapy is not recommended for low-grade gliomas of the cerebral hemisphere in children. An increased risk of late complications and anaplastic changes in the original tumor were observed following radiotherapy [5, 6]. Total or nearly total resection seems to be the best treatment of benign gliomas in children. Residual tumor, in cases of incomplete resection, may be treatable with radiosurgery. Although radiotherapy is an essential part of the multidisciplinary treatment of malignant gliomas, radiation damage is severe in the developing brain [7]. Stereotactic irradiation, therefore, should be considered, especially for young children under 5 years of age. This report describes a role for radiosurgery based on the pathobiology of cerebral gliomas in children, compared with those in adults.

Materials and Methods

Twenty-five patients under 16 years of age with gliomas of the cerebral hemisphere were evaluated clinically. These gliomas were 15% of the pediatric gliomas in our series. The patients' ages ranged from 6 months to 16 years (mean 9.0 years); 12 were male and 13 were female. Neuroimaging studies, including computed tomography (CT) and/or magnetic resonance imaging (MRI), were performed in 16 patients. Surgical specimens were examined histologically, immunohistochemically and ultrastructurally and 9 autopsies were performed.

We classified the childhood gliomas into three groups from histologic, immunohistochemical and ultrastructural findings: differentiated, poorly differentiated and others.

Results

Clinical Characteristics

Clinical manifestations included seizures in 13 patients, headaches in 8 and paresis in 4. Tumors were located in the temporal lobe (7 cases), parietal lobe (6), occipital lobe (3) and frontal lobe (2). Seven patients had tumors involving more than two lobes. Ten patients died (7 within 2 years after treatment). Fifteen patients were alive 1–27 years (mean 8.4 years) following treatment. Most tumors had relatively clear margins on CT and/or MRI and peritumoral edema was slight (fig. 1), even in recurrent cases. Cysts and/or calcifications were seen in 9 tumors.

a b

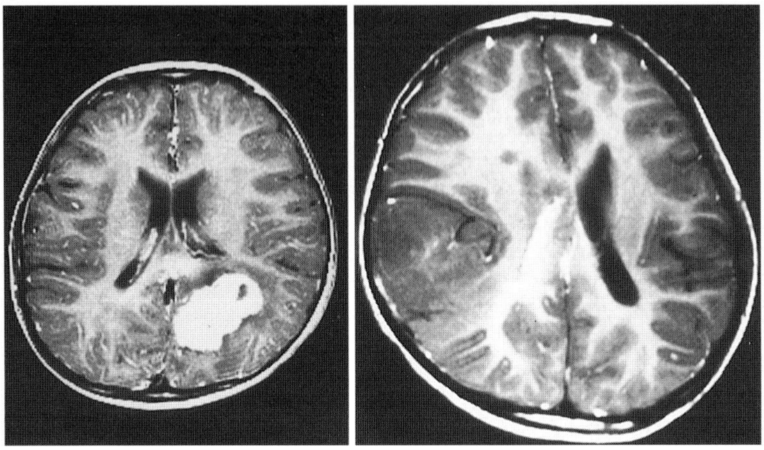

Fig. 1. a T_1-weighted MRI of a 3-year-old girl showing an enhancing lesion (ependymoma) with clear margins in the left occipital lobe. Peritumoral edema is not demonstrated. **b** T_1-weighted MRI of a 9-year-old girl showing a large lesion (glioblastoma) with relatively clear margins in the left parietal lobe. Peritumoral edema is not remarkable.

Histologic, Immunohistochemical and Ultrastructural Findings

Histologic examination showed 10 differentiated gliomas (8 astrocytomas, 1 ependymoma, 1 oligodendroglioma), 10 poorly differentiated gliomas (5 astrocytic, 2 oligodendroglial, 1 ependymal, 2 undifferentiated) and 5 other gliomas (2 giant-cell glioblastomas, 1 glioblastoma, 1 pleomorphic xanthoastrocytoma, 1 gliosarcoma). Most tumor cells were homogeneous but polymorphism was found in some tumors. Glial fibrillary acidic protein (GFAP)-positive cells were detected by immunohistochemistry in relation to the degree of tumor differentiation (fig. 2a–c). Ependymal differentiation of tumor cells was found by ultrastructural studies (fig. 2d).

Differentiated gliomas of the diffuse type with an unclear margin, as found in adults, were encountered infrequently. Most malignant gliomas were composed of poorly differentiated tumor cells, although glial differentiation was detected by immunohistochemistry and electron microscopy. These malignant tumors were expansive, less infiltrative than in adults, and the tumor margins were frequently

---

Fig. 2. a Differentiated glioma (astrocytoma grade 2). HE. ×135. **b** Poorly differentiated glioma composed of small round cells. HE. ×135. **c** Poorly differentiated glioma (astrocytic) with GFAP-positive cells. Immunostaining for GFAP. ×530. **d** Electron microscopy of poorly differentiated glioma (ependymal) showing junctional complex and microvilli. ×26,600.

2a 2b

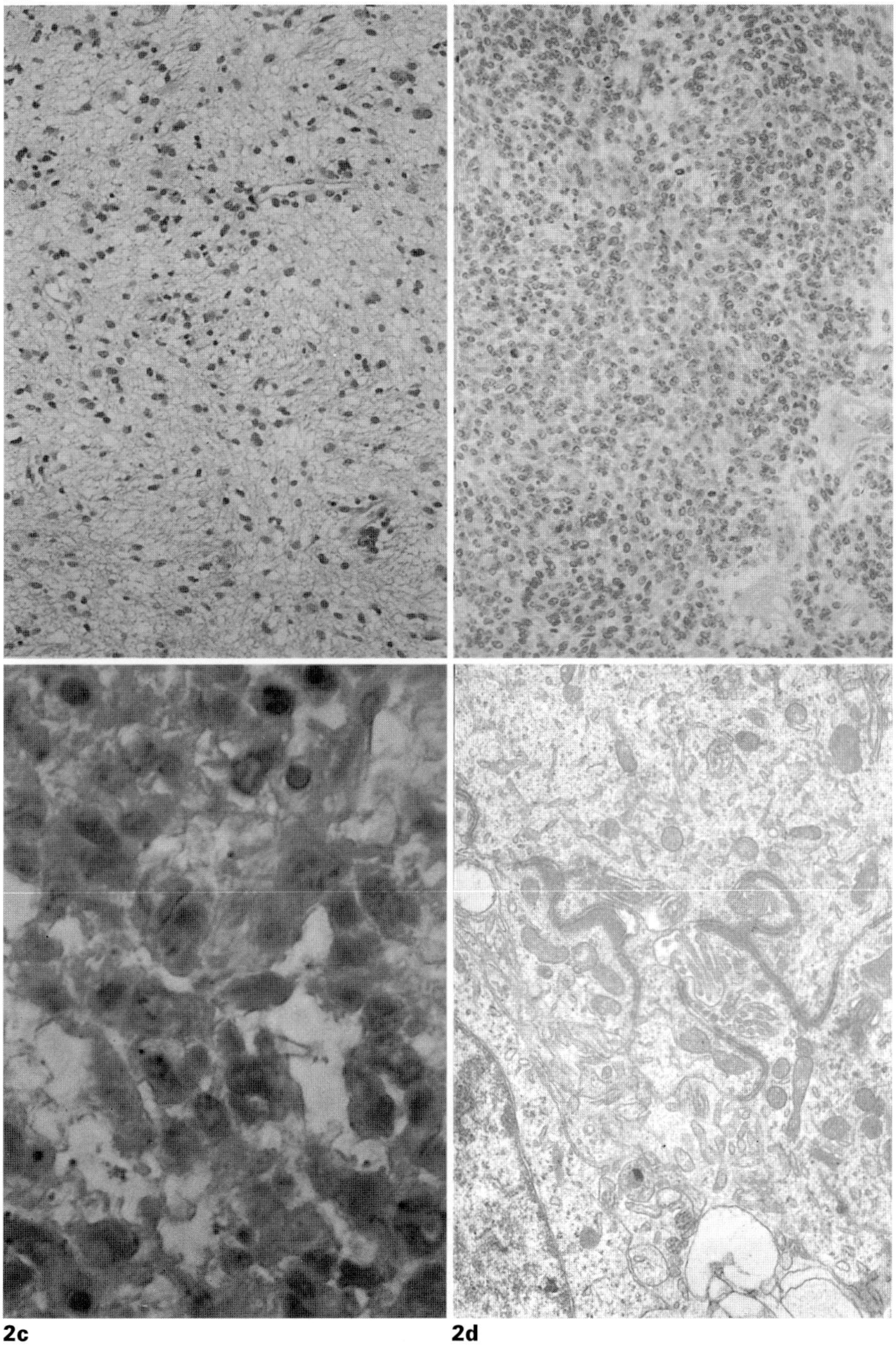

2c 2d

clear. Total surgical removal was possible in some cases as previously reported [8]. Heterogeneity and polymorphism were found in the giant-cell glioblastomas and the xanthoastrocytoma.

Autopsy Findings

The original tumors in the autopsy cases were 5 poorly differentiated, 2 differentiated and 2 other gliomas. Anaplastic or undifferentiated changes were found in 6 tumors (fig. 3a–c) and tumor dissemination and/or metastasis was seen in 7 cases. However, tumor infiltration was not extensive and clear tumor margins were found in some cases (fig. 3d).

Case Reports of Radiosurgery

Two patients with differentiated gliomas were treated by radiosurgery (Gamma Knife) to reduce radiation injuries to the developing cerebral hemispheres.

Case 1. An 8-year-old girl presented with focal seizures. CT revealed a high-density lesion with cystic components in the left occipital lobe. Stereotactic biopsy was performed and the tumor was treated by radiosurgery using a Gamma Knife with 12 Gy at the 40% isodose (fig. 4a). Follow-up neuroimaging studies showed increased size of the tumor (fig. 4b). Near total removal of the tumor was performed 6 months after radiosurgery and histologic examination revealed extensive necrosis of the tumor (astrocytoma grade 2) and thickening of vascular walls (fig. 4c). Anaplastic changes were not observed. The patient received 30 Gy of conventional irradiation following surgical removal and is well, with no recurrence at 5 years.

Case 2. A 3-year-old girl presented with generalized seizures. CT showed a large calcified mass in the left occipital lobe. Following partial removal of the tumor (ependymoma), radiosurgery was performed. The tumor was covered with 9 Gy in the 30% isodose. Near total removal of the tumor was performed at 9 months after radiosurgery, because of the formation of a large cyst (fig. 5a). Surgical specimens showed extensive necrosis of the tumor without anaplastic change (fig. 5b, c). The patient is well without recurrence at 4 years.

Discussion

Pathobiologic characteristics of gliomas in children differ from those in adults. In this series, seizures occurred in 50% of the patients. Seizures at presentation have been reported to have an increased chance of a good prognosis [9].

Fig. 3. a Autopsy specimen from the patient with differentiated glioma shown in figure 2a demonstrating anaplastic changes of the original tumor. HE. × 55. **b** Differentiated glioma (astrocytoma grade 2) at the tumor of surgical resection. HE. × 135. **c** Autopsy specimen showing lack of differentiation in the original tumor. HE. × 135. **d** Autopsy specimen from a patient with giant-cell glioblastoma. The tumor margin is well demarcated and tumor cell infiltration into the surrounding brain is not observed in this area. HE. × 55.

a b

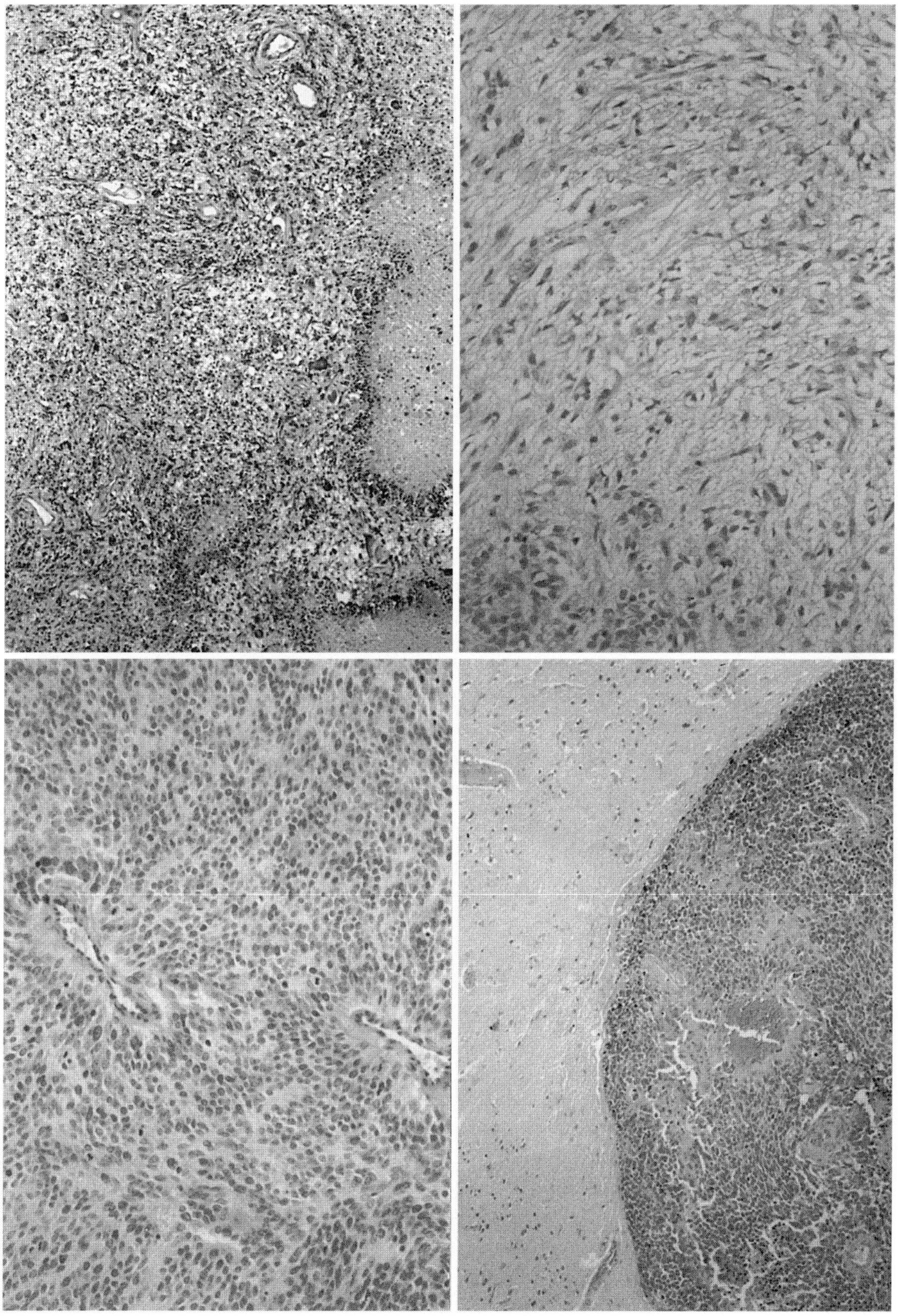

c d

a b c

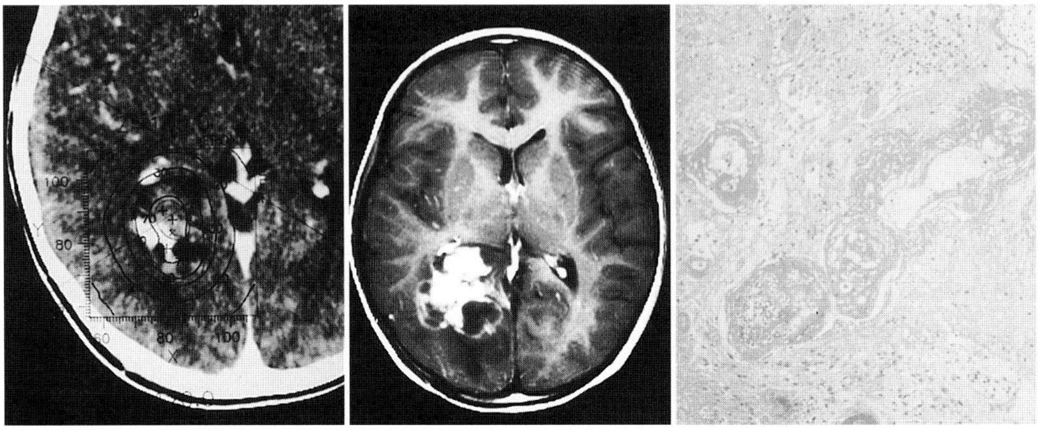

Fig. 4. **a** CT scan during Gamma Knife surgery. The tumor (astrocytoma grade 2) was treated with a 40% isodose of 12 Gy. **b** T_1-weighted MRI 6 months after radiosurgery showing increased size of the tumor. **c** Surgical specimen demonstrating extensive necrosis of the tumor and thickening of vascular walls. HE. × 50.

a b c

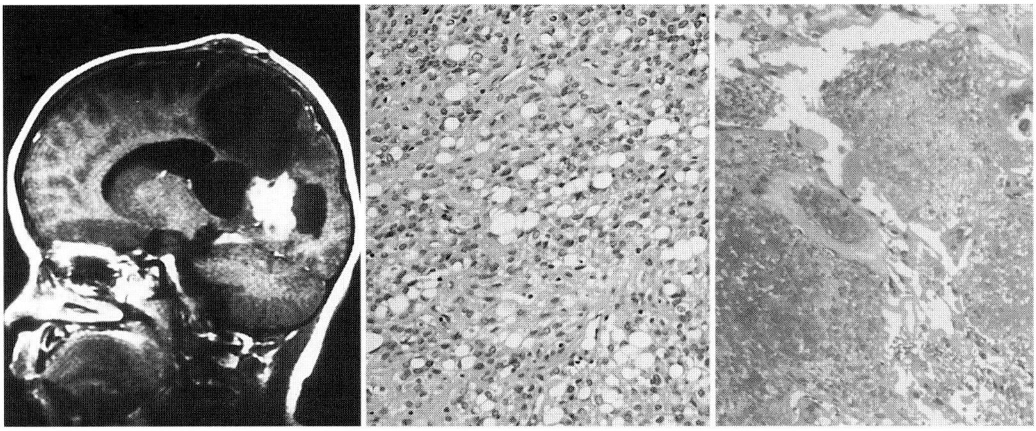

Fig. 5. **a** T_1-weighted MRI 9 months after radiosurgery showing decreased size of the tumor and large cyst formation. **b** Histologic diagnosis, including ultrastructural investigation, was ependymoma at the time of the first operation. HE. × 125. **c** Surgical specimen obtained 9 months after radiosurgery demonstrating extensive necrosis of the tumor. HE. × 125.

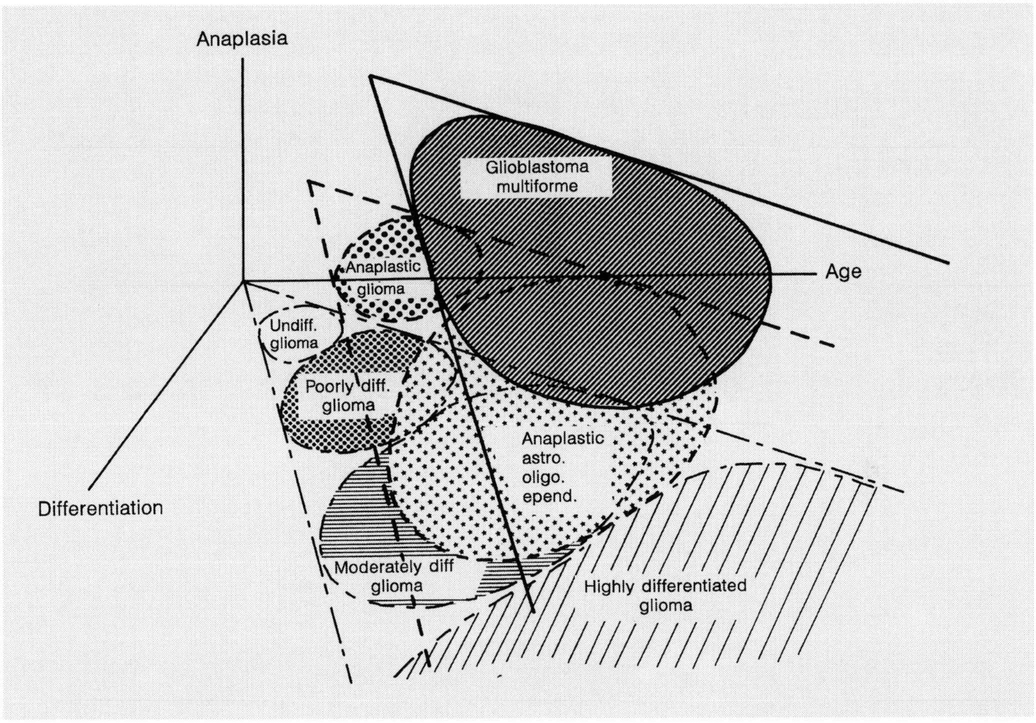

Fig. 6. Schematic representation of the relationships between differentiation, anaplasia and patient age in gliomas.

Not only the tumor site but also the biologic features of the surrounding brain may influence clinical manifestations. Neuroimaging studies showed relatively clear margins in most tumors and only slight peritumoral edema. Cysts and/or calcification were present in 37.5% of tumors, and these were usually benign (differentiated) gliomas, as previously reported [9]. In adult patients, on the other hand, 79 out of 100 recent gliomas were in the cerebral hemispheres, and neuroimaging studies showed irregular margins and perifocal edema in most instances, especially in recurrent cases. There were 25 differentiated tumors, 3 poorly differentiated and 72 anaplastic or glioblastomatous.

We classified the childhood gliomas into three groups on the basis of histologic, immunohistochemical and ultrastructural findings: differentiated, poorly differentiated and others. Differentiated gliomas of the diffuse type with an unclear margin, as found in adults, were rarely encountered. Most malignant gliomas were composed of poorly differentiated tumor cells, although glial differentiation was detected by immunohistochemistry and electron microscopy. These malignant tumors were expansive, less infiltrative than in adults and the tumor margins were

a b c

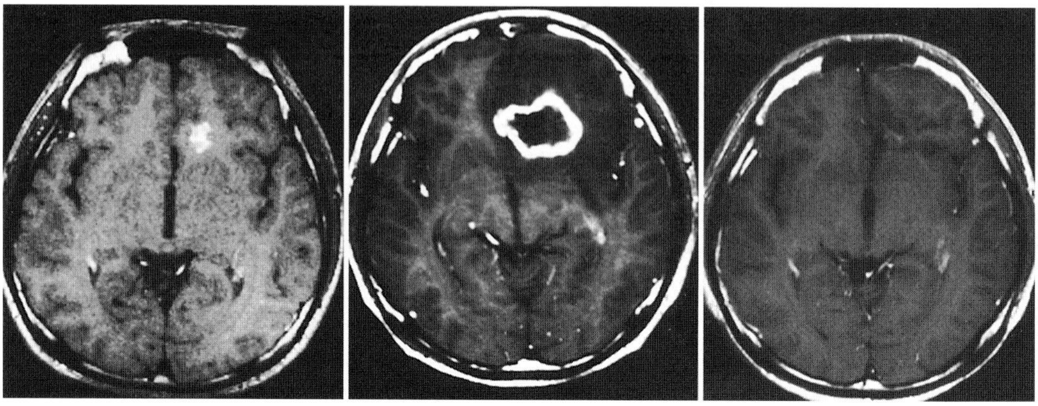

Fig. 7. **a** T_1-weighted MRI of a 15-year-old boy with epilepsy showing an enhancing lesion in the left frontal lobe. The lesion was treated by a Gamma Knife with a 50% isodose of 23 Gy. **b** T_1-weighted MRI 5 months after radiosurgery revealed an increase in the size of the lesion and peritumoral edema. **c** T_1-weighted MRI 12 months later showed a decrease in the size of the original lesion and disappearance of the peritumoral edema.

frequently clear. Total surgical removal was possible in some cases as previously reported [8]. Heterogeneity and polymorphism were found in the giant-cell glioblastomas and the xanthoastrocytoma. The latter is well known as a benign tumor with clear margins [4], and giant-cell glioblastomas have also been shown to have clear margins at autopsy [3]. The relationships between tumor differentiation, anaplasia and patient age are demonstrated in figure 6. Biologic characteristics of gliomas in children may correspond to the neuroimaging findings of relatively clear tumor margins and less to the extent of peritumoral edema. Tumor progression appeared as dissemination and/or metastasis in 77.8% of the autopsy cases.

From the pathobiology of these gliomas, total resection of differentiated gliomas is recommended, and conventional radiotherapy is not recommended for hemispheric, low-grade gliomas in children [6]. Radiosurgery may have a role as a treatment option for differentiated gliomas and may theoretically decrease radiation damage to surrounding brain [10–13]. Small residual tumors following surgery may also be good candidates for radiosurgery. We treated 2 patients with differentiated gliomas with a Gamma Knife. Although surgical removal of the tumor was required in both patients secondary to increasing mass following radiosurgery, surgical specimens showed extensive necrosis of the tumors. No recurrence and no radiation damage to surrounding brain have been recognized to date, although the follow-up period is still short. In case 1, the size of the tumor might have descreased in the ensuing several months even without surgical resection [14]. We experienced one such case involving a calcified lesion in the frontal lobe. Although the histology of the lesion was not verified, the mass increased markedly 5 months after radiosurgery, but decreased 2 months later. Shrinkage of the original lesion was obtained 12 months later (fig. 7). In contrast, cyst formation, as observed in case 2, must be resected because cysts usually increase in size, as shown in acoustic neuromas treated by radiosurgery.

Multidisciplinary treatment should be considered for poorly differentiated gliomas, because of tumor dissemination and metastasis. However, these tumors have less infiltrative potential and relatively clear margins. Radiosurgery may have a role at least to decrease the risk of radiation injury to developing brain [7, 10]. For other infiltrative or diffuse gliomas, infrequent in children, fractionated radiosurgery may be considered as a part of multidisciplinary treatment [15].

In conclusion, gliomas of the cerebral hemisphere in children have different pathobiologic characteristics to those in adults. Poorly differentiated (malignant) gliomas accounted for half the mortality.

References

1 Matson DD: Neurosurgery of Infancy and Childhood, Springfield, Thomas, 1969.

2 Cohen ME, Duffner PK: Brain Tumors in Children: Principles, Diagnosis and Treatment. New York, Raven Press, 1984.

3 Rubinstein LJ: Tumors of the Central Nervous System. Washington, AFIP, 1972.

4 Russell DS, Rubinstein LJ: Pathology of Tumours of the Nervous System, London, Arnold, 1989.

5 Pollack IF, Claassen D, Al-Shboul Q, Janosky JE; Deutsch M: Low-grade gliomas of the cerebral hemispheres in children: An analysis of 71 cases. J Neurosurg 1995;82:536–547.

6 Jenkin D, Greenberg M, Hoffman H, Hendrick B, Humphreys R, Vatter A: Brain tumors in children: Long-term survival after radiation treatment. Int J Radiat Oncol Biol Phys 1995;31:445–451.

7 Inoue HK, Nakamura M, Ono N, Kawashima Y, Hirato M, Ohye C: Long-term clinical effects of radiation therapy for primitive gliomas and medulloblastomas: A role of radiosurgery. Stereotact Funct Neurosurg 1993;61(suppl 1):51–58.

8 Inoue HK, Kunimine H, Zama A, Ono N, Nakamura M: Clinical pathology of primitive gliomas in the cerebrum. Acta Neurochir (Wien) 1986;81:94–99.

9 Shady JA, Black PM, Kupsky WJ, Tarbell NJ, Scott RM, Leong T, Holmes G: Seizures in children with supratentorial astroglial neoplasms. Pediatr Neurosurg 1994;21:23–30.

10 Inoue HK, Kohga H, Nakamura M, Ono N, Kakegawa T, Hirato M, Ohye C, Shibazaki T, Andou Y: Long-term follow-up study of conventional irradiation for brain tumors in children: A role for radiosurgery. Acta Neurochir (Wien) 1994;62(suppl):83–87.

11 Marchese MJ, Chang CH: Malignant astrocytic gliomas in children. Cancer 1990;65:2771–2778.

12 Kestle JR, Hoffman HJ, Mock AR: Moyamoya phenomenon after radiation for optic glioma. J Neurosurg 1993;79:32–35.

13 Voges J, Sturm V, Berthold F, Pastyr O, Schlegel W, Lorenz WJ: Interstitial irradiation of cerebral gliomas in childhood by permanently implanted 125-iodine – Preliminary results. Klin Pädiatr 1990;202:270–274.

14 Wowra B, Schmitt HP, Sturm V: Incidence of late radiation necrosis with transient mass effect after interstitial low dose rate radiotherapy for cerebral gliomas. Acta Neurochir (Wien) 1989;99:104–108.

15 Inoue HK, Hayashi S, Ishihara J, Horikoshi S, Zama A, Hirato M, Shibazaki T, Andou Y, Ohye C: Fractionated Gamma Knife surgery for malignant glioma: Neurobiological effects and FDG-PET studies. Stereotact Funct Neurosurg 1995;64(suppl 1):249–257.

Proc 7th Int Meeting Leksell Gamma Knife® Society,
Island of Lana'i, Hawaii, November 1995
Stereotact Funct Neurosurg 1996;66(suppl 1):288–295

Stereotactic and Functional Neurosurgery

Comparison between Adult and Pediatric Arteriovenous Malformations Treated by Gamma Knife Radiosurgery

T. Tanaka, T. Kobayashi, Y. Kida, H. Oyama, M. Niwa

Department of Neurosurgery, Komaki City Hospital, Komaki, Japan

Key Words

Gamma Knife · Radiosurgery · Arteriovenous malformation · Children · Pediatric

Abstract

More than 290 cases of cerebral arteriovenous malformation have been treated at our hospital by Gamma Knife radiosurgery since May 1991, of which 99 were followed with angiography for 1 year or more. The results from adult and pediatric age groups were compared. There were 70 adults and 23 children. Previous hemorrhage had occurred in 73.7% of the adults and 91.3% of the children. The mean volume of the nidus was similar in both groups: 4.2 cm^3 in adults and 4.8 cm^3 in children. In both groups approximately 70% of the cases fell into Spetzler and Martin grade III. The mean margin dose was 20.0 Gy in the adults and 20.5 Gy in the children. Complete nidus occlusion at 1 year occurred in 45% of the adults and 74% of the children. The rates at 2 years were 81 and 94%, respectively. Complications occurred only in adults and consisted of 2 rebleeds, 1 radiation edema and 1 radiation necrosis. Gamma Knife radiosurgery is considered to be safer and have a higher success rate in children than in adults.

Introduction

There have been many reports about radiosurgery treatment of cerebral arteriovenous malformations (AVMs) since Steiner et al. [1] treated the first patient in 1972 [2–7].

KARGER

E-Mail karger@karger.ch
Fax + 41 61 306 12 34
http://www.karger.ch

1011–6125/96/0665–0288$10.00/0

Takayuki Tanaka, MD
Department of Neurosurgery
Komaki City Hospital
Komaki 485 (Japan)

Table 1. Location of AVM

	Adults	Children
Thalamus	15	6
Basal ganglia	13	3
Frontal lobe	8	1
Temporal lobe	8	1
Parietal lobe	8	4
Occipital lobe	10	4
Other	19	4

A total of 290 cases with AVM have been treated with the Gamma Knife at our hospital between May 1991 and September 1994. Of these, 99 have been followed with angiography for at least 1 year. Some of the patients were adults, some children. A comparison of these two groups is the subject of this report.

Materials and Methods

The 99 patients with AVM were treated by Gamma Knife radiosurgery between May 1991 and September 1994. In 1995, they underwent follow-up angiography, undertaken at least 1 year after treatment. There were 76 adults and 23 children. The age range was 17–70 years (mean 33.3) for the adults and 2–15 years (mean 11.5) for the children.

Results

AVM Characteristics

The locations are specified in table 1. The mean diameter of the nidus was 4.9–38 mm in the adults (mean 17.6 mm) and 8.8–33.3 mm in the children (mean 18.2 mm). The mean volume of the nidus was 4.2 cm^3 in the adults and 4.8 cm^3 in the children.

Clinical Characteristics

Intracerebral hemorrhage had occurred in 56 (73.7%) of the adults and 21 (91.3%) of the children. Of the adults, 19 (25%) had received previous microsurgery, while 5 of the children (22%) had received this treatment. Seven adults (10%) had received previous endovascular embolization as opposed to none of the children. Nine of the adults (12%) had required surgery to relieve cerebrospinal fluid pressure (ventricular drainage or ventriculoperitoneal shunt). On the

Table 2. AVM grade according to Spetzler and Martin [8]

	I	II	III	IV	V
Adults	2	16	50 (66%)	2	6
Children	0	5	17 (74%)	1	0

Table 3. Complete obliteration rates for AVMs

	1 year after treatment	2 years after treatment
Adults	45% (27/60)	81% (42/52)
Children	74% (14/19)	95% (20/21)
Total	52% (41/79)	85% (62/73)

Table 4. Complete AVM obliteration rate related to Spetzler and Martin grade

	Grade	1 year after treatment	2 years after treatment
Adults	II	45% (5/11)	82% (9/11)
	III	44% (19/43)	85% (28/33)
Children	II	75% (3/4)	80% (4/5)
	III	73% (11/15)	100% (16/16)

other hand 8 of the children (35%) had required this form of treatment. One case in each group had received external-beam radiotherapy.

The commonest clinical grading was Spetzler grade III [8], accounting for about 70% of all cases in each group (table 2).

Gamma Knife Treatment

The method used was as previously reported [3, 9]. The mean margin dose was 20.0 Gy in adults and 20.5 Gy in children. The mean maximum dose was 36.8 Gy in both groups. The complete occlusion rate in the adults at 1 year was 45% and in the children 74%. The complete occlusion rate in the adults at 2 years was 81% and in the children, 95% (table 3). The obliteration rate classified according to the Spetzler and Martin classification system is given in table 4. The

Table 5. Complete obliteration rate of AVMs related to size

	Mean diameter	1 year after treatment	2 years after treatment
Adults	<1 cm	88% (7/8)	100% (8/8)
	1–2 cm	47% (16/34)	90% (26/29)
	2–3 cm	29% (4/14)	54% (7/13)
	⩾3 cm	0% (0/4)	50% (1/2)
Children	<1 cm	100% (2/2)	100% (2/2)
	1–2 cm	100% (11/11)	92% (12/13)
	2–3 cm	20% (1/5)	84% (5/6)
	≥3 cm	0% (0/1)	50% (1/2)

obliteration rate was inversely proportional to the size of the malformation (table 5). Complications only occurred in adults. There were 2 post-treatment hemorrhages, 1 radiation-induced edema and 1 radionecrosis.

Illustrative Cases

Case 1 (fig. 1). This 10-year-old boy suffered an intraventricular hemorrhage from an AVM fed by an artery from the left posterior cerebral artery. He was treated with radiosurgery. The maximum dose was 41 Gy and the margin dose was 20 Gy. The nidus had disappeared 12 months after treatment.

Case 2 (fig. 2). This 40-year-old man presented with an epileptic seizure. There was a left parietal AVM fed from the middle cerebral artery. The maximum radiosurgery dose was 40 Gy and the margin dose was 20 Gy. After 12 months, about 90% of the nidus had disappeared, and after 2 years it was completely obliterated.

Discussion

Since the original report of Steiner et al. [1], many good results following Gamma Knife radiosurgery have been reported [2–7]. However, there is little information comparing the results in adults and children.

It has been reported that the rate of intracranial hemorrhage is higher in children than in adults [10, 11]. The current study supports this contention. Yasargil [12] and Mori et al. [13] have reported that many large AVMs are found in children. This was not the case in the present series, though this may be the result of cases selection.

a

b

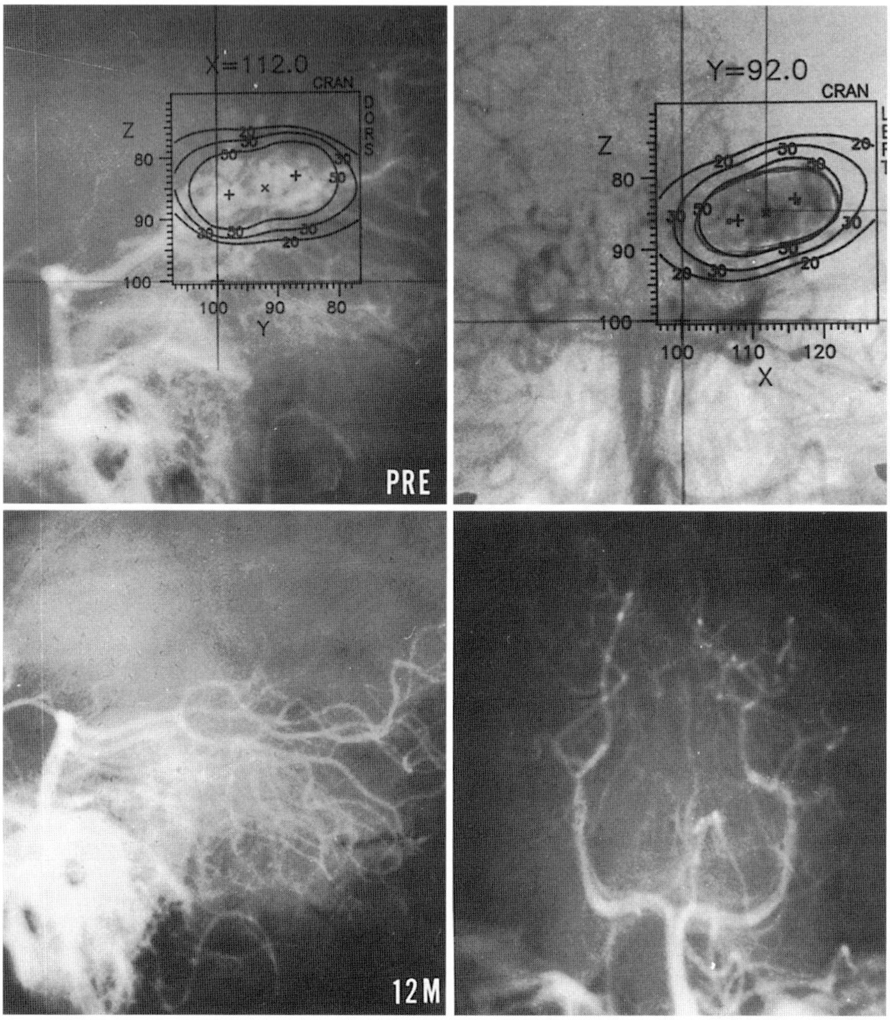

Fig. 1. Angiography of case 1. **a** Anteroposterior and lateral views before radiosurgery, with isodose curves. **b** The nidus had disappeared 12 months after radiosurgery.

Hui et al. [14] have stated that combined therapy with microsurgery, endovascular embolization and radiosurgery is superior to any single modality. In this series, 7 of the adults and none of the children had received preradiosurgery embolization, probably due to the difficulties encountered when performing embolization for many hours under local anesthesia in children. Moreover, the

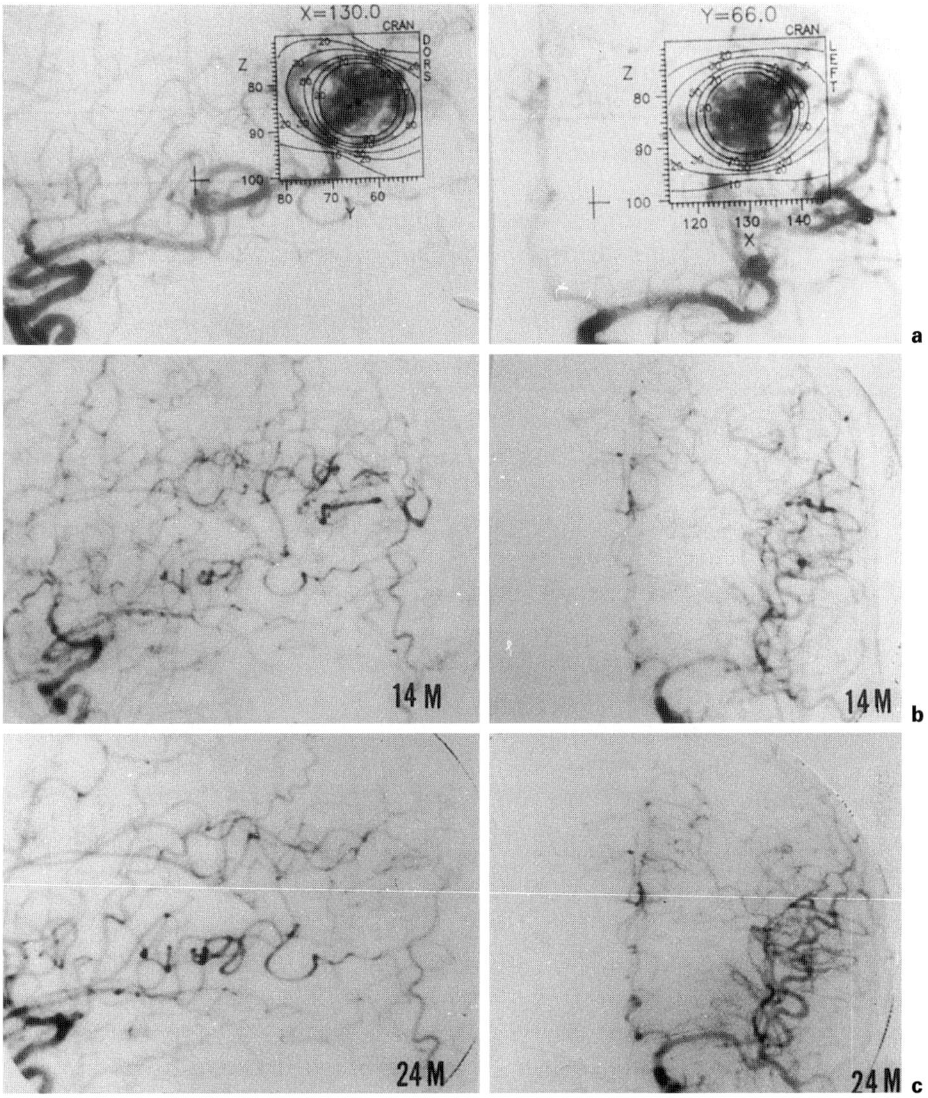

Fig. 2. Angiography of case 2. **a** Anteroposterior and lateral views before radiosurgery, with isodose curves. **b** About 90% of the nidus has disappeared after 14 months. **c** Total obliteration 24 months after treatment.

problems are compounded by the size and fragility of blood vessels in children. Nonetheless, Wisoff and Berenstein [15] have reported the embolization of pediatric AVMs and stated that there was some indication for the method in this age group, particularly for those with larger AVMs.

Maximum and minimum doses were determined using the 3% risk curve of Flickinger et al. [16, 17], taking the AVM location into account as well. The dose did not differ between the adults and the children. Moreover, the doses were very similar to those reported by Lunsford et al. [3], who used a mean margin dose of 21 Gy. Steiner et al. [6] reported a complete obliteration rate of 33.7–39.5% at 1 year and 79–86.5% at 2 years. Lunsford et al. [3] reported an 80% complete obliteration rate at 2 years. Steiner et al. [6] reported that AVMs were more likely to occlude in children than in adults. However, they have no detailed account of the differences in size, dose and obliteration rates in the two groups.

In our material, the obliteration rate in children both at 1 and 2 years was higher than in adults. This could not be related to lesion volume or radiation dose, which were similar for both groups. Nor did it seem to be related to the Spetzler and Martin grade or the size of the lesion. The increased rate of obliteration was observed in all groups except AVMs of 30 mm diameter or more, of which there are too few to draw any valid conclusion. Nonetheless, in both adults and children, AVMs greater than 2 cm diameter had a noticeably lower obliteration rate than smaller lesions.

Steiner et al. [6] reported 3% radiation necrosis after Gamma Knife radiosurgery for AVMs and Lunsford et al. [3] reported 4%. Friedman et al. [18] found a rate of 2.5% using a linear accelerator. In their material, radiation damage was not related to either lesion volume or radiation dose. We used the Flickinger 3% risk curve to determine the dose and observed 1 adult patient (2.6%) with radionecrosis.

Steiner et al. [7] reported an overall rebleed rate of 3.3%. In our series, the rebleed rate, which was restricted to adults, was 2.6%, in keeping with the natural rebleeding rate of these lesions of 2.2–4% [19, 20].

In conclusion, pediatric AVMs may be more likely to respond to radiosurgery by occlusion than those in adults, and there seem to to be fewer complications after radiosurgery in the pediatric age group.

References

1 Steiner L, Leksell L, Greitz T, Forster DMC, Backlund EO: Stereotactic radiosurgery for cerebral arteriovenous malformation: Report of a case. Acta Chir Scand 1972;138:459–464.

2 Altschuler EM, Lunsford LD, Coffey RJ, Bissonette DJ, Flickinger JC: Gamma Knife radiosurgery for intracranial arteriovenous malformations in childhood and adolescence. Pediatr Neurosci 1989; 15:53–61.

3 Lunsford LD, Kondziolka D, Flickinger JC, Bissonette DJ, Jugreis CA, Maitz AH, Horton JA, Coffey RJ: Stereotactic radiosurgery for arteriovenous malformations of the brain. J Neurosurg 1991;75:512–524.
4 Ogilvy CS: Radiation therapy for arteriovenous malformations: A review. Neurosurgery 1990;26: 725–735.
5 Pollock BE, Lunsford LD, Kondziolka D, Maitz AH, Flickinger JC: Patient outcomes after stereotactic radiosurgery for 'operable' arteriovenous malformations. Neurosurgery 1994;35:1–8.
6 Steiner L, Linquist C, Steiner M: Radiosurgery with focused gamma-beam irradiation in children; in Edwards M, Hoffman H (eds): Cerebral Vascular Diseases in Children and Adolescents. Baltimore, Williams & Wilkins, 1989, vol 9, pp 367–388.
7 Steiner L, Lindquist C, Steiner M: Radiosurgery; in Symon L (ed): Advances and Technical Standards in Neurosurgery. Berlin, Springer, 1992, vol 19, pp 40–57.
8 Spetzler RF, Martin NA: A proposed grading system for arteriovenous malformations. J Neurosurg 1986;65:476–483.
9 Tanaka T, Kobayashi T, Kida Y: Gamma Knife treatment for arteriovenous malformations of the brain. Surg Cerebr Stroke (Tokyo) 1992;20:355–358.
10 Fong D, Chan S: Arteriovenous malformations in children. Child Nerv Syst 1988;4:199–203.
11 Kondziolka D, Humphreys RP, Hoffman HJ, Hendrick EB, Drake JM: Arteriovenous malformations of brain in children: A forty year experience. Can J Neurol Sci 1992;19:40–45.
12 Yasargil MG: Children with AVM; in Yasargil MG (ed): Microneurosurgery. Stuttgart, Thieme, 1992, vol 4, pp 393–396.
13 Mori K, Murata T, Hashimoto N, Handa H: Clinical analysis of arteriovenous malformation in children. Child Brain 1980;6:13–25.
14 Hui F, Lasjaunias P: Interventional neuroradiology in the management of pediatric cerebral arteriovenous malformations: Illustrative study of three case reports. Ann Acad Med Singapore 1993;22: 811–817.
15 Wisoff JH, Berenstein A: Interventional neuroradiology; in Edwards M, Hoffman H (eds): Cerebral vascular diseases in children and adolescents. Baltimore, Williams & Wilkins, 1989, pp 139–157.
16 Flickinger JC: An integrated logistic formula for prediction of complications from radiosurgery. Int Radiat Oncol Biol Phys 1989;17:879–885.
17 Flickinger JC, Lunsford LD, Kondziolka D: Dose-volume considerations in radiosurgery. Stereotact Funct Neurosurg 1991;57:99–105.
18 Friedman WA, Bova FJ: Linear accelerator radiosurgery for arteriovenous malformations. J Neurosurg 1992;77:832–841.
19 Brown RD, Wiebers DO, Forbes G, O'Fallon WM, Piepgras DG, Marsh WR, Maciunas RJ: The natural history of unruptured intracranial arteriovenous malformations. J Neurosurg 1988;68:352–357.
20 Ondra SL, Troupp H, George ED, Schwab K: The natural history of symptomatic arteriovenous malformations of the brain: A 24 year follow-up assessment. J Neurosurg 1991;73:387–391.

Proc 7th Int Meeting Leksell Gamma Knife® Society,
Island of Lana'i, Hawaii, November 1995
Stereotact Funct Neurosurg 1996;66(suppl 1):296–301

Stereotactic and Functional Neurosurgery

The Open Gamma Knife Center Concept

S.J. Goetsch, T. Hardy, D. Hodgens, A. Lizarraras, K. Ott, C. Scharfen, H. Tung

San Diego Gamma Knife Center, La Jolla, Calif., USA

Key Words
Gamma Knife · Radiosurgery · Open center · Protocols · Credentials · Certification

Abstract
A freestanding Gamma Knife radiosurgery center has been open for just over 1 year in La Jolla, Calif., USA, located in the grounds of a medium-sized community hospital. The center employs a full-time medical physicist and neurosurgical nurse together with clerical personnel. The neurosurgeons and radiation oncologists are drawn from the entire community and bill their fees separately. Written protocols for each indication to be treated govern patient eligibility and suggested treatment algorithms. Additionally, each patient to be treated is presented in conference, and a treatment strategy (i.e., radiosurgery, craniotomy, conventional radiation therapy) is decided. Twenty new physicians and physicists have begun training to use the Gamma Knife in the first year. Certification must be achieved before a clinician can be the physician of record.

Introduction

A freestanding radiosurgery center operating the Leksell Model U Gamma Knife was opened in a major North American metropolitan center in October 1994. The center is privately owned and located in a medical office building adjoining a major community hospital (Scripps Memorial Hospital, La Jolla, Calif., USA). Gamma Knife radiosurgery patients receive computerized tomography (CT), magnetic resonance imaging (MRI) and/or angiography studies through the hospital radiology center. The frame is situated, the patient is held while planning

KARGER
E-Mail karger@karger.ch
Fax + 41 61 306 12 34
http://www.karger.ch

1011–6125/96/0665–0296$10.00/0

Steven J. Goetsch, PhD
San Diego Gamma Knife Center
9834 Genesee Avenue, Suite 100
La Jolla, CA 92037 (USA)

is performed, and the treatment is carried out within the San Diego Gamma Knife Center (SDGKC). The patient is subsequently admitted to the hospital for overnight observation.

A linear-accelerator-based radiosurgery program had been in operation at this site for 4 years prior to the opening of the Gamma Knife Center. About 100 cases had been treated during its period of use, providing useful experience for some of the original practitioners. It is rarely used since the opening of the SDGKC.

The SDGKC is a limited partnership, not owned by any of the physicians who practice there. The center charges a global fee which bundles the radiological imaging examinations and the overnight hospital observation. Each physician bills his or her professional fee separately.

The personnel at the center include a full-time Director of Medical Physics and a neurosurgical nurse. The physicist had 4 years experience at a major linear-accelerator-based radiosurgery program prior to becoming Director of Medical Physics. The nurse established a neurosurgical nursing program at this hospital and worked with many of the community neurosurgeons. A receptionist who doubles as a data entry operator and billing manager completes the SDGKC personnel.

The center was conceived as a community resource for the city of San Diego, which has a metropolitan population of about 2.5 million people, approximately 1% of the United States population. Intracranial diseases were considered to be sufficiently common to support a dedicated Gamma Knife radiosurgery unit with such a population base. Therefore, the SDGKC was conceived as an 'open' center for all interested neurosurgeons and radiation oncologists in the community, regardless of hospital or group affiliation.

Challenges of an Open Center

Most radiosurgery centers have only a few clinicians involved in treatment. This new concept proposes having many surgeons and radiation oncologists. This poses a number of problems. What candidates are appropriate for Gamma Knife radiosurgery? What should treatment strategies and doses be? How many procedures must a physician perform to attain proficiency? How many cases a year must a physician perform to retain proficiency? How are new physicians to be trained and certified? How are all physicians to be 'policed' to assure that the standards of the new center are always maintained?

A number of answers were supplied to these questions. The first four neurosurgeons and one of the two radiation oncologists attended the traditional Gamma Knife radiosurgery course sponsored by Elekta Instruments in Stockholm. One of these surgeons and the remaining radiation oncologist had treated nearly

Table 1. Patient eligibility for Gamma Knife radiosurgery of metastatic brain tumors

(1) Systemic malignancy documented by tissue diagnosis.
(2) Primary disease under control.
(3) Stereotactic brain biopsy confirmation in patients treated for primary malignancy more than 1 year previously for first evidence of recurrence, or if no tissue diagnosis of the primary.
(4) No more than three known metastatic lesions.
(5) No lesion greater in any one dimension than 3.5 cm.
(6) Karnofsky Performance Status greater than 70 (capable of independent existence).

100 patients using an early linear-accelerator-based radiosurgery technique and were familiar with stereotactic frames, and radiosurgery in particular. These six physicians became the core group, known as the Gamma Knife Committee. Power to grant certification to new members and to determine acceptable candidates for Gamma Knife radiosurgery was given to this group. The full-time medical physicist was also an ex officio member of this group.

Written documentation was given a high priority. A policy and procedure manual was developed which specified the way in which the center was to be governed. The managing partners appointed a Surgical Director and two Medical Directors who organized the committees and made clinically related decisions. Written protocols were soon devised for the following brain disorders: acoustic neuromas, arteriovenous malformations, gliomas, meningiomas, metastatic brain tumors, pineal tumors and trigeminal neuralgia. These documents specified patient eligibility (table 1), treatment paradigms and the interval of follow-up brain imaging studies. They also contained a synopsis of the current literature. The Gamma Knife Committee could overrule these protocols on a case-by-case basis for cogent reasons. Parkinson's disease, epilepsy and intractable-pain patients are not currently accepted for Gamma Knife radiosurgery, but are referred to those of our neurosurgeons who treat these disorders.

Elaborate checklists for operational procedures were also designed and implemented. Detailed physics checklists and procedures are written for everything for daily, weekly and monthly quality assurance checks and included in detailed operational protocols. Each patient is treated in accordance with strict checklists covering all physical, performance and operational details so that no inadvertent exposure can be made. Every coordinate setting is triple-checked before the patient is treated.

Table 2. Certification process for neurosurgeons

(1)	Demonstrated training and experience in stereotactic surgery.
(2)	Completion of a recognized Gamma Knife radiosurgery training course.
(3)	Board certification in neurosurgery.
(4)	Must perform six Gamma Knife radiosurgery cases under the proctoring of a senior neurosurgeon.
(5)	Certification must be voted on by Gamma Knife Committee.

Training of New Personnel

It was expected from the outset that it would be necessary to train additional physicians, physicists and nurses. Due to the number of students, it was thought to be better to begin training on site with an imported faculty, rather than try to send 10–12 people across the globe to Stockholm for training. The first Gamma Knife radiosurgery course ever held outside Stockholm was therefore conducted at Scripps Memorial Hospital in La Jolla, January 16–20, 1995. Ten students attended (all from the San Diego area) with faculty members from Stockholm, Seattle, Los Angeles and San Diego. These students have now begun bringing cases to the SDGKC and some have completed their certification. A second Gamma Knife radiosurgery course was held in La Jolla, October 2–6, 1995, for 12 more students, 10 from San Diego and 2 from outside the state (one from South America).

The SDGKC training course includes 25 contact hours for groups of one or two learners with a fully equipped Hewlett-Packard 9000 series workstation loaded with the latest version of the Leksell GammaPlan software and up to 25 practice patients. The patient cases are taken from previously treated Gamma Knife patients, with the tumor volumes erased and all shots blanked out. Students are given didactic instruction about a given tumor or disorder in the morning lectures and are then guided through several cases in the afternoon under the tutelage of a senior neurosurgeon, radiation oncologist or Elekta personnel.

Separate certification protocols were agreed upon by the original group of neurosurgeons and radiation oncologists. The paradigm for neurosurgeon training is given in table 2. Since the center opened, one neurosurgeon and two radiation oncologists have completed the certification process.

Role of the Gamma Knife Committee

The Gamma Knife Committee, consisting of the six original physicians plus the staff medical physicist, meets in open session each Wednesday evening. All neurosurgeons, radiation oncologists, neurologists, radiologists and medical physicists in the community are welcome to attend. A staff neuroradiologist from the affiliated hospital attends each meeting. As many as 20 specialists have attended these meetings. Continuing Education Units are awarded through Scripps Memorial Hospital. The meetings include case presentation, review of previous patients and additional educational activities. Each patient is presented in a forum similar to a brain tumor conference at a teaching hospital. Each patient's CT, MRI and/or angiographic films are reviewed and compared to written protocols for the indicated disorder. Some patients are recommended by the group to have surgery, some for conventional radiation therapy, some are approved for Gamma Knife radiosurgery and others are counseled to watch and wait. Patients are submitted by Gamma Knife center physicians, community physicians and by the patients themselves. Minutes are kept of these meetings and all patient treatment decisions are recorded.

Educational forums are offered to Gamma Knife center participating physicians on a regular basis. These meetings are also open to the community. SDGKC physicians and the staff physicist frequently give lectures in the community and around the United States. The SDGKC was also an anchor sponsor of the Fifth Annual UCLA Minimally Invasive Therapy of the Brain Workshop.

The Gamma Knife Committee also has the primary role in reviewing quality control and continuous quality improvement in the Gamma Knife center. Any problem cases or complications (morbidity, mortality) are brought before this committee and discussed. The Gamma Knife Committee relies heavily on the medical physicist and neurosurgical nurse to implement quality control at all levels and to maintain high standards at all times. In this sense, they are the 'police' of the SDGKC. This has not been a problem up to the time of writing.

The Gamma Knife Committee also reviews and certifies new users. Each physician must be recertified annually. Minimum requirements for continuing certification include performing at least six Gamma Knife Radiosurgery cases per year and attendance at at least one Gamma Knife Committee meeting per month.

Patient Accession

The center recently completed its first year of operation, coinciding with the treatment of patient number 100. Patients reflect a wide variety of disease indications (fig. 1) with malignant disease predominating slightly. Metastatic disease

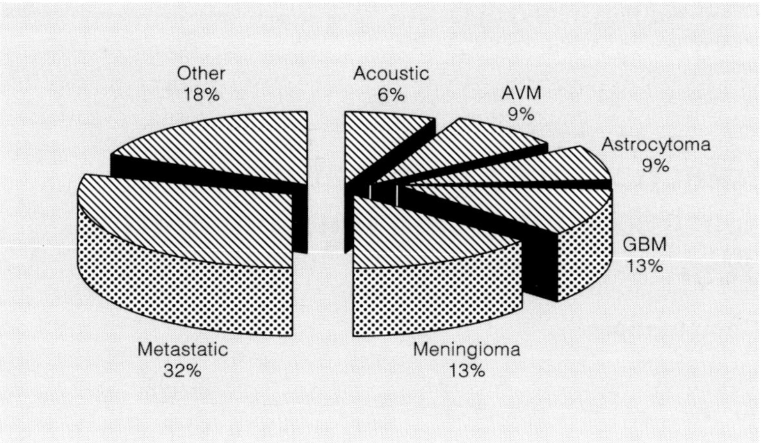

Fig. 1. Distribution of Gamma Knife patients in San Diego. AVM = Arteriovenous malformation; GBM = glioblastoma.

was the leading indication as has been reported in other radiosurgical centers. Meningiomas were the most common benign disease, slightly ahead of arteriovenous malformations.

On 10 treatment days, two patients were treated sequentially, usually with the aid of a second nurse. A physicist has been trained as a backup to the staff physicist, and has successfully treated patients in the latter's absence.

Future Developments

The center is growing rapidly, with eight certified physicians and two certified physicists. A total of 15 more physicians and two physicists are currently in training. This new neurosurgical technology has been made available to nearly every hospital in this community.

Additional open centers are being developed in London, Mexico City, and southern California. Staff at these centers will be trained at SDGKC. The latest multimedia satellite-based and Internet tele-video and tele-radiology communications equipment will be installed at each of these centers. Experience among centers can be shared and difficult cases will be discussed with trained specialists across the globe, from diverse educational and medical backgrounds. The open center concept promises to bring costly and sophisticated neurotechnology to the community hospital level.

Proc 7th Int Meeting Leksell Gamma Knife® Society,
Island of Lana'i, Hawaii, November 1995
Stereotact Funct Neurosurg 1996;66(suppl 1):302–308

Stereotactic and Functional Neurosurgery

Stereotactic Dose Computation and Plan Optimization Using the Convolution Theorem

I. Dose Computation

X. Wu, J.Y. Ting, A.M. Markoe, H.J. Landy, J.A. Fiedler, J. Russell

Department of Radiation Oncology and Department of Neurological Surgery,
University of Miami School of Medicine, Miami, Fla., USA

Key Words

Stereotactic radiosurgery · Leksell Gamma Knife · Dose computation

Abstract

With Leksell Gamma Knife stereotactic radiosurgery, the dose distribution delivered by a specific helmet can be assumed to remain as a fixed-dose distribution when the shot is moved to different locations within the predefined dose calculation matrix. The convolution theorem may be implemented to take advantage of this fact for fast dose computation and plan construction. Using this technique, the shot spatial arrangement is formulated as a convolution kernel, which is theoretically a three-dimensional multi-δ function. The dose distribution is computed by the convolution of this single-shot dose distribution with the shot convolution kernel. To determine the shot arrangement, an ideal dose distribution is generated based upon the target structure. Deconvolution is then applied to find the convolution kernel which best fits the proposed ideal dose distribution. The primary task of this presentation is to focus on and describe in detail the dose computation using the convolution theorem.

Introduction

Treatment planning for stereotactic radiosurgery often involves dose computations for plans using multiple noncoplanar radiation beams, which leads to many rotational and translational matrix transformations. Many efforts have been made toward dedicated stereotactic dose computations [1–5]. The dose computation method presented here takes advantage of a property of the Leksell

KARGER

E-Mail karger@karger.ch
Fax + 41 61 306 12 34
http://www.karger.ch

1011–6125/96/0665–0302$10.00/0

Xiaodong Wu, PhD
Department of Radiation Oncology
University of Miami School of Medicine
P.O. Box 016960
Miami, FL 33101 (USA)

Gamma Knife which allows single-shot dose distributions to be approximated as a fixed distribution, independent of shot location. This assumption holds true only within a limited region, but it is almost always applicable, since tumors treated via stereotactic radiosurgery are always small. Using this assumption, convolution theory can be applied to compute a multiple-shot dose distribution and construct the shot spatial arrangement. To perform this computation, the dose distribution for a single shot is first obtained and stored as a three-dimensional (3D) array. When the shot location is to be determined, another 3D array is generated, which is convolved with the single-shot dose array. A program capable of computing both forward and inverse 3D fast Fourier transforms is used to calculate the composite dose distribution using the convolution theorem. To configure the shot spatial arrangement, an 'ideal' dose distribution must be first constructed, based on the tumor structure and appropriate conformation criteria. If this 'ideal' dose distribution is constructed properly, the deconvolution process generates the useful shot spatial and weighting information. The shot arrangement generated by this deconvolution needs to be filtered and renormalized before it finally fits the desired conformal dose distribution. Two examples are presented to demonstrate the effectiveness of the described algorithm.

Method

Convolution

The convolution of two functions f(r) and g(r), denoted by $f(r)*g(r)$, is mathematically defined by the integral:

$$f(r)*g(r) = \int_{-\infty}^{+\infty} f(\alpha)\cdot g(r-\alpha)d\alpha \tag{1}$$

One aspect of equation (1) which will be of use in this work involves the convolution of a function f(r) with the impulse function $\delta(r - r_0)$, which is defined as follows:

$$\int_{-\infty}^{+\infty} f(r)\cdot\delta(r-r_0)\,dr = f(r_0) \tag{2}$$

As an illustration of equations (1) and (2), figure 1 shows the convolution of f(x) with g(x), assuming

$g(x) = \delta(x - 10) + \delta(x - 25) + 0.7\,\delta(x - 60)$

In this case, convolution amounts merely to 'copying' f(x) at the location of each impulse.

Dose Computation of Multiple Shots

Assuming that the dose distribution from a single shot is $D_0(x, y, z)$, and that a multiple shot arrangement S(x, y, z) can be mathematically expressed as

$$S(x, y, z) = \sum_i w_i\delta(x - x_i, y - y_i, z - z_i)$$

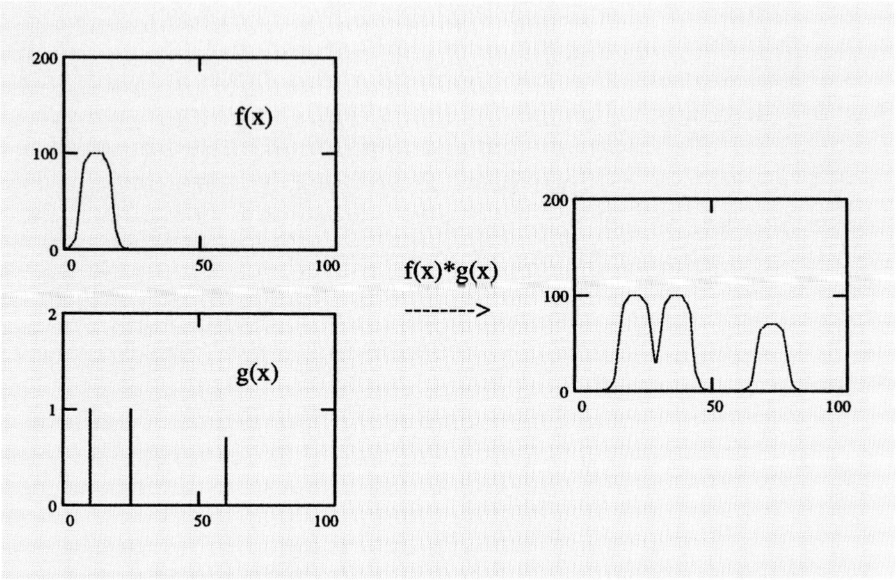

Fig. 1. Copying feature of convolution.

where w_i represents the weight of the ith shot, then the composite dose distribution D(x, y, z) from S(x, y, z) can be computed by the convolution:

$$D(x, y, z) = D_0(x, y, z) * S(x, y, z) = \sum_{l}^{L} \sum_{m}^{M} \sum_{n}^{N} D_0(l, m, n) \cdot S(x - l, y - m, z - n)$$

where L, M, N are extended array dimensions that double the original array size to avoid wraparound error.

The actual computation of the convolution is achieved using the Fourier convolution theorem:

$$D(x, y, z) = \mathcal{F}^{-1}\{\mathcal{F}[D_0(x, y, z)] \cdot \mathcal{F}[S(x, y, z)]\}$$

where $\mathcal{F}^{-1}$ and $\mathcal{F}$ are 3D inverse and forward Fourier transform operators, respectively.

Shot Configuration

Using deconvolution, a treatment plan with multiple shots can be precisely reversed, i.e., S(x, y, z) can be reconstructed by deconvolving D(x, y, z) with $D_0(x, y, z)$. This makes it possible to use deconvolution to assist a treatment plan. Based on tumor contour information and the applied conformal criteria, an 'ideal' dose distribution is constructed as DI(x, y, z). Using deconvolution, we have:

$$S(x, y, z) = \mathcal{F}^{-1}\{\mathcal{F}[DI(x,y,z)] \div \mathcal{F}[D_o(x,y,z)]\}.$$

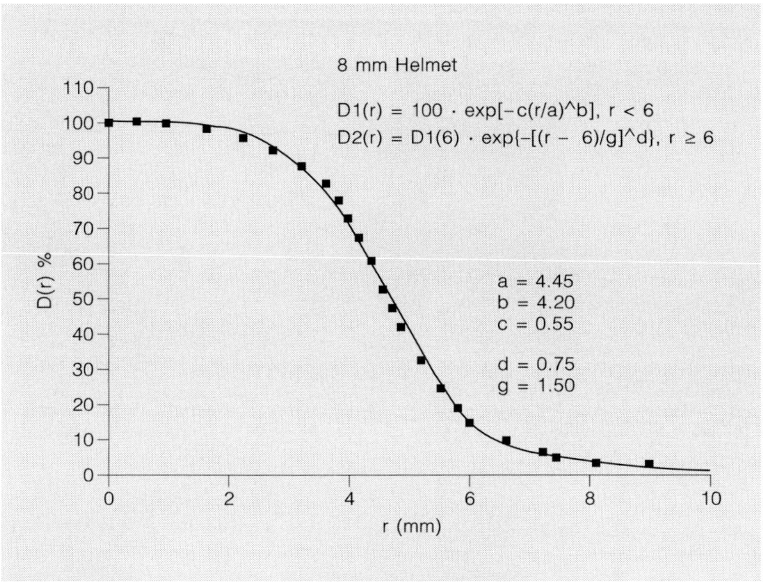

Fig. 2. Two-step radial fitting dose function for the 8-mm helmet.

The critical step in the procedure above is the construction of DI(x, y, z). Depending upon how DI(x, y, z) is specified, S(x, y, z) may contain superfluous information, or may even be completely invalid. Iteration and filtering are required to yield a practical optimized shot arrangement.

Results

Dose Computation Using Convolution Theorem

The example demonstrated here is a seven-shot (equally weighted) treatment using the 8-mm collimator helmet. The 3D dose distribution matrix for a single shot is generated using a two-step radial fitting function (fig. 2), assuming an isotropic distribution. (This is for demonstration purposes only. In reality, the method also works with anisotropic distribution.) The coordinates of each shot are listed in table 1.

The composite dose distributions from the convolution are shown in figure 3 in different x-y planes with associated z values. When the dose values calculated from the convolution method are compared with those obtained using conventional matrix summation methods, they are found to be practically identical.

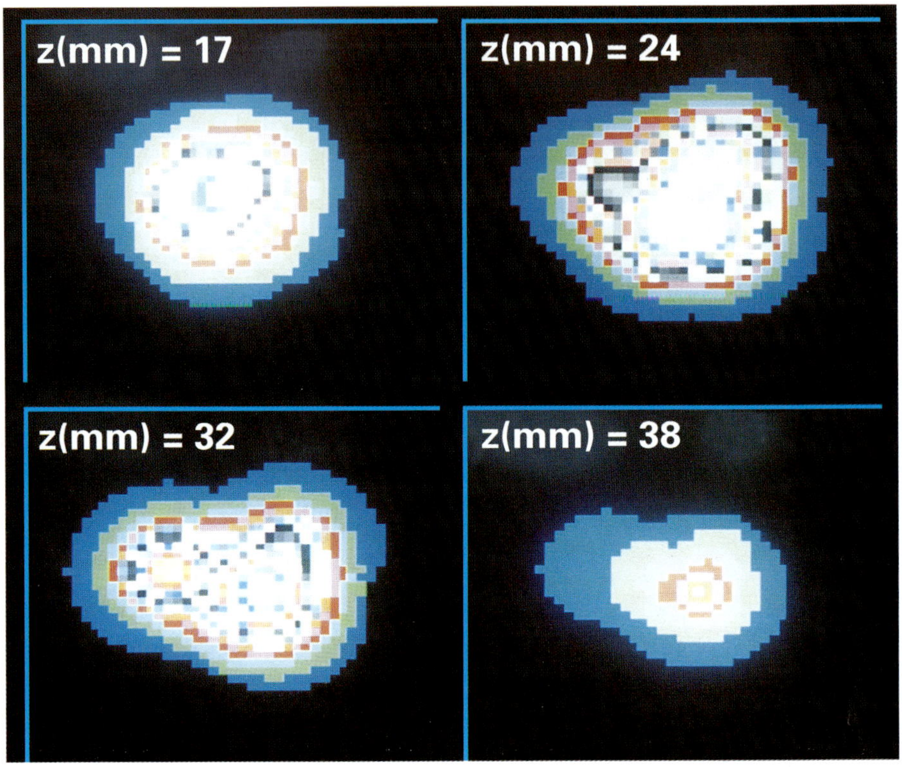

Fig. 3. Dose distributions computed by convolving $D_0(x,y,z)$ and $S(x,y,z)$.

Table 1. Shot coordinates

Shot	x, mm	y, mm	z, mm
1	8.0	3.0	16.0
2	11.0	13.0	19.0
3	5.0	16.0	14.0
4	7.0	12.0	9.0
5	14.0	9.0	10.0
6	9.0	7.0	4.0
7	14.0	15.0	13.0

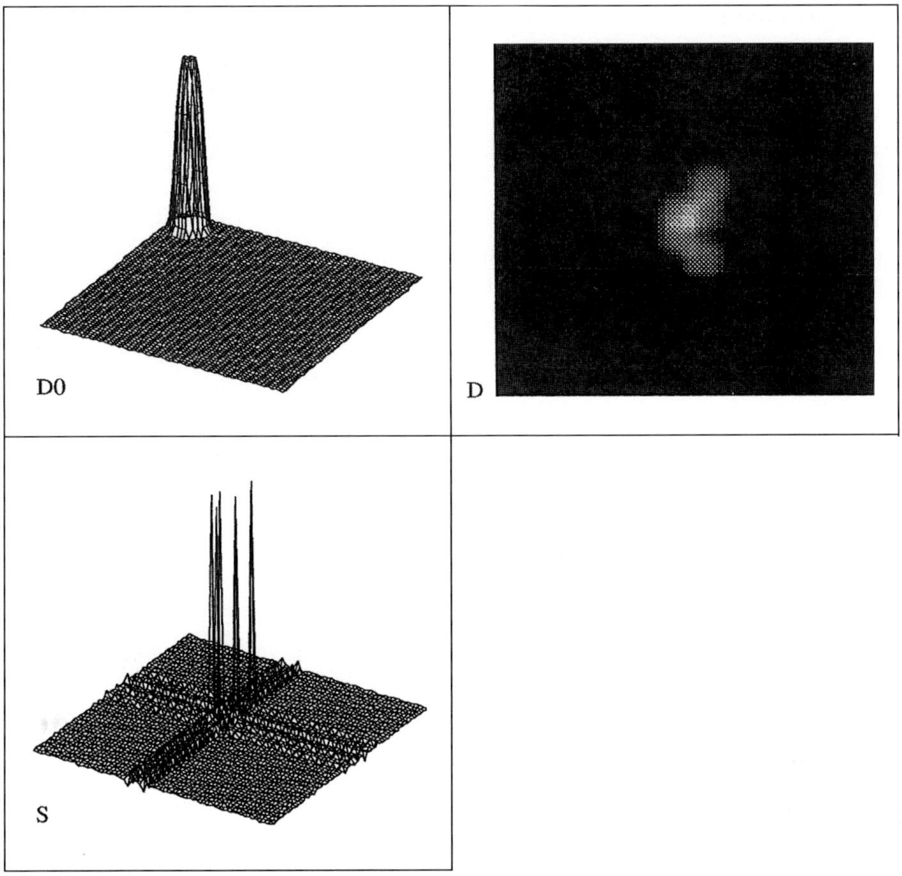

Fig. 4. Shot construction using deconvolution.

Shot Configuration

Figure 4 shows an example of shot construction using deconvolution. S is the shot spatial arrangement obtained by deconvolving the proposed dose distribution D with the single-shot dose distribution D_0. As one can see, many negligibly weighted shots, which will later be filtered out, are generated along with five useful shots.

Discussion

Stereotactic dose computation using convolution theorem simplifies the computational procedure for multiple-shot treatments. Although the method is only suitable for a single helmet, many treatments may indeed be planned with multiple shots from a single helmet. The example shown demonstrates the effectiveness of this algorithm. Since the method begins with a fixed single-shot dose distribution, it can be used to precompute a dose distribution during the planning process before the final dose distribution is computed.

The use of deconvolution to assist optimal treatment planning is a more complicated issue. The example presented in figure 4 indicates the feasibility of the algorithm. A detailed discussion will be provided in the second portion of this study.

References

1 Flickinger JC, Lunsford LD, WU A, Maitz A, Kalend AM, Lindner G: Multiple shot dosimetry for the Gamma Knife. Int J Radiat Oncol Biol Phys 1988;15(suppl 1):161.

2 Flickinger JC, Lunsford LD, Wu A, Maitz A, Kalend AM: Treatment planning for Gamma Knife radiosurgery with multiple isocenters. Int J Radiat Oncol Biol Phys 1990;18:1495–1501.

3 Flickinger JC, Maitz AH, Kalend A, Lunsford LD, Wu A: Treatment volume shaping with selective beam blocking using the Leksell Gamma unit. Int J Radiat Oncol Biol Phys 1990;19:783–789.

4 Stone RA, Smith V, Verhey LJ: Inverse treatment planning for stereotactic radiosurgery. Med Phys 1994;21:920.

5 Wu A, Kalend AM: A new algorithm for Gamma Knife treatment planning system. Stereotactic Radiosurgery Update 1992;217–220.

Proc 7th Int Meeting Leksell Gamma Knife® Society,
Island of Lana'i, Hawaii, November 1995
Stereotact Funct Neurosurg 1996;66(suppl 1):309–319

Stereotactic and Functional Neurosurgery

Electrophysiological Target Localization Is Not Required for the Treatment of Functional Disorders

R.F. Young[a], *S.S. Vermeulen*[b], *P. Grimm*[b], *A. Posewitz*[c]

Departments of [a] Neurosurgery, [b] Radiation Oncology, and [c] Radiation Physics, Northwest Neuroscience Institute and Gamma Knife Center, Northwest Hospital, Seattle, Wash., USA

Key Words

Gamma Knife · Radiosurgery · Functional neurosurgery · Trigeminal neuralgia · Movement disorders · Parkinson's disease · Essential tremor · Chronic pain · Thalamotomy · Pallidotomy

Abstract

A total of 117 patients underwent 124 functional stereotactic procedures with the Leksell Gamma Knife to treat trigeminal neuralgia, movement disorders and chronic pain. Target identification was performed with stereotactic magnetic resonance imaging alone without electrophysiologic localization. Clinical observation of these patients over 1–41 months indicates that the efficacy of the procedure is comparable with that seen with open stereotactic procedures where electrophysiological localization is used. Using current techniques, the complications of functional neurosurgery with the Gamma Knife are nearly nonexistent. We believe that functional neurosurgery can be performed effectively and safely without electrophysiological localization, using the Leksell Gamma Knife.

Introduction

Electrophysiological localization has played an important role in improving the efficacy and safety of functional stereotactic neurosurgery. The addition of single-cell microelectrode recording and microstimulation to the earlier macro-

KARGER

E-Mail karger@karger.ch
Fax + 41 61 306 12 34
http://www.karger.ch

1011–6125/96/0665–0309$10.00/0

Ronald F. Young, MD
Northwest Hospital Gamma Knife Center
1560 N 115th, Suite G 5
Seattle, WA 98133 (USA)

electrode techniques has further refined this method. It also provided an important avenue for research into the pathophysiology of a variety of functional brain disorders such as chronic pain, movement disorders and epilepsy [1, 2]. Leksell's dissatisfaction with the complications and invasive nature of open stereotactic neurosurgical operations led him to develop the Leksell Gamma Knife in the 1950s and 1960s, specifically for the performance of functional procedures. Leksell and his colleagues [3–10] published a number of reports which described their experience with this technique. Recent interest in minimally invasive surgery has led us and others to reexplore the feasibility to the Gamma Knife as a tool for functional neurosurgery, particularly with the advent of modern imaging techniques [11–18]. Since the Gamma Knife is a noninvasive radiosurgical instrument, target localization must also depend on noninvasive techniques, usually magnetic resonance imaging (MRI). Some authors, however, continue to believe that functional neurosurgical operations should be performed only with intraoperative electrophysiological target localization [19–21]. This report describes our experience since June 1992 with functional stereotactic neurosurgery using the Gamma Knife without electrophysiological monitoring.

Material and Methods

This report describes our experience with 124 separate functional stereotactic operations performed with the Leksell Gamma Knife in 117 patients since June 1992. Forty-seven patients underwent unilateral (n = 45) or bilateral (n = 2) medial thalamotomy for treatment of chronic pain. Forty-four patients each underwent a single procedure for the treatment of trigeminal neuralgia. Twenty-five patients underwent unilateral thalamotomy (n = 10), unilateral pallidotomy (n = 11) or bilateal pallidotomy (n = 4) for treatment of movement disorders due to Parkinson's disease, essential tremor or prior strokes. In all except 1 patient, stereotactic MRI scans were performed to localize the targets using the Leksell Model G stereotactic frame. In 1 patient, computed tomography (CT) scanning was employed due to the presence of metallic implants which precluded MRI scanning. Clinical follow-up has been maintained in all patients at intervals of no more than 6 months and usually at 3-monthly intervals. At least one follow-up MRI scan has been obtained in all patients treated for chronic pain or movement disorders to compare the actual final anatomical lesion location with the planned preoperative target coordinates. In 53 patients, it was possible to obtain the follow-up MRI scan at our institution by placing the patient's head within the stereotactic frame with a noninvasive technique, thus allowing the MRI coordinate system and computer anaylsis with GammaPlan to calculate the final target coordinates of the lesions.

A detailed quality assurance program was employed to minimize MRI image distortion [21]. Scans were obtained in a Siemens Magnatom 1.0 Tesla MRI scanner with a high field gradient (15 mT/m), which was regularly examined and adjusted. For each scan, the final position of all visible points of the Leksell Model G stereotactic frame fiducial system was measured to ascertain that the frame was aligned correctly in the scanner head coil. The frame was applied to the patient's head so that the intended target was as close to the center of the stereotactic coordinate system space as possible. Scans were performed using standard T_1 and short TAU inversion recovery techniques in the axial and coronal planes. Duplicate scans in both planes were often obtained with reversal of the phase- and frequency-encoding directions. MRI slice thickness was 3 mm in most cases, but volume acquisition techniques were sometimes used to obtain thinner sections.

Anatomical targets were localized by direct visualization alone for patients with trigeminal neuralgia. In these patients, the target was the proximal portion of the trigeminal nerve root just lateral to its junction with the pons. This could be easily identified in both axial and coronal views [22]. Treatment with the Leksell Gamma Knife was delivered with a single isocenter, 4-mm collimator helmet and a dose maximum of 70 Gy. The isocenter was positioned directly over the trigeminal root so that the 40% isodose line was just anterolaterla to the pontine surface. For patients whose trigeminal neuralgia stemmed from tumors, the radiosurgical treatment was directed at the tumors themselves. Tumor volumes varied from 3.2 to 15.7 cm^3 and radiosurgical doses of 10–20 Gy were prescribed to the 40 or 50% isodose lines.

For patients with movement disorders or chronic pain, the target was localized both by direct visualization and by reference to the Schaltenbrand and Wahren stereotactic atlas [23]. Directly visualized reference points (e.g., anterior and posterior commissures, width of third ventricle, thalamic size, locations of internal capsule, optic tract) were taken into account. Moreover, indirect calculations were performed in which the known relationship of the thalamic nuclear groups was considered and their putative position determined by reference to stereotactic maps adjusted for the characteristics of the particular patient's anatomy (e.g. intercommissural distance).

For pallidotomy, the anteroposterior (Y) coordinate was placed 2–4 mm anterior to the intercommissural point. The lateral (X) and vertical (Z) coordinates were determined by direct visualization of the intended target, the ventral posterolateral globus pallidus. Particularly attention was paid to the location of the subjacent optic tract and the superomedially located internal capsule. Final actual target coordinates were: $X = 21.8 \pm 2.3$ mm lateral to the mid-third ventricle (range 18–27); $Y = 3.0 \pm 0.9$ mm anterior to the intercommissural point (range 2–5), and $Z = 0.8 \pm 2.0$ mm above the intercommissural plane (range 4.5 above to 2.5 below). Lesions were made with a single isocenter exposure using a 4-mm-collimator helmet and radiosurgical dose maxima of 140–160 Gy.

For thalamotomy for movement disorders, the target was the ventral intermedius (VIM) nucleus and the posterior portion of the ventrolateral (VL) nucleus (ventralis oralis posterior, VOP of Hassler [24]). The coordinates were determined with particular reference to the junction between the lateral border of the thalamus and the internal capsule. The intent was to place the lateral margin of the lesion as close as possible to the lateral thalamic borders and the center of the lesion about 7 mm posterior to the mid-commissural point and 3 mm above the intercommissural plane. The radiosurgical technique was identical to that for pallidotomy.

For medial thalamotomy to treat chronic pain, the target and technique have been previously described [15–17]. The radiosurgical method has been modified, however, so that we now utilize only a single isocenter exposure with a 4-mm-collimator helmet and radiosurgical dose maxima of 140–160 Gy. Multi-isocenter exposures with a 4-mm collimator and similar radiosurgical doses in our early experience produced lesions of unpredictable size with potentially serious complications. Doses below 140 Gy are also unpredictable and sometimes produced no visible lesion on follow-up MRI scans.

Results

Our 117 patients underwent a total of 124 Gamma Knife radiosurgical procedures for treatment of functional disorders without electrophysiological target localization. Forty-five patients with trigeminal pain were treated between August 1993 and November 1995. Follow-up periods ranged from 1 to 27 months (mean 14 months). Thirty-four patients exhibited 'idiopathic' trigeminal neuralgia, presumably due to vascular compression at the trigeminal nerve root entry zone. Three patients had multiple sclerosis as the etiology of their trigeminal pain, whereas 8 patients had various types of tumors (meningioma, schwannoma, or acoustic neuromas) as causes of their pain. Seventeen patients had undergone a total of 39 prior surgical treatments (mean 2.3 procedures per patient), whereas 28 patients had had no previous surgical intervention. Twenty-six of the latter patients (91%) had complete or nearly complete pain relief with a latency period of 24 h–3.5 months after treatment. Thirteen patients (76%) who had prior surgical treatment had similar results. Six patients (13%) never had effective pain relief. Only 2 patients (5.1%) who had initial pain relief developed recurrent pain and both are well controlled on Tegretol, whereas they were not controlled prior to Gamma Knife treatment. Of the 8 patients whose trigeminal neuralgia was due to tumors, 6 (75%) are currently pain free. No patient suffered any complication of the treatment. Only 1 patient, a woman who had undergone prior partial surgical removal of a trigeminal schwannoma, developed any increase in preexisting facial sensory loss, and no patient with normal facial sensation developed any new sensory loss on the face.

Ten patients underwent unilateral VL/VIM thalamotomy for the control of tremor due to Parkinson's disease, essential tremor or post-stroke tremor. On the other hand, 15 patients underwent unilateral (n = 11) or bilateral (n = 4) pallidotomy for treatment of rigidity, bradykinesia, akinesia or Sinemet-induced dyskinesias related to Parkinson's disease. Eight of 10 patients who underwent thalamotomy (80%) had complete or nearly complete resolution of tremor with a latency period of 3–11 months following the procedure. In addition, pallidotomy relieved bradykinesia or rigidity in 77% of patients who exhibited this symptom. It relieved symptoms in all patients who exhibited dyskinesias, but was successful in only 45% of those who were akinetic. No patient in either the thalamotomy or pallidotomy groups experienced any identifiable complication of these procedures. No hemiparesis, sensory loss, visual field defects or other neurological symptoms due to the procedures were seen. On the other hand, of the 20 patients treated for Parkinson's disease, 5 (25%) developed some progression of their parkinsonism not related to their Gamma Knife treatment. The most common example was the onset of bradykinesia and gait disturbance in a patient previously successfully treated for tremor.

Forty-seven patients with chronic pain due to a variety of causes underwent a total of 51 separate Gamma Knife medial thalamotomies between July 1993 and November 1995. Forty-three patients underwent a unilateral procedure, 2 patients underwent a second unilateral procedure to enlarge a prior gammathalamotomy, and 2 patients underwent bilateral medial thalamotomies. Pain was assessed using a visual analog scale (VAS), an assessment of medication usage and an evaluation of the capacity of the patient to function in the activities of daily living, including employment. Of 47 patients, 29 (61%) showed an at least 50% reduction in VAS pain intensity estimates, utilized minimal or no narcotic analgesics and showed concomitant significant gains in their abilities to function in daily living. Twenty-three patients underwent thalamotomy using a two- (21 patients) or three- (2 patients) isocenter technique and of these, 5 (21.7%) developed neurological complications related directly to the treatment. In all patients, the complications were due to lesions which became much larger than expected at intervals from 4 to 9 months following the procedure. In no cases were the complications due to anatomically misplaced lesions. Typical complications included hemiparesis, hemisensory loss, dysphasia and involuntary movements. In 1 patient who developed a very large lesion, headache, nausea, vomiting and diplopia also developed. One patient underwent a bilateral medial thalamotomy. Both lesions were made with the two-isocenter technique, with 3 months between lesions and this patient died of radiation necrosis 14 months after the first lesion. In the other 4 patients who developed complications, the neurological symptoms cleared completely or nearly completely in several months, with concomitant shrinkage of the radiographically demonstrated lesions. In 1 patient, hemiparesis and dysphasia persist 18 months after the original procedure. No patient who underwent a medial thalamotomy with the single-isocenter technique developed any delayed neurological deficit.

Follow-up MRI scans were performed at 3-month intervals in patients who underwent thalamotomy or pallidotomy. Since no anatomical lesion was expected and no neurological complications developed following treatment of trigeminal neuralgia, routine follow-up scans were obtained only in those patients treated for tumors. Calculations were made of the original preoperative stereotactic X, Y, and Z target coordinates, and these were compared to the coordinates of the estimated lesion center as identified on postoperative scans. The estimates of lesion coordinates were made by a radiation physicist (A.P.) without knowledge of the preoperative values. Maximum differences between calculated and actual target coordinates were usually 1 mm or less and never exceeded 1.5 mm.

Thalamotomy lesions made with the single-isocenter technique were generally spherical. They first became visible as early as 1 month following the procedure, as low-density regions on T_1-weighted MRI scans. By 3 months, the lesions were clearly visible and enhanced with intravenous gadolinium on T_1-weighted

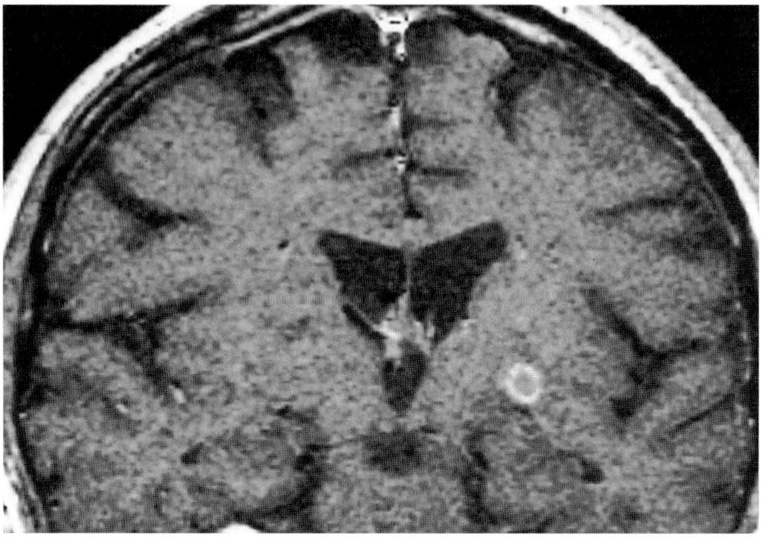

1

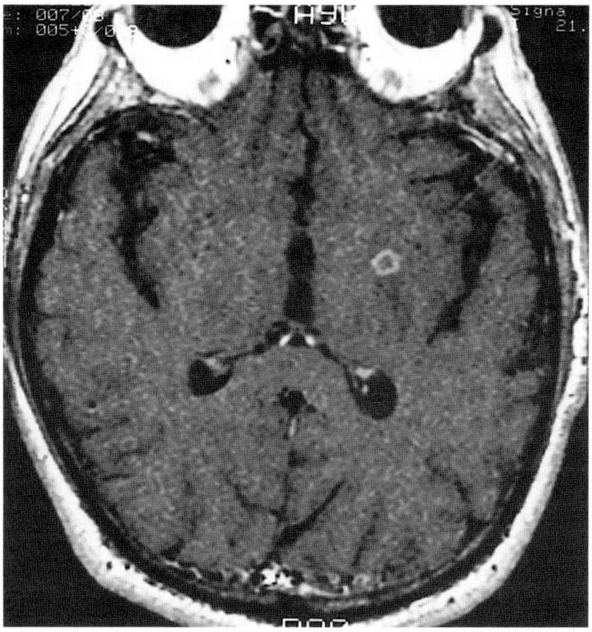

2

Fig. 1. T_1-weighted coronal plane, gadolinium-enhanced MRI scan 3 months following left pallidotomy with the Gamma Knife in a patient with Parkinson's disease. The patient has been followed for 27 months after the lesioning procedure and has excellent control of bradykinesia and contralateral tremor.

Fig. 2. T_1-weighted axial plane gadolinium-enhanced MRI scan. Same patient as in figure 1.

scans (fig. 1, 2). On T_2-weighted scans, an area of increased signal intensity of variable size surrounded the lesion and at times extended into adjacent structures such as the internal capsule. No associated neurological symptoms were noted, however. Lesions usually reached their maximum volumes at about 6–9 months following the procedure and then gradually decreased in size.

Lesions made with the two- or three-isocenter technique had a bilobed or trilobed appearance but generally followed the same time progression as single-isocenter lesions. In 5 patients, the lesions which developed were much larger than expected with extensive diffuse surrounding signal changes seen as low-attenuation regions on T_1-weighted scans and as extensive high signal intensity on T_2-weighted scans. All of these lesions eventually decreased in size and in some cases were barely visible by 18–24 months following the procedures.

The pallidotomy lesions are an excellent example of the use of stereotactic MRI scanning to adjust target coordinates to an individual patient's brain configuration and to calculate the accuracy of the technique as described above. Our stereotactic pallidotomy coordinates were: $X = 21.8 \pm 2.3$ (female 20.9, male 22.86) with a range of 18–27 mm; $Y = 3.0 \pm 0.9$ anterior to the midcommissural point with a range of 2–5 mm; $Z = 0.8 \pm 2.0$ above the commissural plane.

Discussion

Electrophysiological localization has been an important aspect of overall functional stereotactic target localization virtually from the inception of human stereotactic surgery. The addition of microelectrode recording in the early 1960s and microstimulation have added significantly to the information gained from macrostimulation and macroelectrode recording. Until the advent of MRI scanning, no functional targets within the brain could be directly visualized, and thus the anatomical localization of functional targets was dependent upon calculations relative to certain reference points, most commonly the anterior and posterior commissures, and/or the foramen of Monro. Some additional anatomical guidance was obtained from observations of, for instance, third ventricular width and length which could be used to expand or contract brain maps obtained from stereotactic atlases. If either ventriculography or CT scanning is used for target approximation, we agree that electrophysiological target localization is needed for most functional neurosurgical operations. The necessity for electrophysiological localization varies with the disease being treated and with the specific target within the brain. MRI scanning localizes the trigeminal root very precisely, and for this target it would appear that electrophysiological localization is unneccessary. Our results with radiosurgical treatment of trigeminal neuralgia directed at the trigeminal sensory root near the pons demonstrates an efficacy which is very similar to that reported for either microvascular decompression or any of the percutaneous procedures. Given the small size of the anatomical target in the trigeminal nerve root and the equally small size of the effective radiation field generated by the Gamma Knife with the 4-mm-collimator helmet, the high success rate in relieving trigeminal neuralgia would seem to attest to the accuracy of this MRI-directed functional radiosurgical procedure. Long-term follow-up will be required to assess the recurrence rate of trigeminal neuralgia after radiosurgical treatment. It is very clear, however, that the morbidity of the radiosurgical technique is far lower than with any of the other surgical approaches. In addition, a small but definite mortality rate with the other surgical procedures is absent with radiosurgery.

Perhaps electrophysiological localization has been most strongly supported in the treatment of movement disorders, notably Parkinson's disease, essential tremor and post-stroke tremor. The electrophysiological signature of the VIM thalamic nucleus is well known, yet a survey by Laitinen [25] in 1985 of 12 prominent stereotactic neurosurgeons around the world yielded a wide disparity in preferred targets. Our personal contact with many neurosurgeons who perform functional stereotactic surgery indicates that most rely on macrostimulation as their only form of electrophysiological target localization in spite of the presumably greater accuracy of microelectrode localization [26]. This preference indicates some of the drawbacks of electrophysiological target localization, including (1) significant increases in the length and cost of the surgical procedures; (2) increased morbidity related to multiple electrode penetrations and the occasional occurrence of an intracerebral hematoma; (3) misleading responses to stimulation by patients who are sedated or who are distracted by headache due to intracranial air, and (4) brain shifts which occur due to cerebrospinal fluid leakage, particularly in older patients with cerebral atrophy.

In a recent publication by Dogali et al. [27], in which a pallidotomy target was localized by both microelectrode and macroelectrode techniques, 'postoperative MRI scans confirmed the placement of all lesions within ± 1 mm of preoperatively planned targets.' Given this accuracy of preoperatively planned targets, using a technique virtually identical with ours, the value of intraoperative electrophysiological target localization must be questioned.

The advent of stereotactic MRI scanning and direct visualization of targets for functional neurosurgery has reduced and perhaps eliminated the need for electrophysiological target localization. The potential errors in MRI stereotactic localization due to a variety of factors have been addressed in several previous reports [22, 28–31]. A careful quality assurance program is required to minimize MRI distortion. As we have demonstrated in this report, such methods result in actual lesion locations which rarely vary by more than 1 mm from the intended target site, based on detailed comparisons of preoperative target coordinates and postoperative stereotactic measurements of lesion locations. More importantly, the clinical results confirm the safety and accuracy of functional lesions in the treatment of movement disorders. Our rates of tremor control with thalamotomy, and control of bradykinesia, rigidity and Sinemet-induced dykinesias with pallidotomy approximate very closely the rates of control with more traditional functional stereotactic procedures which employ intraoperative electrophysiologic target localization and radiofrequency lesioning [28, 32–34]. No patient in our experience has developed any complication of the method using a single-isocenter, 4-mm-collimator helmet and radiosurgical dose maxima of 140–160 Gy.

Our experience in the performance of radiosurgical medial thalamotomy for the treatment of chronic pain also suggests that the efficacy is similar to that reported for radiofrequency medial thalamotomy [35, 36]. Our target localization was based on our own prior reports of abnormal, spontaneous, high-frequency neuronal activity in the medial thalamus of certain patients with chronic pain [37]. Unfortunately, not all patients with chronic pain appear to exhibit this abnormal activity, and, since no other reliable electrophysiological signature of the medial thalamus exists, even radiofrequency lesioning procedures in the medial thalamus may depend only on anatomical target localization.

Our experience with medial thalamotomy suggests that multi-isocenter lesions (two or three) made with a 4-mm-collimator helmet and radiosurgical dose maxima of 140–160 Gy are not safe. Nearly 25% of patients who underwent medial thalamotomy with this technique developed both radiographic evidence of lesions much larger than expected and concomitant adverse neurological consequences. One death and 1 apparently permanent neurological deficit resulted from this technique, so it is no longer employed. Even with the multi-isocenter technique, however, no patient suffered any adverse consequences due to misplacement of the lesion. Only when very large lesions were seen with significant radiographic changes in surrounding brain were any adverse clinical symptoms seen. It is unclear at this time whether multi-isocenter techniques at lower radiosurgical doses will produce more reliable lesions.

One disadvantage of radiosurgical techniques is the latency period between the procedure and the desired clinical effect. This period may vary from as little as 24 h for trigeminal neuralgia to as long as 6–9 months or more for the relief of movement disorders or chronic pain. Since the latter two are chronic diseases, the latency period seems a small price to pay for reducing the invasive nature of the overall procedure.

Justifiable concerns are often raised about the possibility that functional radiosurgical procedures may induce long-delayed deleterious effects such as the induction of tumors. Although such occurrences have never been recorded to this point with any radiosurgical procedure, the possibility is certainly not excluded.

Conclusions

Functional stereotactic neurosurgery may be accomplished with a high degree of safety and accuracy without the need for electrophysiological target localization. Target coordinates must be determined using stereotactic MRI scans with exquisite attention to quality assurance protocols to minimize the potential for MRI image distortion. Radiosurgical lesions of appropriate size and location may be safely made with the Leksell Gamma Knife using a 4-mm-collimator helmet, a single isocenter and radiosurgical dose maxima of 140–160 Gy. Lesions made with the same collimator system and similar radiosurgical doses and a multi-isocenter technique are, we believe, dangerous and are not recommended. Whether multi-isocenter lesions may be made more safely with lower doses is unclear at this time.

Finally, the efficacy of functional lesions made with the Gamma Knife approximates that for radiofrequency lesioning. We believe that functional neurosurgery with the Gamma Knife, within the guidelines described in this report, and without electrophysiological target localization, is a reasonable alternative to open radiofrequency lesioning techniques.

References

1 Albe-Fessard D, Arfel G, Guiot G: Activités électriques charactéristiques de quelque structure cerébral chez l'homme. Ann Chir 1963;17:1185–1214.

2 Tasker RR, Kiss ZHT: The role of the thalamus in functional neurosurgery. Neurosurg Clin N Am 1995;6:73–104.

3 Leksell L: The stereotactic method and radiosurgery of the brain. Acta Chir Scand 1951;102:316–31.

4 Leksell L: Cerebral surgery: Gamma thalamotomy in two cases of intractable pain. Acta Chir Scand 1968;134:585–595.

5 Leksell L: Stereotactic radiosurgery in trigeminal neuralgia. Acta Chir Scand 1971;37:311–314.

6 Leksell L, Backlund EO: Stereotactic gamma capsulotomy; in Hitchcock ER, Ballantine HT Jr, Meyerson BA (eds): Modern Concepts in Psychiatric Surgery. Amsterdam, Elsevier/North Holland, 1979, pp 213–216.

7 Steiner L, Forster D, Leksell L, Meyerson BA, Boethius J: Gammathalamotomy in intractable pain. Acta Neurochir (Wien) 1980;52:173–184.

8 Wennerstrand J, Ungerstedt U: An anatomical study of gamma-radiolesions. Acta Chir Scand 1970;136:133–137.

9 Forster DMC, Leksell L, Meyerson BA, Steiner L: Gammathalamotomy in intractable pain; in Janzen R, Keidel WE, Herz A, Steichele C (eds): Pain: Basic Principles – Pharmacology and Therapy. Thieme, Stuttgart, 1972, pp 194–198.

10 Leksell L: Stereotactic radiosurgery. J Neurol Neurosurg Psychiatry 1983;46:797–803.

11 Rand RW, Jacques DB, Melbye BG, Copcutt BG, Levenick MN, Fisher MR: Leksell Gamma Knife treatment of tic douloureux. Stereotact Funct Neurosurg 1993;61(suppl):93–102.

12 Rand RW, Jacques DB, Melbye BG, Copcutt BG, Fisher MR, Levenick MN: Gamma Knife thalamotomy and pallidotomy in patients with movement disorders: Preliminary results. Stereotact Funct Neurosurg 1993;61(suppl):65–92.

13 Barcia-Salorio JL, Rodan T, Herandez G, Lopez-Gomez L, Roldan P: Radiosurgical treatment of epilepsy. Appl Neurophysiol 1985;48:400–403.
14 Lindquist C, Kihlström L, Hellstrand E: Functional neurosurgery – A future for the Gamma Knife? Stereotact Funct Neurosurg 1991;57:72–81.
15 Young RF, Jacques DS, Rand RW, Copcutt BG: Medial thalamotomy with the Leksell Gamma Knife for treatment of chronic pain. Acta Neurochir Suppl (Wien) 1994;62:105–110.
16 Young RF, Jacques DS, Rand RW, Copcutt BG: Technique of stereotactic medial thalamotomy with the Leksell Gamma Knife for treatment of chronic pain. Neurol Res 1995;17:59–65.
17 Alterman RL, Kall BA, Cohen H, Kelly PJ: Stereotactic ventrolateral thalamotomy: Is ventriculography necessary? Neurosurgery 1995;37:717–722.
18 Bakay RE: Comment on Alterman RL, et al: Stereotactic ventrolateral thalamotomy: Is ventriculography necessary? Neurosurgery 1995;37:717–722.
19 Bakay RAE: Comment on Otsuki T, et al: Stereotactic gamma-thalamotomy with a computerized brain atlas: Technical case report. Neurosurgery 1994;35:767.
20 Kelly PJ: Comment on Ostuki, et al: Stereotactic gamma-thalamotomy with a computerized brain atlas: Technical case report. Neurosurgery 1994;35:767.
21 Young RF, Posewitz A: Accuracy of stereotaxis. J Neurosurg 1996;84:303–304.
22 Kondziolka D, Lunsford LD, Flickinger JC, Young RF, Vermeulen SS, Duma CM, Jacques DB, Rand RW, Regis J, Peragut JC, Epstein MH, Lindquist C: Stereotactic radiosurgery for trigeminal neuralgia: A multi-institution study using the gamma unit. J Neurosurg, in press.
23 Schaltenbrand G, Wahren W: Atlas for Stereotaxy of the Human Brain. Stuttgart, Thieme, 1977.
24 Hassler R: Architectonic organization of the thalamic nuclei; in Schaltenbrand G, Walker AE (eds): Stereotaxy of the Human Brain: Anatomical, Physiological and Clinical Applications, ed 2. New York, Thieme-Stratton, 1982, pp 140–180.
25 Laitinen LV: Brain targets in surgery for Parkinson's disease: Results of a survey of neurosurgeons. J Neurosurg 1985;62:346–351.
26 Burcheil KJ: Thalamotomy for movement disorders. Neurosurg Clin North Am 1995;6:55–72.
27 Dogali M, Fazzini E, Kolodny E, Eidelberg D, Sterio D, Devinsky O, Beric A: Stereotactic ventral pallidotomy for Parkinson's disease. Neurology 1995:45:753–761.
28 Alexander E III, Kooy HM, Van Herk M, Schwartz M, Barnes PD, Tarbell N, Mulkern RV, Holupka EJ, Loeffler JS: Magnetic resonance image-directed stereotactic neurosurgery: Use of image fusion with computerized tomography to enhance spatial accuracy. J Neurosurg 1995;83:271–276.
29 Alexander E III, Mulkern RV, Loeffler JS: Response. J Neurosurg, in press.
30 Sumanaweera TS, Adler JR Jr, Napel S: Characterization of spatial distortion in magnetic resonance imaging and its implications for stereotactic surgery. Neurosurgery 1994;35:696–704.
31 Jankovic J, Cardoso F, Grossman R, Hamilton WJ: Outcome after stereotactic thalamotomy for parkinsonian, essential, and other types of tremor. Neurosurgery 1995;37:680–687.
32 Laitinen LV: Pallidotomy for Parkinson's disease. Neurosurg Clin North Am 1995;6:105–112.
33 Laitinen LV, Hariz MI: Movement disorders; in Joumans JR (ed): Neurological Surgery, ed 4. Philadelphia, Saunders, 1996, pp 3575–3609.
34 Young RF: Intracranial procedures for pain management; in Apuzzo MLG (ed): Brain Surgery: Complication Avoidance and Management. New York, Churchill Livingstone, 1993, pp 1497–1508.
35 Young RF: Stereotactic surgical ablation for pain relief; in Rengachary SS, Wilkins RH (eds): Neurosurgical Operative Atlas. Baltimore, Williams & Wilkins, pp 177–188.
36 Tasker RR: Thalamotomy. Neurosurg Clin North Am 1990;1:841–864.
37 Rinaldi PC, Young RF, Albe-Fessard D, Chodakiewitz J: Spontaneous neuronal hyperactivity in the medial and intralaminar thalamic nuclei of patients with deafferentation pain. J Neurosurg 1991;74:415–421.

Proc 7th Int Meeting Leksell Gamma Knife® Society,
Island of Lana'i, Hawaii, November 1995
Stereotact Funct Neurosurg 1996;66(suppl 1):320–328

Stereotactic and Functional Neurosurgery

Lesion Size following Gamma Knife Treatment for Functional Disorders

G.M. Friehs[a], G. Norén[a], C. Ohye[d], C.M. Duma[b], R. Marks[b], J. Plombon[c], R.F. Young[c]

[a] Department of Neurosurgery, Brown University, Providence, R.I.,
[b] The Good Samaritan Hospital, Gamma Knife Center, Los Angeles, Calif., and
[c] Northwest Hospital Gamma Knife Center, Seattle, Wash., USA;
[d] Department of Neurosurgery, Gunma University School of Medicine, Maebashi, Japan

Key Words

Gamma Knife · Functional disorders · Parkinsonism · Pain · Thalamotomy · Pallidotomy

Abstract

In this study we investigated the reproducibility and consistency of the size of radiosurgical lesions produced for functional disorders. The T_1 gadolinium-enhanced magnetic resonance (MR) images of 56 patients treated for parkinsonism, pain, or other functional diseases were used to measure 140 lesion sizes at various times after radiosurgical treatment (1–26 months, mean: 11.3 months). Only the 4-mm collimator was used to create the lesions. The maximum dose ranged from 110 to 180 Gy (mean: 145 Gy). In 42 cases (78%), one isocenter was used to create the lesion. Thirteen lesions (20%) were created with two isocenters and in 1 case, three isocenters were used. Lesions were detectable on MR images as early as 30 days after treatment. The maximum lesion volume was reached after 6–12 months and ranged from nondetectable to more than 4,000 mm^3. Larger lesion volumes were strongly associated with the use of more than one isocenter. In addition, maximum doses of 160 Gy or more increased the likelihood of producing lesions larger than expected. It is therefore concluded that the use of the Gamma Knife for the treatment of functional disorders is safest when single-isocenter shots with the 4-mm collimator and a maximum dose of less than 160 Gy are used.

KARGER

E-Mail karger@karger.ch
Fax +41 61 306 12 34
http://www.karger.ch

1011–6125/96/0665–0320$10.00/0

Gerhard M. Friehs, MD
Department of Neurosurgery, Brown University
Rhode Island Hospital, 2 Dudley Street,
MOB Suite 555
Providence, RI 02905 (USA)

Table 1. Patient indications and Gamma Knife procedures

Indication	Procedure	n	%
Parkinsonism	lateral thalamotomy	18	32
	pallidotomy	10	18
Pain	medial thalamotomy	27	48
Dystonia	thalamotomy	1	2
Total		56	100

Introduction

Although the Gamma Knife was originally designed for the treatment of functional disorders, the precise role and value of radiosurgery for these indications have not been clearly determined. In this context, one of the major concerns has been the question of consistency and reproducibility of lesion size, given recent reports about unexpectedly large lesion sizes using an 8-mm collimator [1] or multiple-isocenter shots with the 4-mm collimator [2, 3].

To shed light on this matter, we conducted a retrospective study in which we measured lesion sizes created with the Gamma Knife for the treatment of functional disorders. The purpose of this study was to see if lesion volumes were predictable and reproducible and to determine if age, sex, maximum target dose, and number of isocenters were predictors of lesion volume.

Materials and Methods

Sixty-nine patients (36 males, 33 females) were initially enrolled into the study protocol. Their ages ranged from 35 to 89 years for males and 37–81 years for females with a mean age at time of treatment of 66.9 years for both sexes. The patients were followed radiographically for 8–724 days with a mean follow-up period of 203 days.

The indications for treatment are listed in table 1. The vast majority of patients underwent treatment for parkinsonism or pain with a radiosurgical medial or lateral thalamotomy. All lesions analyzed were placed in various deep brain nuclei, so all data points represent target regions in the gray matter. Lesions placed in white matter structures such as the anterior internal capsule were not included in this analysis.

Only the 4-mm-collimator helmet was used. The lesions were created using one (78%), two (20%), or three (2%) isocenters. The maximum dose ranged from 110 to 180 Gy with a mean maximum dose of 145 Gy. Plugging was required in only 3 patients.

Only patients with postoperative magnetic resonance imaging (MRI) were included in this study. In 56 patients (81.2%), the MRI was performed using T_1-weighted gadolinium-enhanced imaging techniques. Occasionally, additional MRI series were performed (i.e. T_2-weighted, T_1-weighted without contrast or others). However, these additional images were infrequent and therefore could not be used in our analysis.

The lesion size, which was defined as the maximum extension of the gadolinium-enhanced area in the X, Y, and Z directions, was measured. The volume of the enhancement was approximated using the following formula:

$$V = \frac{4\pi}{3} \times \left(\frac{X+Y+Z}{6}\right)^3$$

The data in our analysis were therefore gathered from 140 lesions measured in 56 patients. Statistical analysis was limited to descriptive statistics. In this paper we present our preliminary results for a small patient population. Thus, we have purposefully avoided significance tests such as group comparisons or regression analyses which will be published once the complete data set is accumulated and analyzed.

Results

When plotting the lesion volume against the number of isocenters (fig. 1), a clear tendency towards increasing volumes is seen in lesions created with more than one isocenter. Single-isocenter lesions cluster around volumes of 200 mm^3, with few outliers, corresponding to a lesion diameter of approximately 7 mm. When looking at two- or three-isocenter lesions, the average volume becomes much larger, as expected. However, the variance also increases, resulting in a reduction in the predictability of lesion volumes. Again, few outliers are noted with lesion volumes exceeding 4,000 mm^3. Since most of our data are based on the use of single-isocenter shots, and since multiple isocenters are almost never used anymore for functional radiosurgery, the remaining results only take single-isocenter lesion volumes into consideration.

Figure 2 depicts the lesion volume of single-isocenter shots as a function of time. When looking at the development of lesion volumes over time, the maximum volume is reached 6–9 months after radiosurgical treatment. Outliers did not occur before 6 months or after 12 months postoperatively. Over a period of 12–24 months, the gadolinium-enhanced regions decrease in volume and finally completely disappear.

There was no correlation between the patient's age and lesion volume, suggesting that age is not a predictor of larger lesion size (fig. 3). Also, outliers were not related to any specific age group and, therefore, could not be predicted by age.

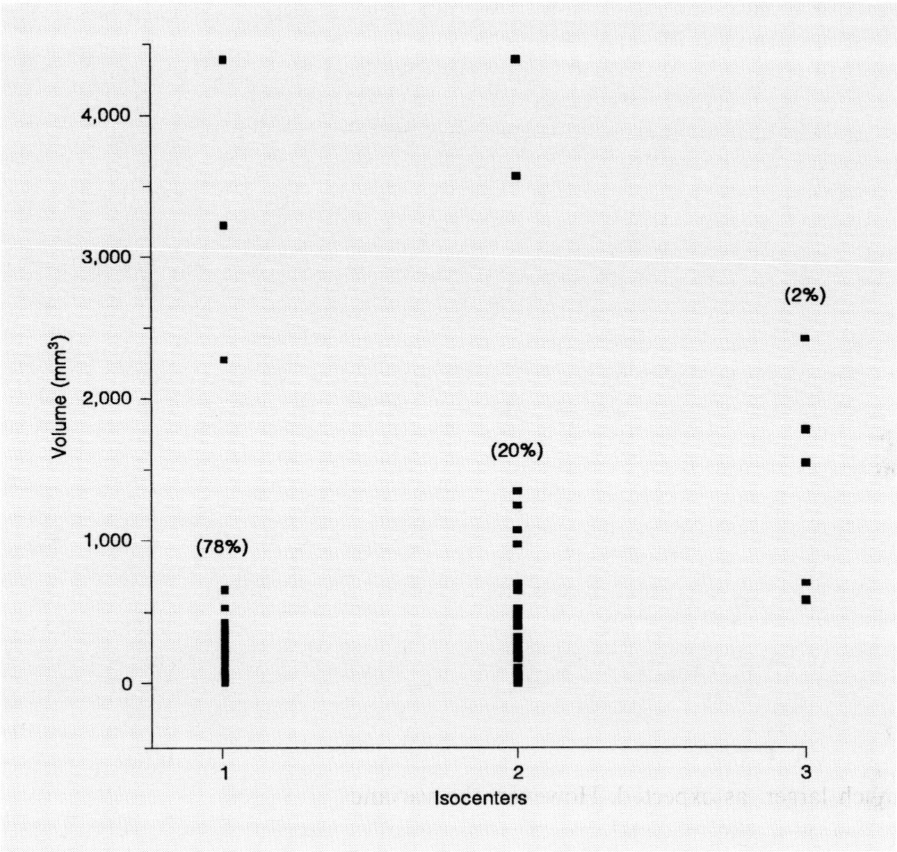

Fig. 1. Lesion volume plotted as a function of the number of isocenters. There was a clear association between larger lesion volumes and more isocenters. This relational increase was not linear. Note that the unpredictability of unexpectedly large lesion volumes increases when more than one isocenter is used. The percentages indicate the proportion of lesions created with that isocenter configuration.

Figure 4 shows the lesion volume as a function of sex. For graphical purposes, the extreme volume outliers are ignored. The mean volume with standard deviations is depicted as a diamond. As can be seen, lesion volumes had a tendency to be smaller in women than in men (around 150 versus 210 mm^3).

When plotting the maximum dose against the lesion volume, a positive correlation can be seen (fig. 5). Higher maximum doses were clearly associated with larger lesion volumes. It was also interesting to find that all outliers with very large lesion volumes were associated with maximum doses of 160 Gy or more.

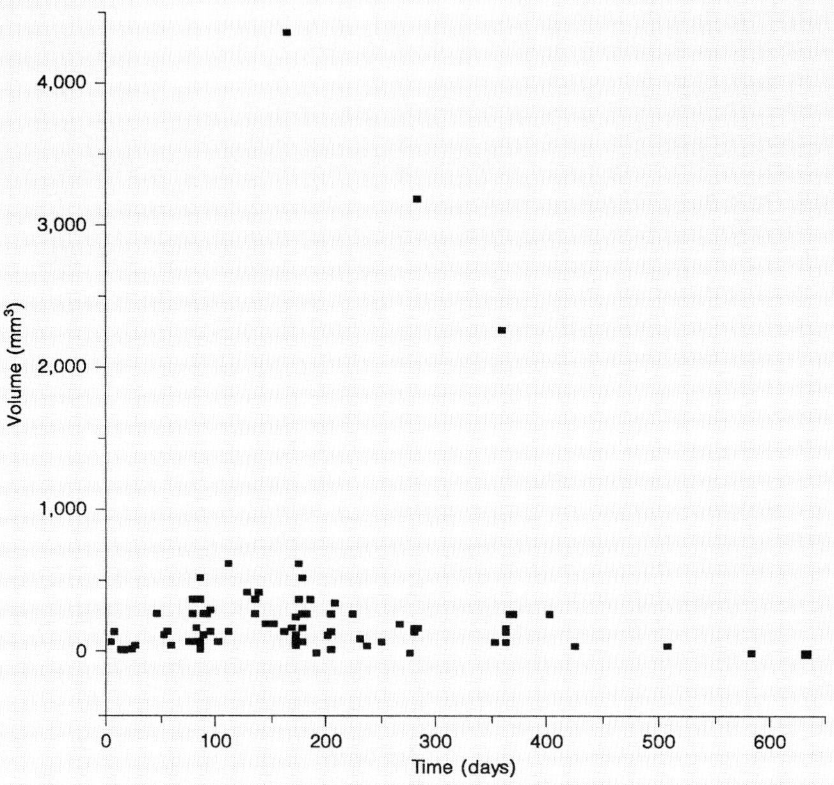

Fig. 2. Lesion volume as a function of time. Maximum lesion sizes were reached after 100–200 days. Before and after that, the volume is small and sometimes undetectable.

Discussion

Radiosurgical treatment of functional disorders is not a novel idea. The Gamma Knife was designed by Lars Leksell with that purpose in mind. The original treatments performed and reported by Leksell himself showed that radiosurgical creation of brain lesions was possible [4]. Although the results of these initial experiments were good and the complication rate was low, it has to be realized that the treatments were conducted with a prototype version of the Gamma Knife and a collimator helmet that is not available anymore. Therefore, the results cannot be directly applied to today's treatment planning.

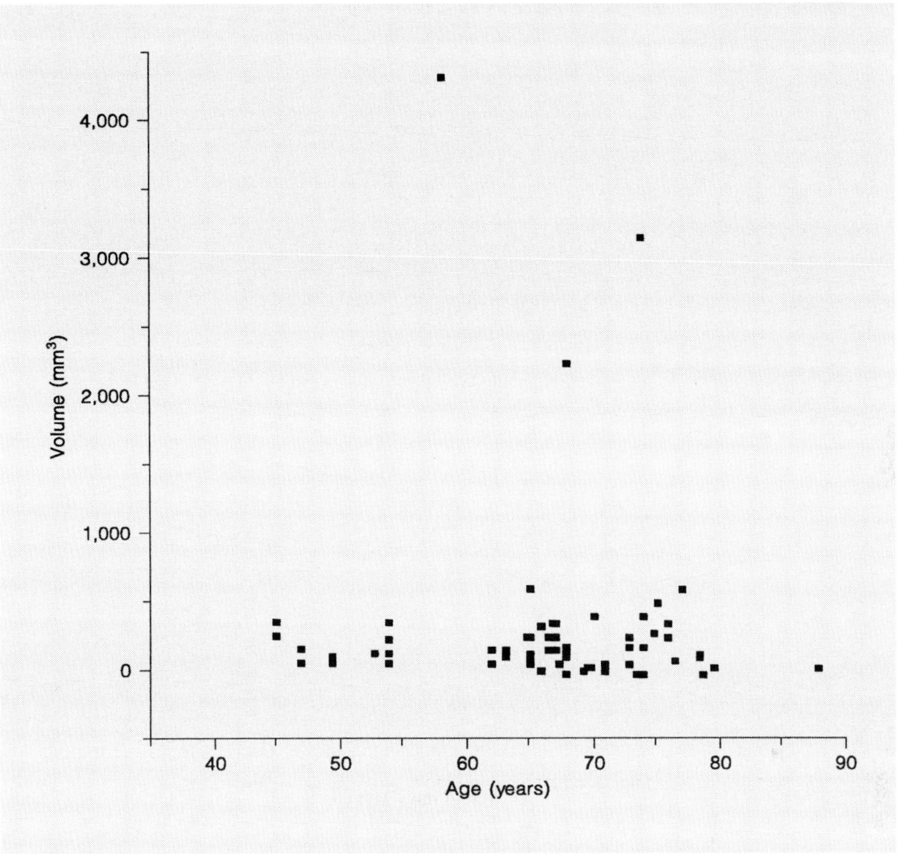

Fig. 3. Lesion volume plotted against patient age. No correlation was seen, and thus older age was not a predictor of large lesion volumes.

More recently, several Gamma Knife centers have started performing radiosurgical treatments for functional disorders. Reports from the literature to date include patients successfully treated for parkinsonism [5–7], intractable pain [3], obsessive-compulsive disorder [8], dystonia [9], trigeminal neuralgia [10], and epilepsy [11, 12]. Except for tic douloureux and epilepsy, small lesions in gray matter nuclei or white matter tracts are necessary. Since neurophysiological target verification is not possible with radiosurgery, one has to rely on anatomical target localization and predictable lesion volumes, in order to treat successfully and limit complications. Although the lesion size can be estimated given certain treatment parameters, there have been recent reports warning about considerable vari-

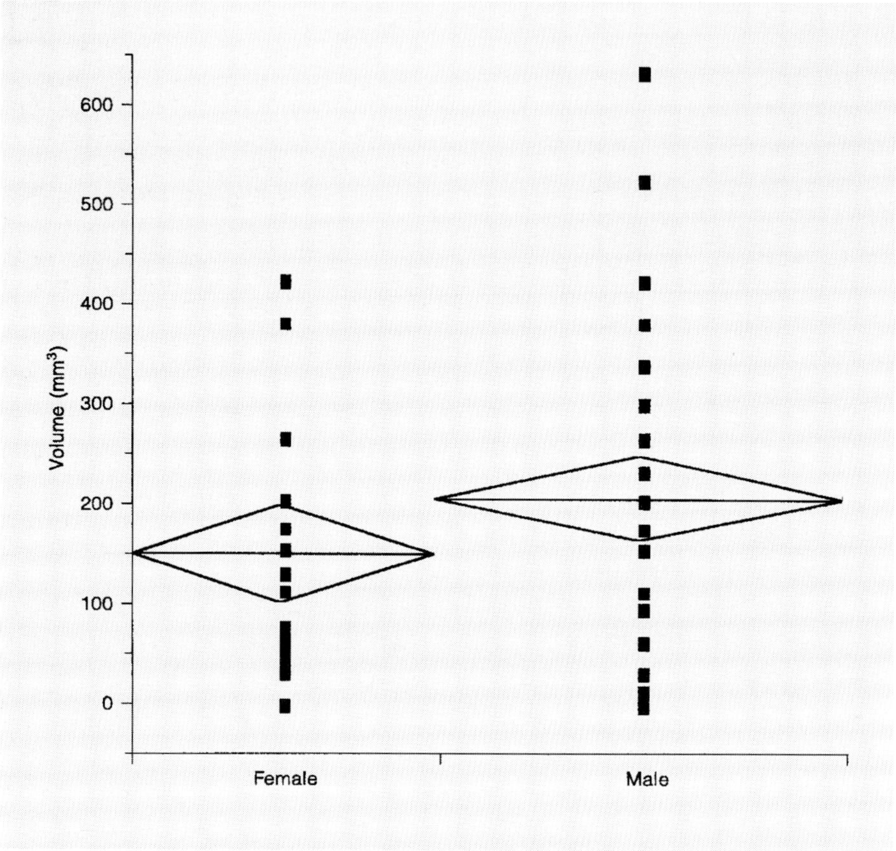

Fig. 4. Lesion volume as a function of sex. The diamonds indicate the mean ± SD. There was a tendency for female patients to have smaller volumes than males (about 150 mm^3 versus 210 mm^3). Note that the y-axis scale is different to that in the other figures; the outliers have been omitted.

ations between expected and actual lesion volume [2, 3]. Therefore, the current retrospective analysis of lesion volumes in patients treated radiosurgically for functional disorders was conducted to assess how consistent and predictable functional lesions were in human brains.

In conclusion, we found the lesion volumes to be reasonably predictable with an occasional chance of unexpectedly large lesions. The occurrence of outliers was strongly associated with the number of isocenters. Furthermore, every outlier occurred with maximum doses of 160 Gy or more. There was no association with

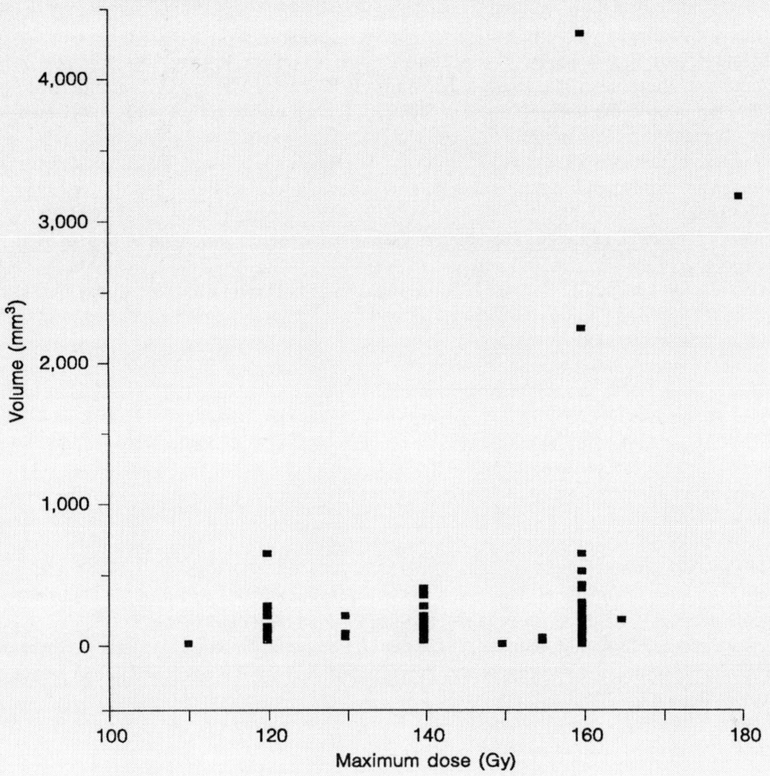

Fig. 5. Correlation of maximum dose with lesion volume. There is a positive correlation, and all outliers occurred with maximum doses of 160 Gy or more. Below that dose, lesion volumes are very consistent.

the age of the patient, and there was a tendency for women to have smaller lesion volumes than men. It is therefore concluded that Gamma Knife treatment for functional disorders in gray matter is safest when a single-isocenter, 4-mm-collimator shot is used with a maximum dose of less than 160 Gy. The final and complete analysis of this multicenter study will answer the question of gender difference and will allow us to give mean values, variances and confidence intervals for expected lesion volumes.

References

1 Lindquist C, Steiner L, Hindmarsh T: Gamma Knife thalamotomy for tremor: Report of two cases; in Steiner L (ed): Radiosurgery: Baseline and Trends. New York, Raven Press, 1992, pp 237–243.

2 Lindquist C, Hindmarsh T, Kihlström L, Mindus P, Steiner L: MRI and CT studies of radionecrosis development in the normal brain; in Steiner L (ed): Radiosurgery: Baseline and Trends. New York, Raven Press, 1992, pp 237–243.

3 Young RF, Vermeulen SS, Grimm P, Posewitz AE, Jacques DB, Tand RW, Copcutt BG: Gamma Knife thalamotomy for the treatment of persistent pain. Stereotact Funct Neurosurg 1995;64(suppl 1):172–181.

4 Steiner L, Forster D, Leksell L, Meyerson B: Gammathalamotomy in intractable pain. Acta Neurochir 1980;52:173–184.

5 Friehs GM, Ojakangas CL, Pachatz P, Schröttner O, Ott E, Pendl G: Thalamotomy and caudatotomy with the Gamma Knife as a treatment for parkinsonism with a comment on lesion sizes. Stereotact Funct Neurosurg 1995;64(suppl 1):209–221.

6 Hirato M, Ohye C, Shibazaki T, Nakamura M, Inoue HK, Andou Y: Gamma Knife thalamotomy for the treatment of functional disorders. Stereotact Funct Neurosurg 1995;64(suppl 1):164–171.

7 Rand RW, Jacques DB, Melbye RW, Copcutt BG, Fisher MR, Levenick MN: Gamma Knife thalamotomy and pallidotomy in patients with movement disorders: Preliminary results. Stereotact Funct Neurosurg 1993;61(suppl 1):65–92.

8 Kihlström L, Guo WY, Lindquist C, Mindus P: Radiobiology of radiosurgery for refractory anxiety disorders. Neurosurgery 1995;36:294–302.

9 Kwon Y, Whang CJ: Stereotactic Gamma Knife radiosurgery for the treatment of dystonia. Stereotact Funct Neurosurg 1995;64(suppl 1):222–227.

10 Régis J, Manera L, Dufour H, Porcheron D, Sedan R, Peragut JC: Effect of the Gamma Knife on trigeminal neuralgia. Stereotact Funct Neurosurg 1995;64(suppl 1):182–192.

11 Régis J, Peragut JC, Rey M, Samson Y, Levrier O, Porcheron D, Régis H, Sedan R: First selective amygdalohippocampal radiosurgery for 'mesial temporal lobe epilepsy'. Stereotact Funct Neurosurg 1995;64(suppl 1):193–201.

12 Whang CJ, Chang JK: Short term follow-up of stereotactic Gamma Knife radiosurgery in epilepsy. Stereotact Funct Neurosurg 1995;64(suppl 1):202–208.

Proc 7th Int Meeting Leksell Gamma Knife® Society,
Island of Lana'i, Hawaii, November 1995
Stereotact Funct Neurosurg 1996;66(suppl 1):329–332

Stereotactic and Functional Neurosurgery

Stereotactic Gamma Thalamotomy for the Treatment of Parkinsonism

Li Pan, Jia-Zhong Dai, Bin-Jiang Wang, Wei-min Xu, Liang-fu Zhou, Xing-Rong Chen

Shanghai Gamma Knife Hospital and Shanghai Hua Shan Hospital, Shanghai Medical University, Shanghai, P.R. China

Key Words

Gamma Knife · Radiosurgery · Parkinson's disease · Thalamotomy

Abstract

From September 1994 to June 1995, eight patients with intractable parkinsonism underwent gamma thalamotomy in our hospital. All of these patients were male, with an average age of 59.3 years. The duration of the disease from initial diagnosis was 2–10 years (mean 6.8 years). All had failed or had serious side effects with antiparkinsonian medicine. Seven cases had tremor-dominant symptoms, while the other had mainly rigidity. Six cases had bilateral symptoms. Computed tomography or magnetic resonance imaging (MRI) was undertaken prior to treatment in all cases to exclude focal brain lesions. Stereotactic MRI was taken with the Leksell frame in place and both T_1- and T2-weighted images were obtained. The targets were located in the area of Vim/Voa/Vop based on the Schaltenbrand atlas. In seven cases, two plugged 4-mm-collimator shots were used. The maximum dose was 160 Gy in six cases and 180 Gy in one case. In another case, a single 4-mm-collimator shot was used, and a maximum dose of 160 Gy was delivered to the target center. The border of the internal capsule was outside the 20–30% isodose line. We intended the 50% isodose line to have an oval-shaped region with the use of two shots and should correspond to the shape of Vim. Follow-up data were available for six patients (mean: 4.5 months, range: 2–9 months). Tremor disappeared in three cases and improved in the other three. In one of these six cases, the tremor disappeared just 3 days after gamma thalamotomy. Rigidity improved in four of these six cases. In only one patient, treated with a maximum dose of 180 Gy, was there any contralateral limb weakness, which developed 3 months after treatment and has been recovering gradually. Follow-up MRI T_2-weighted images in this case showed that the diameter of the lesion was larger than intended and there was a region of diffuse edema in the thalamus and upper brain stem. No other complications occurred in this series.

KARGER

E-Mail karger@karger.ch
Fax + 41 61 306 12 34
http://www.karger.ch

1011–6125/96/0665–0329$10.00/0

Li Pan, MD, PhD
Department of Neurosurgery
Shanghai Gamma Knife Hospital
Shanghai Medical University, 518 Wu Zhong Road (E)
Shanghai 200233 (P.R. China)

Introduction

The concept of radiosurgery was devised by Professor Lars Leksell in 1951 [1] and the first Gamma Knife unit was installed in Stockholm in 1967. However, only five cases with movement disorders were treated with gamma thalamotomy from 1968 to 1970 [2]. New computerized imaging techniques such as computed tomography (CT) and magnetic resonance imaging (MRI) render the brain anatomy visible. By the end of 1994, 155 cases of Parkinson's disease had been treated by stereotactic gamma thalamotomy worldwide. The Gamma Knife (Elekta Instruments, Stockholm, Sweden) was introduced to China in 1993. Almost 1 year later, we began to treat parkinsonism with gamma thalamotomy in our hospital.

Material and Methods

From September 1994 to June 1995, eight patients with parkinsonism were selected for gamma thalamotomy. All were males aged from 36 to 68 years (mean 59.3 years). The duration of the disease from initial diagnosis to date of treatment was 2–10 years (mean 6.8 years). All the patients had either not responded to antiparkinsonian medication or had suffered serious side effects from it. In seven patients, tremor was the dominant symptom. The other patient had primarily rigidity. Six cases had bilateral symptoms. CT and/or MRI were performed before treatment, to exclude focal lesions of the brain.

The stereotactic frame was applied under local anesthesia. The base lines of the frame were adjusted to be parallel with Twining's line, according to landmarks on X-ray films taken prior to frame application. Stereotactic MRI midsagittal scans were taken first. The anterior and posterior commissures were identified on these films. Then, 3 mm-thick trans-axial and coronal sections were taken through the region of the intended target. The target point was calculated and corrected in relation to the Schaltenbrand atlas. Two shots with plugged 4-mm collimators were used. A maximum dose of 160 Gy was used in six cases. One patient with two 4-mm shots received a maximum dose of 180 Gy. Another patient was treated with a single 4-mm shot. In this case, the maximum dose at the target center was again 160 Gy. The border of the internal capsule was outside the 20–30% isodose lines. We intended that the oval outline of the 50% isodose produced with two shots would correspond to the shape of the Vim nucleus.

Follow-up data were available for six patients, of whom four had follow-up CT or MRI. The duration of follow-up ranged from 2 to 9 months (mean: 4.5 months) after treatment.

Results

Clinical examination of the six cases showed that three were free of tremor in their contralateral limbs. In one case, the tremor had resolved only 3 days after gamma thalamotomy. The remaining three patients had varying degrees of improvement in their tremor. Rigidity improved in four of the six patients, but none became normal.

Four cases had CT or MRI scanning after treatment, and radionecrosis could always be seen at the target site. However, the size of these lesions varied, even though the maximum dose had been the same. Mild to moderate edema was seen around the lesions in all but the one patient who had received a maximum dose of 180 Gy.

Contralateral limb weakness was observed in one of the patients, 3 months after gamma thalamotomy. This was the first patient to be treated. A relatively large grid size (1.8 mm) and two shots and a high center dose (180 Gy) were used in this case. Follow-up MRI 6 months after treatment showed that the diameter of the lesion was larger than intended. Moreover, there was diffuse edema in the area of the thalamus and the upper part of the brain stem. The patient is recovering gradually and has remained free of tremor in his contralateral limb. No other complications occurred in our series.

Discussion

Many patients have benefited from antiparkinsonian medicine in recent decades. However, in some cases the treatment is ineffective and in others the side effects may be intolerable. Thus, there remains a need for stereotactic neurosurgery or radiosurgery. All cases in our series belonged to the category of failed medical treatment.

In the early days of Gamma Knife surgery, gamma thalamotomy with a somewhat different target was used to treat intractable pain. It was found that a maximum dose of 150 Gy was required to produce a consistent clinically useful lesion in normal brain [3, 4]. In our series, a dose of 160 Gy was prescribed in each case save one. However, we found that the response to gamma thalamotomy varied from case to case, even though the maximum dose was the same. In one of the four cases where follow-up MRI was taken, the diameter of the radionecrosis was less than intended. Moreover, the clinical result was somewhat disappointing. A similar reaction pattern to Gamma Knife radiosurgery has been reported by Lindquist et al. [5]. The reason is unclear. The brains of different individuals may have different radiosensitivity. Another reason could be that different conditions in different individuals could alter the radioresponsiveness of the brain.

Stereotactic MRI has been found to be a reliable imaging method for target localization of tumors and arteriovenous malformations. High-resolution MRI is also very useful for defining a functional target. With the GammaPlan Dose Planning system it is more convenient to define the midpoint of the AC-PC line accurately using the stereotactic midsagittal or reconstructed sagittal images. Furthermore, survey and mapping functions included in GammaPlan help to transmit the target coordinates to the stereotactic frame. The dose planning procedure is much easier and more accurate than before. At same time, important structures such as the internal capsule can be visualized by imaging, and damage can be avoided by adjusting the target point [5].

Complications occurred in only one patient in our series, perhaps as a result of the high maximum dose (180 Gy). Another factor which should be emphasized is the grid size used for the dose planning matrix. In this case, the grid was too coarse (1.8 mm). We later repeated the dose planning with a grid size of 0.7 mm, and found that the treatment time was reduced by about 10 min, suggesting that this patient might have received 180 Gy plus 10–14 Gy. Much effort should be spent to ensure that this factor is taken into account, especially in the treatment of functional disorders.

In conclusion, gamma thalamotomy would seem to be a safe and effective modality for the treatment of selected cases with parkinsonism. Further studies should be continued.

References

1 Leksell L: The stereotactic method and radiosurgery of the brain. Acta Chir Scand 1951;102:316–319.
2 Lindquist C, Kihlström L, Hellstrand E: Functional neurosurgery: A future for the Gamma Knife? Stereotact Funct Neurosurg 1991;57:72–81.
3 Steiner L, Forster D, Leksell L, Meyerson BA, Boethius J: Gamma thalamotomy in intractable pain. Acta Neurochir (Wien) 1980:52:173–184.
4 Lindquist C, Hindmarsh T, Kihlström L, Mindus P, Steiner L: MRI and CT studies of radionecrosis development in the normal human brain; in Steiner L (ed): Radiosurgery: Baseline and Trends. New York, Raven Press, 1992, pp 245–253.
5 Lindquist C, Steiner L, Hindmarsh T: Gamma Knife thalamotomy for tremor: Report of two cases; in Steiner L (ed): Radiosurgery: Baseline and Trends. New York, Raven Press, 1992; pp 237–243.

Proc 7th Int Meeting Leksell Gamma Knife® Society,
Island of Lana'i, Hawaii, November 1995
Stereotact Funct Neurosurg 1996;66(suppl 1):333–342

Stereotactic and Functional Neurosurgery

Gamma Thalamotomy for Parkinsonian and Other Kinds of Tremor

C. Ohye, T. Shibazaki, M. Hirato, H. Inoue, Y. Andou

Department of Neurosurgery, Gunma University School of Medicine, and
Hidaka Hospital, Maebashi, Japan

Key Words

Gamma Knife · Radiosurgery · Thalamotomy · Parkinson's disease · Tremor · Essential tremor

Abstract

On the basis of our experiences with selective ventralis intermedius thalamotomy with microrecording, certain cases of tremor with Parkinson's disease (PD, six cases), intentional tremor (one case) and essential tremor (one case) were treated by Gamma Knife. In all cases, 140–150 Gy were irradiated using 4-mm collimators. Three different strategies were used. (1) Gamma thalamotomy as the primary surgical treatment. (2) As a secondary treatment, irradiation of the symmetric point of the contralateral selective thalamotomy. (3) Extension of the previous thalamotomy. For the first three cases (all PD), a special plug pattern (100 plugs) was used, but was not employed for the later cases. No acute untoward effects were noted, and overall there appeared to be a reduction in tremor. The time course of tremor reduction varied from case to case, from about 5–6 months to 1 year.

Introduction

Although gamma thalamotomy has a long history [1], the application of the Gamma Knife to functional disorders is far less developed than in other fields, such as the treatment of arteriovenous malformations (AVMs) and benign tumors. At the time of writing, a number of cases with Parkinson's disease have been treated by Gamma Knife, but the results have been variable and in some cases disappointing [2–5], probably because the thalamic target is not visible and it is not easy to determine its location.

KARGER

E-Mail karger@karger.ch
Fax + 41 61 306 12 34
http://www.karger.ch

1011–6125/96/0665–0333$10.00/0

Chihiro Ohye, MD
Department of Neurosurgery
Gunma University School of Medicine
3-39 Showa-machi
Maebashi, Gunma 371 (Japan)

Some time ago, we developed selective thalamotomy with microrecording for various kinds of tremor, especially for parkinsonian tremor. We have found that the most lateral part of the nucleus ventralis intermedius (Vim) is the target of choice for consistent, long-lasting arrest of tremor of whatever kind [6, 7]. Thus, if this target can be determined using magnetic resonance imaging (MRI) or computed tomography (CT), and with reference to a standard atlas of the human thalamus [8], it should be possible to use the Gamma Knife for tremor surgery. Certainly, in this situation a selective lesion is difficult to achieve, with the result that some radiation will unavoidably be delivered to a zone ouside the target of choice.

This article presents preliminary experience with gamma thalamotomy for eight cases of tremor.

Subjects and Methods

Eight patients with tremor were treated with the Gamma Knife (table 1). There were six cases with Parkinson's disease and two with tremor (one developed intention tremor after thalamic hemorrhage due to AVM and the other was a case with essential tremor). In three of the cases with parkinsonism (cases 1, 3 and 6), the radiosurgery was the primary surgical treatment. In these cases, the target was invisible and we relied on a standard brain atlas and MR images. We now know the optimal area to be coagulated for a tremor case: the most lateral portion of the thalamic Vim nucleus. The dosimetry was performed to cover this region without damaging the internal capsule and the sensory relay nucleus of the thalamic ventralis caudalis nucleus. The central dose was located approximately 7–8 mm anterior to the posterior commissure and 4–5 mm medial to the lateral border of the thalamus, as delineated on MRI. It was also 4–5 mm above the level of the intercommisural line (see fig. 1). Special care was taken to ensure that the 30% isodose line did not extend laterally, in order to avoid high-dose radiation affecting the internal capsule and the sensory relay nucleus of the thalamic ventralis caudalis. The dose planning was changed from the fourth patient in order to reduce the time the patient must lie in the Gamma Knife. A single shot was used, aimed at a target 4 mm anterior to the posterior commissure, 4–5 mm medial to the lateral border of the thalamus in MRI and 4–5 mm above the level of the intercommissural line. The size of the smallest collimator (4 mm) makes it virtually unavoidable that the target center is placed more medially and anteriorly than is usual for thalamotomy, because with the smallest collimator available, the 50% isodose diameter may be almost 10 mm. In our early cases (cases 1–3), we used a special plugging pattern to obtain spherical dosimetry curves, aimed especially at limiting the lateral spread of radiation. This pattern plugged 100 collimators, which resulted in a long radiation time (almost 3 h in the first 3 cases, table 1). To save time, later in the series (cases 4–8), a single unplugged 4-mm collimator was used.

For the other three cases with Parkinson's disease (cases 2, 5 and 7), gamma irradiation was a secondary procedure. All these patients had already undergone an operation performed on one side using stereotactic coagulation guided by microrecording. None had residual tremor originating from the operated side. In these cases, the target point was determined to be as symmetrical as possible with the contralateral one, as depicted on MRI (fig. 2). Thus the selection of the target point was much easier in these cases. Even so, the

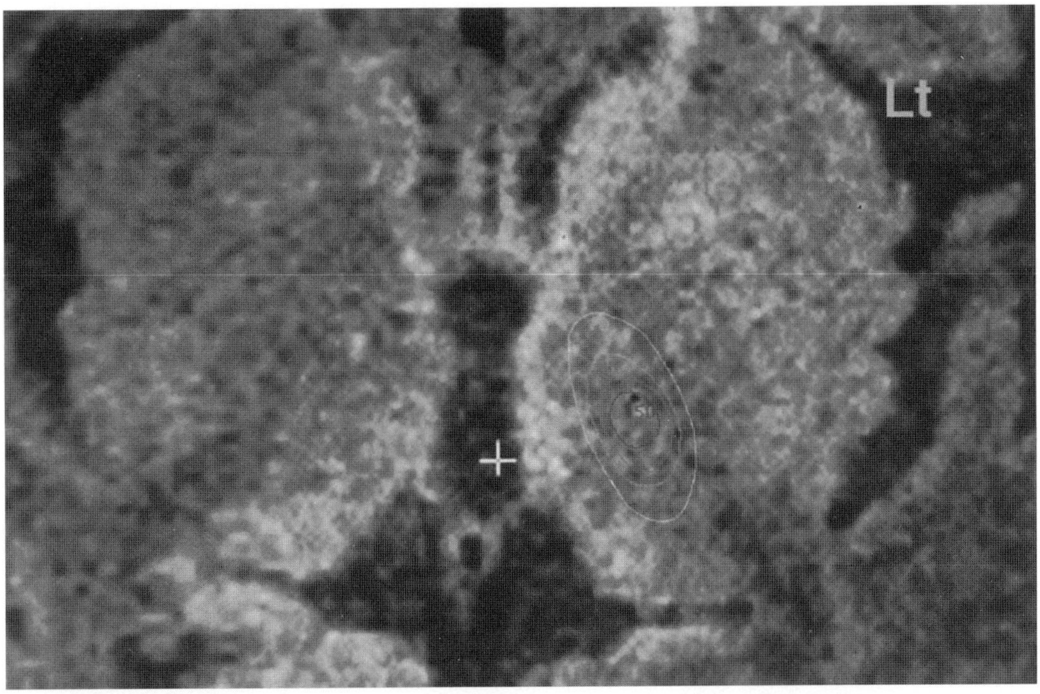

Fig. 1. Dosimetry of gamma Vim thalamotomy on a horizontal MRI section in case 1. A special plugging pattern was used and a spherical isodose curve was obtained.

Table 1. Patients treated with gamma thalamotomy

No.	Patient	Age	Sex	Diagnosis	Operation date	Side	Central dose Gy	Edge dose Gy	Edge isodose %	Shots	Radiation time, min
1	S.M.	71	F	PA	8 Sep 1993	L	150	75.0	50	1	136.7
2	Z.F.	51	M	PA	13 Apr 1994	R	150	90.0	60	2	211.9
3	M.T.	78	M	PA	22 Jun 1994	L	150	75.0	50	1	137.9
4	Y.M.	22	M	intention tremor	2 Aug 1994	R	150	75.0	50	1	74.2
5	K.M.	61	M	PA	7 Sep 1994	R	150	75.0	50	1	75.0
6	Z.T.	77	M	PA	31 May 1995	R	150	75.0	50	1	85.2
7	H.O.	61	M	PA	5 Jul 1995	R	140	70.0	50	1	80.8
8	T.K.	70	F	essential tremor	4 Oct 1995	L	140	70.0	50	1	81.2

PA = Parkinson's disease.

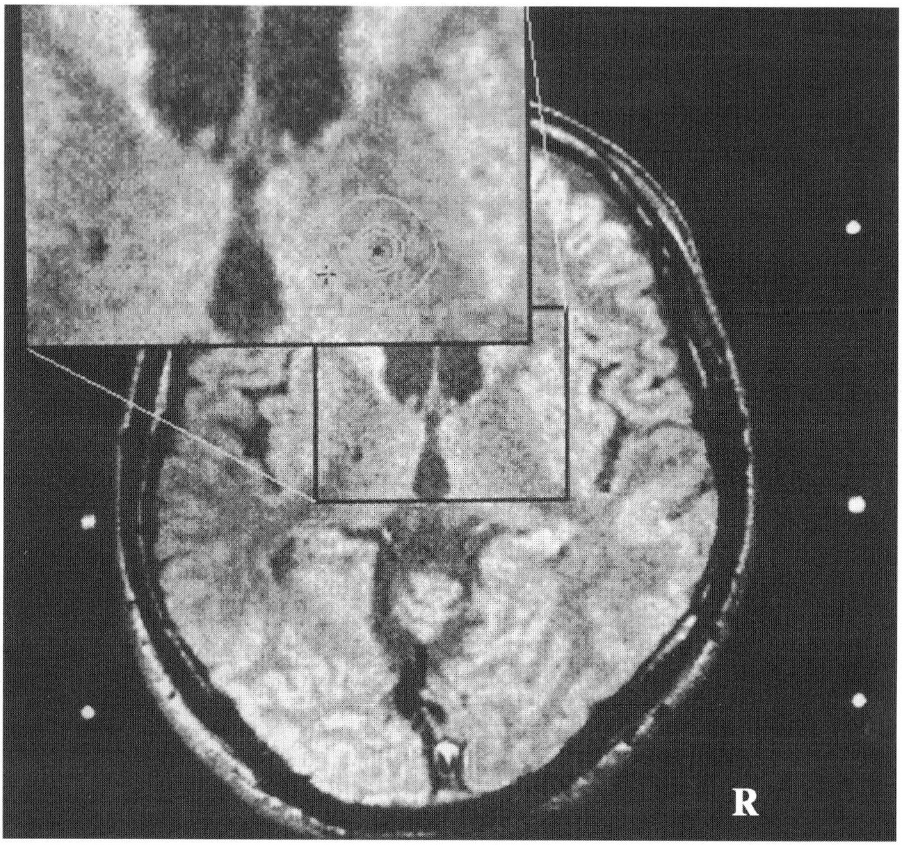

Fig. 2. Dosimetry at a symmetrical thalamic point (right Vim) in reference to the previous open thalamotomy (left Vim) on MRI in case 5. In this case, no plugging pattern was used, only a 4-mm collimator. The corresponding isodose curve is almost oval in shape.

center of the dosimetry was inevitably still slightly anterior and medial to the normal situation, for the same reasons described above for the previous cases.

For case 4 with intention tremor, which developed after thalamic hemorrhage due to an AVM, gamma irradiation had already been performed in another clinic 2 years previously. The posthemorrhagic thalamic lesion was visible on MRI and occupied the medial and ventral part of the thalamus and probably extended more ventrally to invade the mesencephalon. The patient had gradually developed intention tremor starting about 2 months after the hemorrhage. Because of this lesion, he had slight paresthesia in the affected limb. Dose planning was performed so as to cover the anterolateral part of the existing lesion. From this case on, we used a single 4-mm collimator without a plugging pattern.

In the last case (case 8), with essential tremor, the usual stereotactic thalamotomy had not been as successful as desired. The tremor was not completely arrested because the atro-

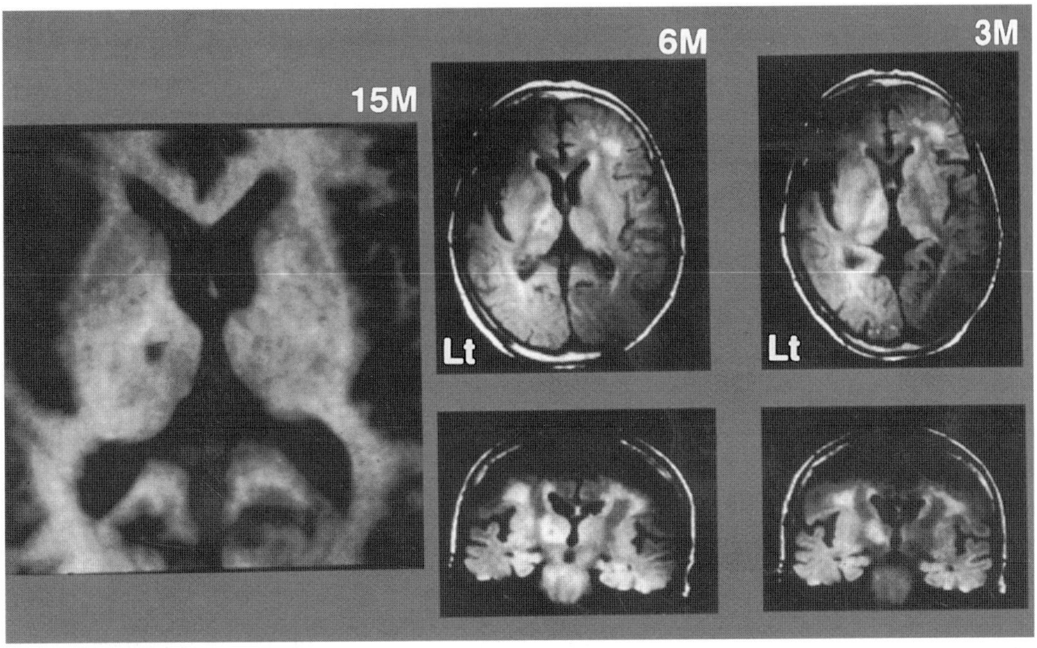

Fig. 3. Time sequential changes of an irradiated area on MRI in case 1. Images at 3, 6 and 15 months after gamma thalamotomy.

phied brain shifted several millimeters during surgery (there was excess flow of cerebrospinal fluid and the coagulation did not cover the intended region, even though the location of the coagulation had been physiologically controlled. The tremor reduced substantially to begin with, but recurred after a week. The patient had difficulty in using the hand. For these reasons, gamma thalamotomy with the 4-mm collimator was planned with the aim of expanding the lesion posteriorly.

Since the radiation lasted for more than 1 h, an intermission of 5–10 min was taken in all cases, as necessary.

Results

After gamma irradiation, periodic clinical and MRI examinations were performed to identify any clinical and morphological changes.

Case 1

The first patient, an elderly lady, had continuous bilateral tremor at rest. There were no neurological changes, not even in the tremor, until about 1 year had elapsed after treatment. MRI (the T_2 image was more clear) at 3 and 6 months after irradiation showed quite exten-

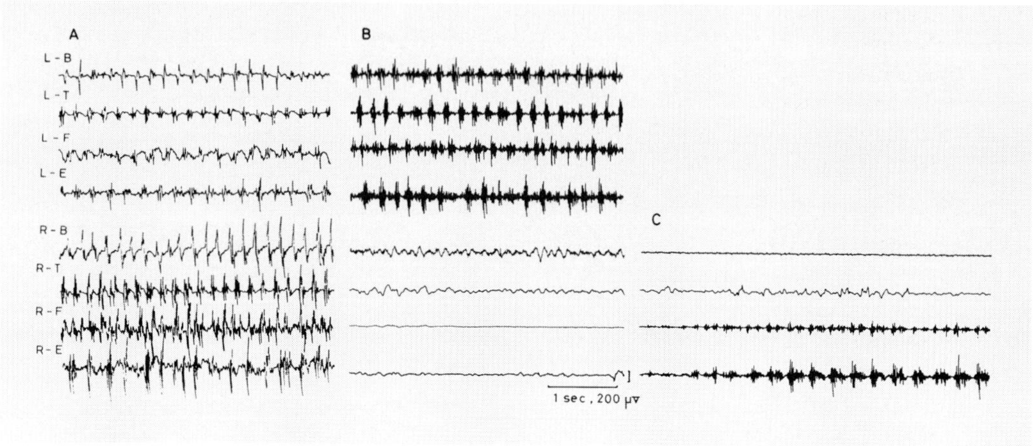

Fig. 4. EMGs showing change in tremor in case 1. **A** Before thalamotomy. Bilateral continuous tremor was marked. L = Left; R = right; B = biceps; T = triceps; F = flexors; E = extensors. **B** After gamma thalamotomy (15 months). Tremor was seen only on the left (nonoperated) side. **C** During mental task (calculation in this case, 100 – 7).

sive changes in the thalamic target zone, extending to the internal capsule and apparently to the globus pallidus (fig. 3). However, later, the damaged region became concentrated into a punched-out lesion at the lateral border of the supposed thalamic Vim nucleus (fig. 3). At an early stage, we were anxious that some unexpected side effect such as motor paresis or paresthesia might appear. However, no such symptoms or signs were ever observed. After 1 year, she noticed that her tremor had become less marked in amplitude, and within several months, the resting tremor had disappeared almost completely. Nonetheless, temporary oscillation during intentional action was retained (fig. 4). She was satisfied with the result, saying that her daily life was much facilitated, because her tremor-free right hand was easier to use. Because she had continuous resting-type tremor on the other side (left hand), we were planning to perform right-sided gamma thalamotomy, but unfortunately she died suddenly in June 1995 (about 2 years after left-sided gamma thalamotomy) probably due to a stroke (the precise cause of death was not determined).

Case 2

This patient also suffered from Parkinson's disease, but had been treated with a left-sided thalamotomy about 2 years before and had no tremor at all in his right extremities. In spite of this, resting tremor had gradually developed in his left side. Gamma thalamotomy was planned, referring the target to the previous contralateral thalamotomy lesion. A symmetrical point was chosen as a new target. This case was exceptional in our series in that two isometric centers were placed dorsoventrally to each other, to mimic the previous contralateral coagulative lesion, which extended in a dorsoventral direction. A total of 150 Gy was given, and a plugging pattern was used. The postoperative period was uneventful for almost a year. MRI showed an apparently well-localized radiation lesion at the lateral border of the supposed location of the Vim, extending slightly more medially and ventrally.

In this case, the posttreatment course was different from that of the first case, in which an expanding lesion was observed in the early postirradiation period. The tremor did not change much until 1 year after radiation, when it gradually decreased to some extent. In addition, the patient noticed that the tremor was much less in an extended posture. At the time of writing, 15 months have passed with a further decrease in the tremor. Thus, in this case, reduction of tremor started with a longer delay interval and a slower time course than in case 1.

Case 5

This patient with parkinsonian resting tremor is another interesting case. He too had been previously operated on one side (left Vim) about 2 years earlier, with complete arrest of tremor. However, his left arm began to shake, and the tremor attained a considerable severity. For this case also, gamma irradiation was planned to place a lesion symmetrical with the previous, contralateral, thalamic coagulation. The plugging pattern was not used. A total of 150 Gy were given using the 4-mm collimator. Interestingly, the tremor began to reduce at 3 months after irradiation, and at 6–9 months, practically no tremor was seen. No paresis or paresthesia appeared. Consequently, his release from tremor was smooth, and after 1 year he is now doing quite well.

Case 3

This was a 78-year-old man with Parkinson's disease of which the major disturbance was tremor. Because he was old and a poor risk for open thalamotomy, gamma thalamotomy was performed. In this case, 150 Gy were delivered using the plugging pattern. The target was located in the lateral part of the left Vim as in case 1. Unfortunately, he fell out of the follow-up study because he lived in a remote region. When we had communication recently from his family, he was already dead. The cause was unclear, being diagnosed as some kind of cerebrovascular disorder.

Case 4

This patient was a young man with a right thalamic AVM to which gamma irradiation had been performed in another center several years previously. About 1 year after the treatment he noticed intention tremor of his left arm. Neuroimaging revealed a thalamic lesion due to hemorrhage, which occupied the medial and ventral part of the thalamus extending even more ventrally. Gamma thalamotomy for tremor was planned to cover a slightly anterior and lateral part of the previous lesion. Until 1 year after irradiation, he noticed no change in the tremor or in other neurological signs. However, later, the intention tremor gradually reduced in amplitude and frequency, making it much easier for him to use his left hand. He is now studying without problems.

Cases 6, 7 and 8

For the remaining three patients (two cases with Parkinson's disease and one case with essential tremor), gamma Vim thalamotomy was done recently using the 4-mm collimator, and delivering a dose of 140 Gy. For case 6, gamma thalamotomy was the primary treatment. For case 7, a contralateral Vim coagulation thalamotomy had already been performed and a symmetrical target point was chosen. Case 8 had had a Vim thalamotomy on the same side with an unsatisfactory result. The previous lesion was extended posteriorly with gamma thalamotomy. To date all three cases are under follow-up observation. No acute side effects have been observed.

Discussion

It has long been known that the selection of the target point is of primary importance in the field of functional neurosurgery. The basis for our gamma thalamotomy for tremor cases derives from our long series of selective Vim thalamotomies with microrecording. Physiologically guided thalamotomy clearly showed that the optimal target for consistent, reproducible tremor alleviation is the lateral part of the thalamic Vim nucleus. Theoretically, tremor of any kind could be treated effectively, either by a radiofrequency lesion or by gamma irradiation. Thus, after several trials of gamma thalamotomy for thalamic pain with a visible target [9], we started with Parkinson's disease, mainly with tremor. Thereafter, the indication was extended to intention and essential tremor. Nonetheless, it should be noted that our target determination had two different strategies: a non-visible target was determined from a standard atlas, and a visible target was patterned after a conventional lesion shown on MRI. Certainly, for the latter cases, as in cases with thalamic pain, the target determination was much easier than for cases without a visible target. Fortunately, in both situations, the results observed so far have been promising.

Use of the Gamma Knife for functional disorders faces two difficulties which need to be solved. One is target determination, as discussed above. The other is how to localize the irradiated volume as intended. For the treatment of tremor, this is particularly important, because our selective Vim thalamotomy requires only a small coagulation of about 40–60 mm^3 [10]. However, the currently available Gamma Knife cannot achieve such a small irradiation volume, and the high-dose region is inevitably larger than necessary. It should also be remembered that the closer the target approaches the lateral border of the Vim, the greater the risk of a high radiation dose to the internal capsule. The 10% isodose line (15 Gy in the case of a 150-Gy central dose) was deemed to be without danger and should not extend far beyond the confines of the thalamus. In practice, it is difficult to cut off the lateral margin as much as required without using a special plugging pattern. This may be the most difficult problem to be solved to our satisfaction. Our tentative solution is to place the target center more medially, thereby deviating from the ideal target. In this regard, some technical improvement should be urged.

Our results demonstrated two different courses of tremor improvement, as shown schematically in figure 5. There may be a relatively short interval to tremor arrest (6 months) or a more prolonged period of a year or more. Although the same dose was used in all cases, the reaction or susceptibility of the individual

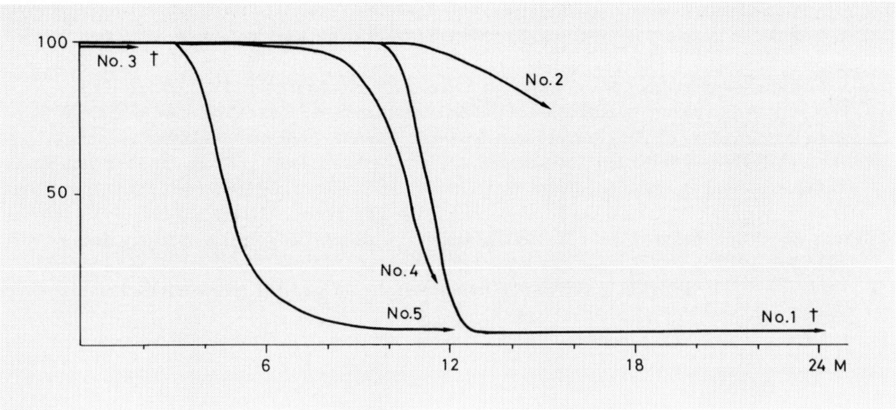

Fig. 5. Time sequential changes in tremor after gamma thalamotomies in case 1–5. Case 3 died 2 months after irradiation. Three other cases (6–8) were too early to estimate and are omitted from this figure.

brain seems to vary from case to case [11, 12]. Moreover, the course of MRI changes was individual for each case. It is not possible at present to predict the course of clinical and imaging changes. A long interval between radiation and clinical improvement could be another disadvantage of gamma thalamotomy. However, tremor itself is not a life-threatening condition, and the patient can tolerate waiting without any major problems.

At all events, our results indicate that gamma thalamotomy for tremor is possible. It can give a consistent favorable and safe outcome, provided it is carefully used as selective thalamotomy.

References

1 Leksell L: Cerebral radiosurgery. I. Gamma thalamotomy in two cases of intractable pain. Acta Chir Scand 1968;134:585–595.

2 Lindquist C, Steiner L, Hindmarsh T: Gamma knife thalamotomy for tremor. Report of two cases; in Steiner L (ed): Radiosurgery: Baseline and Trends. New York, Raven Press, 1992, pp 315–331.

3 Otsuki T, Jokura H, Takahashi K, Ishikawa S, Yoshimoto T, Kimura M, Yoshida R, Miyazawa T: Stereotactic γ-thalamotomy with a computerized brain atlas: Technical case report. Neurosurgery 1994;35:764–768.

4 Rand RW, Jaques DB, Melbye RW, Copcutt BG, Fisher MR, Levenick MN: Gamma knife thalamotomy and pallidotomy in patients with movement disorders: Preliminary results. Stereotact Funct Neurosurg 1993:61:65–92.

5 Friehs GM, Ojakangas CL, Pachatz P, Schröttner O, Ott E, Pendl G: Thalamotomy and caudatotomy with the gamma knife as a treatment for parkinsonism with a comment on lesion sizes. Stereotact Funct Neurosurg 1995;64(suppl 1):209–221.

6 Ohye C: Selective thalamotomy for movement disorders: Microrecording stimulation, techniques and results; in Lunsford LD (ed): Modern Stereotactic Surgery. Boston, Nijhoff, 1988.
7 Ohye C, Shibazaki T, Hirai T, Kawashima Y, Hirato M, Matsumura M: Tremor-mediating thalamic zone studied in humans and in monkeys. Stereotact Funct Neurosurg 1993;60:136–145.
8 Hassler R: Architectonic organisation of the thalamic nuclei; in Schaltenbrandt G, Wahren W (eds): Atlas for Stereotaxy of The Human Brain. Stuttgart, Thieme, 1977, pp 140–180.
9 Hirato M, Ohye C, Shibasaki T, Nakamura M, Inoue HK, Andou Y: Gamma knife thalamotomy for the treatment of functional disorders. Stereotact Funct Neurosurg 1995;54(suppl 1):164–171.
10 Hirai T, Miyazaki M, Nakajima H, Shibazaki T, Ohye C: The correlation between tremor characteristics and predicted volume of effective lesions in stereotaxic Vim-thalamotomy. Brain 1983; 106:1001–1018.
11 Larsson B: Radiobiological fundamentals in radiosurgery; in Steiner L (ed): Radiosurgery: Baseline and Trends. New York, Raven Press, 1992, pp 3–14.
12 Kihlström L, Guo WY, Lindquist C, Mindus P: Radiobiology of radiosurgery for refractory anxiety disorders. Neurosurgery 1995;36:294–302.

Proc 7th Int Meeting Leksell Gamma Knife® Society,
Island of Lana'i, Hawaii, November 1995
Stereotact Funct Neurosurg 1996;66(suppl 1):343–348

Stereotactic and Functional Neurosurgery

Trigeminal Neuralgia Radiosurgery: The University of Pittsburgh Experience

D. Kondziolka, J.C. Flickinger, L.D. Lunsford, M. Habeck

Departments of Neurological Surgery, Radiation Oncology and the Center for Image-Guided Neurosurgery, University of Pittsburgh, Pa., USA

Key Words

Trigeminal neuralgia · Pain · Gamma Knife · Radiosurgery

Abstract

The results of Gamma Knife stereotactic radiosurgery in the management of 51 patients who had typical trigeminal neuralgia were evaluated at the University of Pittsburgh. In all cases, a 4-mm isocenter was targeted at the proximal nerve at the root entry zone. The target dose varied from 60 to 90 Gy. Forty-four patients (86%) had undergone prior surgery. The mean follow-up after radiosurgery was 9.6 months (range, 2–29 months). The initial response rate was 86%. At the last follow-up, 19 patients (37%) had excellent control (pain free), 21 (41%) had good control (50–90% relief), and 11 (21%) had failed treatment. No patient developed further sensory loss or deafferentation pain. A maximum radiosurgery dose ≥70 Gy was associated with a significantly greater chance for complete pain relief. Using magnetic resonance imaging stereotactic targeting, the proximal trigeminal nerve is an appropriate anatomic target for radiosurgery. Gamma Knife radiosurgery is a useful additional surgical approach in the management of medically or surgically refractory trigeminal neuralgia.

Introduction

The results from two patients who had radiosurgery for trigeminal neuralgia were reported in 1971 by Lars Leksell [1]. In patients treated through the 1970s and early 1980s, stereotactic irradiation of the trigeminal ganglion was per-

KARGER

E-Mail karger@karger.ch
Fax +41 61 306 12 34
http://www.karger.ch

1011–6125/96/0665–0343$10.00/0

Douglas Kondziolka, MD, MSc, FRCS(C)
Presbyterian University Hospital
University of Pittsburgh Medical Center, Suite B-400
200 Lothrop Street
Pittsburgh, PA 15213–2582 (USA)

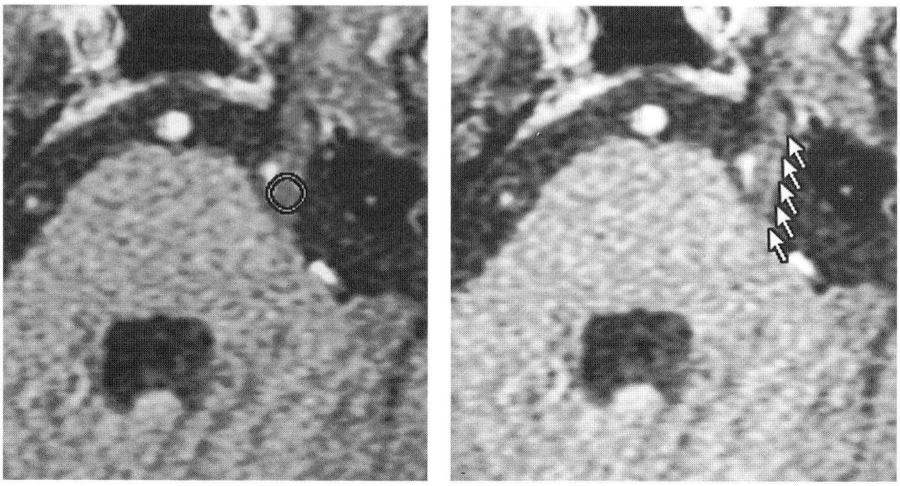

a b

Fig. 1. Axial MR image (volume acquisition, 1-mm slice interval) showing the left trigeminal nerve at radiosurgery with preliminary isoceter planning (**a**), and delineation of the nerve from the pons to Meckel's cave (**b**).

formed, usually at low doses. Rand et al. [2] reported 12 patients who had radiosurgery of the ganglion using 4- and 8-mm collimators and maximum doses between 57 and 75 Gy. Although some patients responded, they concluded that the ganglion was probably not appropriate as a primary radiosurgery target. We evaluated our results after the use of a uniform surgical technique using a dose-escalation approach to trigeminal neuralgia radiosurgery.

Materials and Methods

Patients were accepted for stereotactic radiosurgery (n = 51) if they had typical trigeminal neuralgia. No patient had constant or dysesthetic pain, or anesthesia dolorosa. The mean patient age was 64 years (range, 21–89). Forty-four patients had undergone prior surgery, and the mean number of prior procedures performed per patient was 2.7 (range, 1–8). There were 30 females and 21 males. Three patients had multiple sclerosis.

Radiosurgery Technique

All patients had Gamma Knife radiosurgery using the Leksell Gamma Unit (Elekta Instruments, Atlanta, Ga., USA). High-resolution stereotactic magnetic resonance imaging (MRI) was performed using short TR spoiled-grass volume acquisition images at 1-mm intervals [3]. We identified the trigeminal nerve in its course from the pons to Meckel's cave (fig. 1). The GammaPlan dose planning system was used for calculation. Stereotactic coordi-

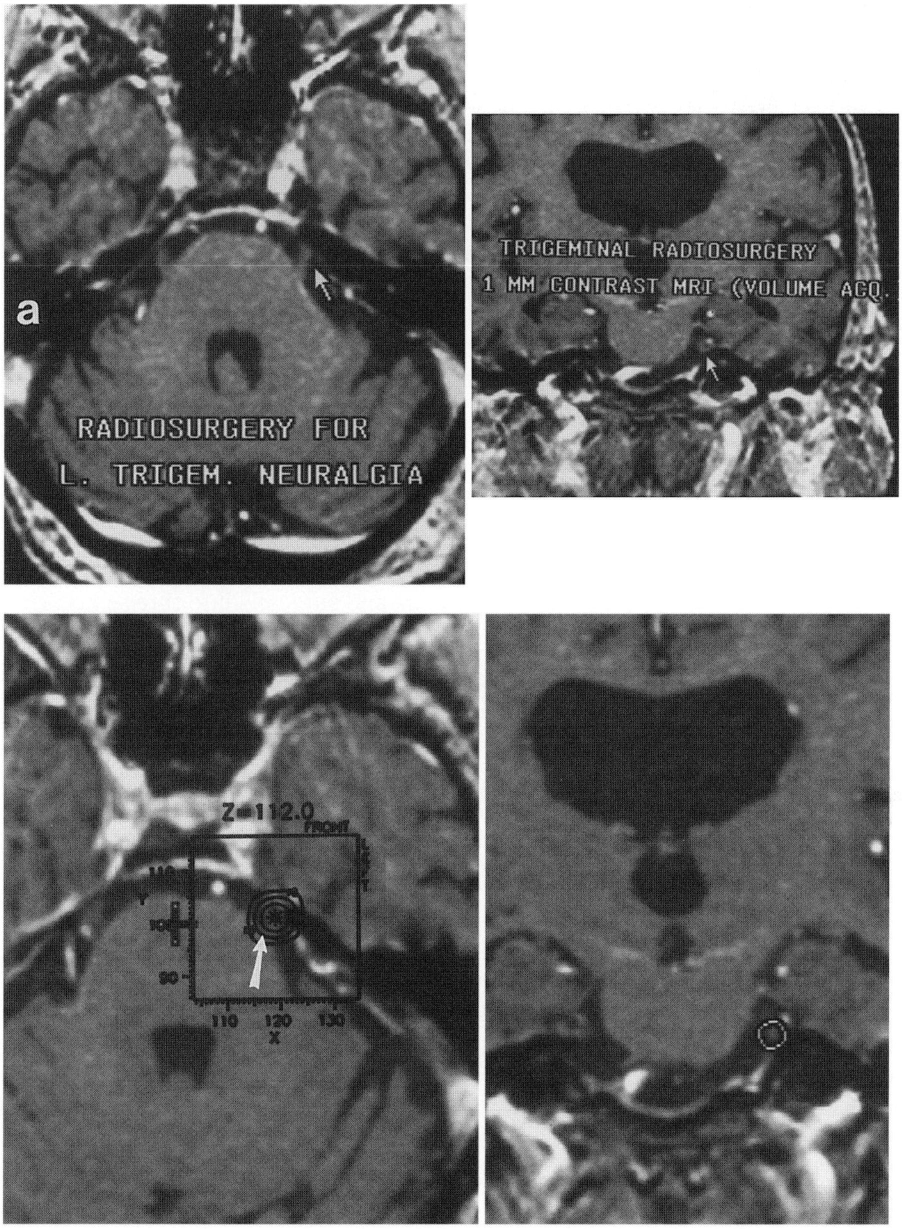

a

b

Fig. 2. a Axial and coronal MR images showing identification of the left trigeminal nerve for radiosurgery. **b** A single 4-mm isocenter was used for irradiation of the nerve, so that the 20% isodose reached the brain stem surface (arrow). A maximum dose of 70 Gy was administered.

nates were calculated for a single 4-mm isocenter, 2–4 mm anterior to the junction of the trigeminal nerve and pons, so that the brain stem surface was irradiated with usually no more than the 20–30% isodose (fig. 2). A range of maximum radiosurgical doses was selected between 60 and 90 Gy. The initial patients were treated according to a dose-escalation protocol (5 patients per dose) beginning at 60 Gy and proceeding to 70 and 80 Gy. The number of patients treated per dose was: 60 Gy, n = 5; 65 Gy, n = 1; 70 Gy, n = 25; 80 Gy, n = 19, and 90 Gy, n = 1. After an intitial evaluation of results showed that a dose ≥70 Gy was associated with better outcomes, we uniformly used 70 and 80 Gy for this condition, although 1 patient was treated at 90 Gy. We continue to study the higher dose range for its possible relationship to faster pain relief and longer-term pain control. All patients were discharged within 24 h. Patients were studied with regard to the degree of pain relief, sensory symptoms and the need for further surgical therapy. Actuarial calculation of pain relief durability was performed using the product-limit method of Kaplan and Meier. Multivariate analysis of response rates was performed using the proportional hazards model of Cox.

Results

Pain Relief

Relief of pain was coded by the patients and surgeons into three categories. These included poor response or failure (0 to <50% improvement), good response (50–90% improvement), and pain free (excellent response). Criteria for improvement included both a reduction in both the frequency and the severity of the pain. Mean follow-up after radiosurgery was 9.6 months (range, 2–29 months). At the last follow-up, 19 patients were excellent (37%), 21 (41%) were good and in 11 (21%), the treatment had failed. Four of the nonresponding patients had an initial good response. Patients with more than three prior procedures had a higher failure rate (7/18 versus 4/33; p = 0.04).

Pain Response and Dose

A maximum dose of ≥ 70 Gy was associated with a significantly better result than a dose of 60 Gy (p = 0.04). When a dose ≥70 Gy was used (n = 45), 19 patients were excellent (42%), 18 were good (40%) and 8 did not respond (17%). Two of 3 patients with multiple sclerosis had a good result at the last follow-up.

Complications

No patient in this series developed an increase in facial paresthesia or decreased sensation after radiosurgery. There was no other morbidity related to treatment.

Discussion

We selected the proximal trigeminal nerve and root entry zone as the irradiation target rather than the gasserian ganglion for two resons: (1) the proximal nerve can be well identified on imaging as it traverses the cerebrospinal fluid of the posterior fossa, and (2) the nerve as a single structure can be irradiated with a small volume of energy (4 mm collimator). In addition, we believe that the portion of the nerve nearer the brain stem is myelinated by oligodendrocytes, and therefore likely to be more sensitive to irradiation than the distal nerve, which is myelinated by Schwann cells. The accuracy of MRI-based small-volume targeting was first evaluated in a comparison with computed tomography imaging [3], in animal models [4], and in the clinical management of small tumors with the 4-mm collimator [5].

Although preliminary information on dose was available [6, 7], we developed a dose-stratification regimen to try to identify a dose-response relationship for trigeminal nerve irradiation. Consecutive patients were irradiated in groups of 6 beginning at 60 Gy. When analysis of a multicenter study became available, we then used 70 Gy as the lowest maximum dose for trigeminal neuralgia patients [3]. Although the results in this study were not as good for patients that had undergone more than three prior surgeries, this does not mean that a radiobiological difference in nerve response existed in these patients. Such patients may have a more refractory and disabling form of trigeminal neuralgia, as noted by poorer results after any type of treatment in patients that had previously undergone surgery.

Stereotactic radiosurgery is perhaps the least invasive procedure for trigeminal neuralgia. It is an especially attractive option for elderly patients or for those with concomitant medical problems. Although early on we reserved this technique mainly for patients with recurrent pain after prior surgery, we have used radiosurgery as primary management for patients with significant cardiac or respiratory problems, or those using anticoagulant medications. Because of a latency interval to relief (usually 1–8 weeks), we do not use radiosurgery for patients with severe pain that hinders eating or drinking. Rather, it is deemed suitable for medically refractory pain that is disabling but not critical.

Radiosurgery for trigeminal neuralgia is not new, but significant modifications in technique have led to improved results. We believe that MRI-based small-volume irradiation of the proximal trigeminal nerve at doses of 70–90 Gy can be an effective management strategy for medically or surgically refractory trigeminal neuralgia.

References

1 Leksell L: Stereotaxic radiosurgery in trigeminal neuralgia. Acta Chir Scand 1971:37:311–314.
2 Rand W, Jacques DB, Melbyer W, Copcutt B, Levenick M, Fisher M: Leksell Gamma Knife treatment of tic douloureux. Stereotact Funct Neurosurg 1993;61:93–102.
3 Kondziolka D, Lunsford LD, Flickinger JC, Young RF, Vermeulen S, Duma C, Jacques D, Rand R, Regis J, Peragut J, Epstein M, Lindquist C: Stereotactic radiosurgery for trigeminal neuralgia: A multi-institutional study using the gamma unit. J Neurosurg 1996;84:940–945.
4 Kondziolka D, Linskey ME, Lunsford LD: Animal models in radiosurgery; in Alexander E, Loeffler J, Lunsford LD (eds): Stereotactic Radiosurgery. New York, McGraw-Hill, 1993, pp 51–64.
5 Ogunrinde OK, Lunsford LD, Flickinger JC, Kondziolka D: Cranial nerve preservation after radiosurgery for small acoustic tumors. Arch Neurol 1995;52:73–79.
6 Leksell L: Stereotactic radiosurgery. J Neurol Neurosurg Psychiatry 1983;46:797–803.
7 Lindquist C, Kihlström L, Hellstrand E: Functional neurosurgery – A future for the Gamma Knife? Stereotact Funct Neurosurg 1991;57:72–81.

Proc 7th Int Meeting Leksell Gamma Knife® Society,
Island of Lana'i, Hawaii, November 1995
Stereotact Funct Neurosurg 1996;66(suppl 1):349–356

Stereotactic and Functional Neurosurgery

Long-Term Follow-Up of Stereotactic Gamma Knife Radiosurgery in Epilepsy

C.J. Whang, Y. Kwon

Department of Neurological Surgery, Asan Medical Center, Seoul, Korea

Key Words

Epilepsy · Focal cerebral lesion · Radiosurgery

Abstract

From June 1990 to May 1995, 31 patients with epilepsy were treated by stereotactic Gamma Knife radiosurgery at the Asan Medical center. The effect of radiosurgery for epilepsy was assessed in 23 patients followed for longer than 1 year. The seizures were medically intractable in all patients: generalized in 13 cases, complex partial in 6 cases and partial in 4 cases. The duration of epilepsy ranged from 1 to 25 years, with a mean of 11.6 years. Electroencephalography and magnetic resonance imaging (MRI) were performed in all patients to identify and localize the seizure focus. The lesions on MRI were nonprogressive and less than 2.0 cm in diameter. At follow-up, 12 patients had an excellent result (class I according to Engel's classification). In 3 of these patients, antiepileptic medication was discontinued. In a further 2 patients, the seizure frequency decreased (class II and III). In the remaining 9 patients, the frequency of seizures was unchanged (class IV). Radiation-induced edema did not seem to affect the outcome with respect to seizure control. The role of radiosurgery in the treatment of epilepsy is still unclear. It is premature to draw any definite conclusions about its efficacy for intractable epilepsy in our series. However, even this small group certainly suggests the possibility of a new safe treatment method in selected patients.

Introduction

The use of advanced neuroimaging techniques has resulted in an increase in the number of patients with intractable epilepsy who are found to be harboring a focal cerebral lesion. Surgical resection of the lesion with or without removal of

KARGER

E-Mail karger@karger.ch
Fax + 41 61 306 12 34
http://www.karger.ch

1011–6125/96/0665–0349$10.00/0

C. Jin Whang, MD, FACS
Department of Neurological Surgery
Asan Medical Center
388-1 Poongnap-Dong, Songpa-Ku
Seoul 138-040 (Korea)

Table 1. Patient characteristics

Sex	
Male	19
Female	4
Age, years	
Mean	33.2
Range	10–50
Type of epilepsy	
Generalized	13
Complex partial	6
Partial	4
Duration of epilepsy, years	
Mean	11.6
Range	1–25

the surrounding epileptogenic cortex may render patients seizure free. However, even with the development of modern anesthetic and surgical techniques, surgical resection may pose a significant risk, especially for those lesions located in deep or eloquent regions. Some reports demonstrate improvements of epilepsy after radiosurgery. Stereotactic radiosurgery for epileptic patients with arteriovenous malformations (AVMs) or low-grade gliomas has been shown to effectively reduce the associated seizure attacks [1–6]. An experimental study with cats with experimentally induced focal seizures showed improvement of electroencephalography (EEG) traces and brain maps following irradiation [7]. Gamma Knife radiosurgery has been proven to be a safe, noninvasive and simple procedure. We have evaluated the efficacy of Gamma Knife radiosurgery in the treatment of patients with chronic seizures, secondary to focal cerebral lesions of various types.

Material and Methods

We report 23 patients (19 men and 4 women) with a focal cerebral lesion on magnetic resonance imaging (MRI) who underwent Gamma Knife radiosurgery between June 1990 and May 1995 and who have been followed for more than 1 year. The mean age of the group was 33.2 years, ranging from 10 to 50 years. Thirteen patients had partial attacks with secondary generalized tonic-clonic seizures. Six patients had complex partial seizures, and 4 patients had simple partial seizures. The duration of the epilepsy ranged from 1 to 25 years, with a mean duration of 11.6 years (table 1). Seizures were the only neurologic symptoms in this series and none of the patients had neurologic deficts. All patients had been treated with antiepileptic medication either with a single agent or with combinations of various kinds for at least 6 months before the condition was considered medically intractable.

Table 2. Localization methods for seizure focus

MRI	small <2 cm diameter nonprogressive lesion no mass effect	
Examples	signal change (T_2-weighted)	n = 7
	hippocampal atrophy	n = 3
	calcification	n = 5
	gadolinium enhancement	n = 3
	AVM	n = 5
EEG	scalp and nasopharyngeal ictal and interictal continuous video EEG monitoring	

Table 3. Radiosurgery dosimetry

	Volume mm^3	Margin isodose, %	Margin dose, Gy	Center dose, Gy	Number of isocenters
Mean	2,433	51.9	22.9	44.6	2.1
Range	30–6,983	45–70	10–50	20–100	1–6

All patients underwent MRI and scalp-recorded EEG asleep and awake. Some patients underwent prolonged video EEG monitoring, when the scalp EEG did not give a clear indication of the location of the epileptic focus. The focal cerebral lesion on MRI was shown to be nonprogressive for at least 6 months. All of these lesions were less than 2.0 cm in diameter. The lesions showed no mass effect and no surrounding edema. Calcification and gadolinium enhancement were observed in some cases and not in others. T_2-weighted images showed signal changes in some patients (table 2). The relationship between lesion and the seizures in a given case was determined by the clinical semiology of the seizures, EEG and video EEG monitoring.

All patients in this series were treated with the Leksell Gamma Knife with 201 Co-60 sources. The mean treatment volume was 2,433 mm^3 (range 30–6983 mm^3). The mean margin dose was 22.9 Gy (range 10–50 Gy). The isodose line placed at the margin of the target varied between 45 and 70% (table 3). The postoperative follow-up has been for more than 1 year (mean 30.5 months, range 14–54 months). The clinical outcome was categorized according to Engel's outcome classification [8] (table 4): class I = seizure free; class II = rare seizure activity (less than three seizure episodes per year); class III = worthwhile improvement (worthwhile seizure reduction, prolonged seizure-free intervals), and class IV = no worthwhile improvement.

Table 4. Outcome classification according to Engel

Class	Definition		
I	seizure free	A	completely seizure free after surgery
		B	aura only after surgery
		C	some seizures after surgery, but seizure free for at least 2 years
		D	atypical generalized convulsion only if antiepileptic drugs withdrawn
II	rare seizure ('almost' seizure free)	A	initially seizure free but has rare seizures now
		B	rare seizures after surgery
		C	more than rare seizures but rare seizures for at least 2 years
		D	nocturnal seizures only, which cause no disability
III	worthwhile improvement	A	worthwhile seizure reduction
		B	prolonged seizure-free intervals amounting to less than half the follow-up period but not less than 2 years
IV	no worthwhile improvement	A	significant seizure reduction
		B	noappreciable change
		C	seizures worse

Results

Gamma Knife radiosurgery was performed in 31 patients. The effects of the radiosurgery were investigated in 23 patients who were followed for more than 1 year. The clinical outcome was evaluated every 6 months after radiosurgery. The outcome during the first 6 months was: 3 patients in class I, 2 patients in class II, 0 patients in class III and 18 patients in class IV. At the 12-month follow-up, the outcome had improved. One of the class II patients at the 6-month follow-up and 5 of the class IV patients had become class I at 12 months. A further 2 class IV patients became class III. Thus, the outcome at the 12-month follow-up was: 9 patients in class I, 1 patient in class II, 2 patients in class III and 11 patients in class IV. One of the class III patients and 1 of the class IV patients had become class I, 18 months after radiosurgery. Another patient rose from class IV to class I at the 24-month follow-up. The study indicated that 12 of the 23 patients had reached class I during the mean follow-up period of 37.3 months. One patient had reached class II in 17 months. One patient had reached class III after 25 months.

Table 5. Long-term follow-up results (n = 23)

Case No.	Seizure type	Duration years	Lesion volume mm^3	Margin dose Gy	Margin isodose %	Results at intervals				
						6 mo	12 mo	18 mo	24 mo	42 mo
1	p	9	1,800	20	50	IV	IV	IV	IV	IV
2	GTC	22	1,200	50	50	IV	I	I	I	I
3	GTC	10	30	50	50	I	I	I	I	I
4	GTC	3	2,040	22	45	IV	I	I	I	I
5	CPS	15	4,200	25	50	IV	I	I	I	I
6	CPS	4	1,012	30	70	IV	III	I	I	I
7	P	4	3,927	25	50	I	I	I	I	I
8	GTC	1	3,230	25	60	IV	IV	I	I	
9	GTC	1	3,024	20	50	IV	I	I	I	
10	GTC	7	2,380	15	50	IV	III	III	III	
11	GTC	22	5,148	10	50	IV	IV	IV	IV	
12	CPS	5	1,440	28	50	IV	IV	IV	I	
13	P	14	256	20	70	IV	I	I	I	
14	CPS	17	720	25	50	II	II			
15	CPS	12	2,646	20	50	IV	IV	IV		
16	GTC	6	2,268	15	50	IV	IV	IV		
17	GTC	17	1,989	15	50	IV	IV	IV		
18	P	9	5,880	28	50	IV	IV	IV		
19	CPS	23	2,268	15	50	IV	IV	IV		
20	GTC	25	6,983	10	50	IV	IV	IV		
21	CPS	17	3,240	15	50	II	I	I		
22	CPS	9	224	25	50	IV	I			
23	GTC	15	63	20	50	IV	IV			

GTC = Generalized tonic-clonic; CPS = complex partial seizure; mo = months; p = partial seizure.

Nine patients remain in class IV at a mean follow-up time of 25 months (range 15–61 months) (table 5).

Three of the class I patients have had their antiepileptic medication discontinued successfully and have remained seizure-free for 7, 22 and 43 months. The correlation of the lesion with the outcome of radiosurgery is summarized in table 6. The class I patients included all types of the structural lesions treated except hippocampal atrophy. The patients with hippocampal atrophy could not receive more than 10 Gy to the target margin for fear of damaging the optic tract. The location of the lesion on MRI, duration of epilepsy, age at radiosurgery and neuroimaging changes during follow-up MRI were not predictive of seizure out-

Table 6. MRI findings

	Patients	Results			
		I	II	III	IV
Signal change (T_2-weighted)	7	4	1		2
Hippocampal atrophy	3				3
Calcification	5	4			1
Gd enhancement	3	2			1
AVM	5	2			2
Total	23	12		1	9
Follow-up period, months					
Mean		37.3	17	25	25
Range		15–68		15–61	

come. No patient developed new neurological deficits. Two patients developed asymptomatic perilesional edema shown on MRI, but this finding was temporary. The frequency of seizures decreased significantly at 12 months after Gamma Knife radiosurgery (fig. 1).

Discussion

There are a few reports on the efficacy of radiosurgery for seizures associated with AVMs and low-grade gliomas. Steiner et al. [6] reported that 41 (69.4%) patients became seizure free or were significantly improved after Gamma Knife radiosurgery. Steinberg et al. [5] reported a 63% improvement in seizures in 35 AVM patients treated with helium ion radiosurgery. Heikkinen et al. [3] noted improvement in 55% of 29 symptomatic epileptic patients with AVMs treated with proton beam irradiation. The proposed mechanism is that the scarce degenerated pacemaker neurons around the AVM may be sensitive to radiation, so the positive effect on epilepsy may be seen with or without angiographic cure.

Rossi et al. [4] treated 15 patients with low-grade cerebral gliomas with stereotactic interstitial irradiation and 8 (53%) became seizure free, while 6 (40%) experienced a marked amelioration of their seizures. Two possible mechanisms were suggested to explain the antiepileptic effect. The first was that the epileptogenic action of the tumor was lowered due to a reduction in tumor mass. The second suggested explanation was that the epileptogenicity of the cerebral neurons mixed with the neoplastic cells in the neighborhood of the tumor was directly

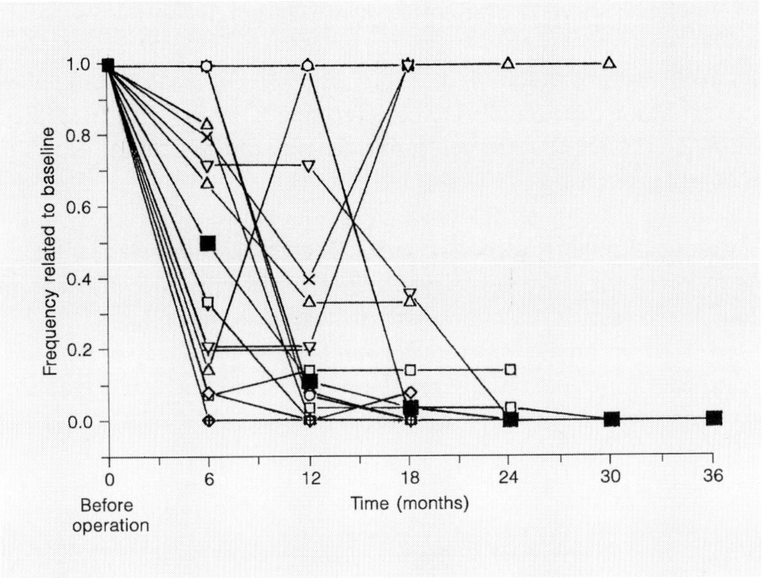

Fig. 1. Seizure frequency. The frequency of seizures was decreased after 6 months, and markedly decreased after 12 months. The solid squares represent the median.

affected by the radiation. In our series, the first mechanism is not possible but the second one could be. Casino et al. [2] noted that following stereotactic lesionectomy for foreign-tissue lesions and intractable partial epilepsy, 17 of 23 patients had a significant reduction in seizures with a long-term follow-up of 48.5 months.

The reasons which have led to the treatment of focal epilepsy with radiosurgery are the following [4]: (1) there is clinical evidence that focal irradiation may be beneficial in the clinical evolution of such attacks – as shown with the AVMs and low-grade gliomas; (2) as Elomaa [9] proposed, radiosurgical treatment of epilepsy may have its effect through nonsynaptic mechanisms of epileptogenesis, and (3) low-dose radiation does not produce the sequelae that are sometimes associated with the extirpation of epileptic foci.

There have been few reports about what radiation dose to an epileptic focus will produce satisfactory control of seizure activity. Low-dose radiation was recommended by Bracia-Salorio et al. [1, 7] because of the absence of the sequelae which sometimes follow the surgical extirpation of epileptic foci and because of the very specific action of ionizing radiation on epileptic neurons. An irradiation dose of 10–15 Gy may reduce cortical activity [10], but the optimal radiosurgical dose is still unknown. Many hypotheses may therefore be formulated. Epileptic neurons may be hypersensitive to irradiation, or irradiation may induce synaptic neoformation [7].

Since the mechanism of radiation in improving epilepsy remains unknown, and the optimal radiation dose remains to be determined, further clinical studies, and longer follow-up are required to determine the role of the Gamma Knife in the treatment of epilepsy.

In conclusion, the efficacy of stereotactic Gamma Knife radiosurgery in the treatment of intractable epilepsy secondary to focal cerebral lesions was evaluated in 23 patients followed for more than 1 year. Twelve patients had an excellent result and 2 had improvement. In 9, there was no change in the epilepsy.

It is too early to draw any definite conclusion about the efficacy of radiosurgery in the treatment of intractable epilepsy. However, from the results with this small series, it certainly seems to offer a possible new safe therapeutic opportunity.

References

1 Barcia-Salorio JL, Roldan P, Hernandez G: Radiosurgical treatment of epilepsy. Appl Neurophysiol 1985;48:400–403.

2 Cascino GD, Kelly PJ, Sharbrough RW: Long-term follow-up of stereotactic lesionectomy in partial epilepsy. Epilepsia 1992;46:17–20.

3 Heiikkinen ER, Konnov B, Melnikov L: Relief of epilepsy by radiosurgery of cerebral arteriovenous malformations. Stereotact Funct Neurosurg 1989;53:157–166.

4 Rossi GF, Scerrati M, Roselli R: Epileptogenic cerebral low-grade tumors: Effects of interstitial stereotactic irradiation on seizures. Appl Neurophysiol 1985;16:127–132.

5 Steinberg GK, Fabrikant JI, Marks MP: Stereotactic heavy-charged-particle Bragg-peak radiation for intracranial arteriovenous malformations. N Engl J Med 1990;323:96–101.

6 Steiner L, Lindquist C, Adler JR: Clinical outcome of radiosurgery for cerebral arteriovenous malformations. J Neurosurg 1992;77:1–8.

7 Bracia-Salorio JL, Vanaclocha V, Cerda M: Response of experimental epileptic focus to focal ionizing radiation. Appl Neurophysiol 1987;50:359–364.

8 Engel J Jr: Outcome with respect to epileptic seizures. In Engel J Jr (ed): Surgical Treatment of the Epilepsies. New York, Raven Press, 1992, pp 553–579.

9 Elomaa E: Focal irradiation of the brain: An alternative to temporal lobe resection in intractable focal epilepsy. Med Hypotheses 1988;6:501–503.

10 Monnier M, Krupp P: Action of gamma radiation on electrical brain activity; in Haley T, Snider R (eds): Response of the Nervous System to Ionizing Radiation. New York, Academic Press, 1962, pp 607–620.

Proc 7th Int Meeting Leksell Gamma Knife® Society,
Island of Lana'i, Hawaii, November 1995
Stereotact Funct Neurosurg 1996;66(suppl 1):357–364

Stereotactic and Functional Neurosurgery

A Comparison of Craniotomy and Gamma Knife Charges in a Community-Based Gamma Knife Center

K. Ott

San Diego Gamma Knife Center, Scripps Memorial Hospital, La Jolla, Calif., USA

Key Words

Gamma Knife · Managed care · Craniotomy · Health care · Treatment expenses

Abstract

The hospital charges for all craniotomies and transsphenoidal procedures were gathered for a 4-year period from a single, non-profit hospital serving San Diego, Calif., USA. Of the individuals in this community, 65% are covered by a variety of managed health care programs which have greatly discounted hospital receipts on a per diem or capitated payment basis. A total of 104 operative cases were identified. Forty-six patients (44%) were judged to have been eligible for Gamma Knife surgery. The average hospital charge for intracranial surgery on Gamma-Knife-eligible individuals was 14% greater than the nominal Gamma Knife surgery charge would have been. The complication rate for treated Gamma-Knife-eligible individuals was 15% including blindness in one eye after removal of a tuberculum sella meningioma, and hemiplegia following a delayed postoperative hemorrhage after arteriovenous malformation resection in another patient. Actual hospital net receipts were 55% of charges and probably approached the true hospital cost per procedure. When these hospital receipts were compared to the estimated cost per procedure of Gamma-Knife surgery, Gamma Knife surgery had a 30% cost advantage over surgical resection.

KARGER

E-Mail karger@karger.ch
Fax + 41 61 306 12 34
http://www.karger.ch

1011-6125/96/0665-0357$10.00/0

Kenneth Ott, MD, FACS
Surgical Director
San Diego Gamma Knife Center
501 Washington Street, Suite 700
San Diego, CA 92103 (USA)

Introduction

There is a lack of information comparing the hospital charges for surgical resection with those of Gamma Knife surgery charges for treatment of specific neurological diagnoses. Previous comparisons from the University of Pittsburgh for a limited variety of surgical diagnoses indicated that the hospital charges for a craniotomy may be twice those for radiosurgery [1, 2]. A more recent study of the theoretical cost-effectiveness of surgical resection versus Gamma Knife stereotactic radiosurgery in the treatment of single brain metastases by Rutigliano et al. [3] indicates Gamma Knife radiosurgery to have a lower total cost per procedure (US$ 22,743 versus US$ 30,461; all costs cited hereafter will be in US$). This assessment used modeled craniotomy and radiosurgery costs based upon Medicare cost and charge databases and a survey of costs from several Gamma Knife units. In this theoretical assessment, surgical resection charges are one-third greater than those of radiosurgery.

There is less information regarding linear accelerator (LINAC)-based stereotactic radiosurgery charges and costs. A recent charge comparison of LINAC radiosurgery and surgery for brain metastasis yielded total hospital charges nearly threefold greater than charges for radiosurgery at the University of Wisconsin [4].

The San Diego Gamma Knife Center was established on the campus of a 250-bed community hospital in October 1994. The hospital has no academic affiliation but operates an active private practice neurosurgical and spinal service, performing nearly 950 operations per year. The Gamma Knife Center replaced a LINAC-based stereotactic radiosurgery program, which had carried out 103 procedures over the previous 33 months.

Over the past 5 years, San Diego has seen a rapid penetration of managed medical care serving the 2.8 million people who live in San Diego County. There has been, pari passu, a corresponding reduction of indemnity fees for service health care plans. Currently, 65% of individuals are in managed care programs, nearly two-thirds of whom are covered by capitated health maintenance organization plans. The penetration of managed care into the health care industry of San Diego has posed a challenge to the establishment of a Gamma Knife surgery program in our community.

This study compares the actual hospital charges and net receipts for a variety of intracranial diagnoses with Gamma Knife surgery charges and costs. Additionally, hospital charges were analyzed in further detail in an effort to determine the ability of physicians to impact the hospital charges by improving cost-effective practice patterns.

Table 1. Summary of 104 craniotomies and transsphenoidal surgeries in a community-based hospital, 1991–1994

Operation/disease	Gamma Knife	
	ineligible	eligible
Supratentorial craniotomies		
Nonmeningioma	20	6
Meningioma	15	12
Arteriovenous malformation	10	3
Transsphenoidal hypophysectomy	9	7
Infratentorial craniotomies		
Nonmeningioma	3	2
Meningioma	1	4
Acoustic neuroma	0	12
Total	58	46

Material and Methods

The hospital medical and accounting records of all patients undergoing nontrauma craniotomies and transsphenoidal surgery were reviewed for the years 1991 through 1994. The eligibility for potential Gamma Knife surgery was determined for each patient after a review of the history and physical examination, imaging data, operative and pathology reports. Eligibility was determined from protocols for Gamma Knife radiosurgery developed by the staff surgeons of the San Diego Gamma Knife Center. The hospital charges and net receipts for each patient were obtained as were details of the charges for individual hospital charge centers such as surgery, pharmacy, intensive care/recovery room, room fee, laboratory, radiology, supplies and in-hospital rehabilitation. The length of stay and complications were noted. Hospital charges contained the costs of complications.

The charges and costs of Gamma Knife surgery were obtained from the San Diego Gamma Knife Center as well as a published survey of Gamma Knife sites [3].

Results

There were 104 craniotomies and transsphenoidal procedures carried out by six neurosurgeons for the 4-year period of the study. This included 66 supratentorial and 22 infratentorial craniotomies and 16 transsphenoidal hypophysectomies (table 1). Forty-six patients (44%) could have been treated by stereotactic radiosurgery. Among the eligible conditions were 5 of 8 metastases, 1 of 5 glioblastomas, 7 of 16 pituitary tumors and all 12 acoustic neuromas.

Table 2. Charges and receipts for Gamma-Knife-ineligible patients

Operation/disease	Charges US$	Receipts US$
Supratentorial craniotomies		
Nonmeningioma	23,101	13,842
Meningioma	51,557	22,322
Arteriovenous malformation	29,194	8,994
Transsphenoidal hypophysectomy	10,820	2,902
Infratentorial craniotomies		
Nonmeningioma	31,888	8,312
Meningioma	80,111	80,077
Acoustic neuroma		
Average	31,042	14,391

The average hospital charges for all 104 patients were $ 28,438, while the average receipts were $ 14,174. The 58 patients who were considered ineligible for Gamma Knife surgery consumed more hospital resources than the eligible individuals. This was reflected in greater charges ($ 31,042) and a longer length of stay (9.2 ± 1.1 days). However, the average receipts were only $ 14,391 (table 2). The average for the 46 Gamma-Knife-eligible individuals were $ 25,149 in charges, 5.3 days length of stay and $ 13,894 in receipts (tables 3, 4). Although the ineligible patients generated $ 5,893 more in charges, this resulted in only $ 497 in greater receipts. There were wide variations in charges, receipts and lengths of stay when the data were subdivided by diagnosis. For example, the average hospital charge for craniotomy for meningioma in ineligible patients was $ 51,557, net $ 22,322, and the length of stay was 13.6 days. On the other hand, the charge for transsphenoidal surgery was $ 10,820, net $ 2,902, and the length of stay was 2.8 days.

The overall surgical complication rate was 22%. One death occurred in a Gamma-Knife-ineligible patient admitted hemiplegic after a hemorrhage into a large metastatic deposit. Most complications were minor and reversed rapidly. One Gamma-Knife-eligible patient with a tuberculum sella meningioma was unilaterally blind after surgery. Another Gamma-Knife-eligible patient became hemiplegic following a delayed hemorrhage after the removal of an arteriovenous malformation. Her hospital charges were $ 204,421 and receipts $ 142,083, which does not include subsequent rehabilitation hospitalization and readmission for a cranioplasty. The complication rate for Gamma Knife radiosurgery in ineligible patients was 28%, and for eligible patients it was 15%.

Table 3. Charges and receipts for Gamma-Knife-eligible patients

Operation/disease	Charges US$	Receipts US$
Supratentorial craniotomies		
Nonmeningioma	19,710	10,739
Meningioma	20,611	9,284
Arteriovenous malformation	83,228	50,620
Transsphenoidal hypophysectomy	7,853	4,773
Infratentorial craniotomies		
Nonmeningioma	15,089	9,339
Meningioma	25,529	14,447
Acoustic neuroma	29,547	12,740
Average	25,149	13,894

Table 4. Summary of length of stay for 104 craniotomy and transsphenoidal hypophysectomy patients

Operation/disease	Gamma Knife	
	ineligible, days	eligible, days
Supratentorial craniotomies		
Nonmeningioma	6.9	4.4
Meningioma	13.6	4.2
Arteriovenous malformation	10.6	31
Transsphenoidal hypophysectomy	2.8	2.2
Infratentorial craniotomies		
Nonmeningioma	6.0	8.5
Meningioma	9.0	5.6
Acoustic neuroma		5.7
Average	9.2	5.3
SD	1.1	4.5
Median	6.0	4.0

An analysis of individual cost centers revealed that nearly two-thirds of the hospital bill was generated by charges from surgery, pharmacy, intensive care/recovery room and room fees (fig. 1, 2). Gamma-Knife-eligible patients had greater operating room charges. For both groups, the majority of charges were 'front loaded': the major portion of the total hospital charge occurred within the first 2 or 3 days of hospitalization.

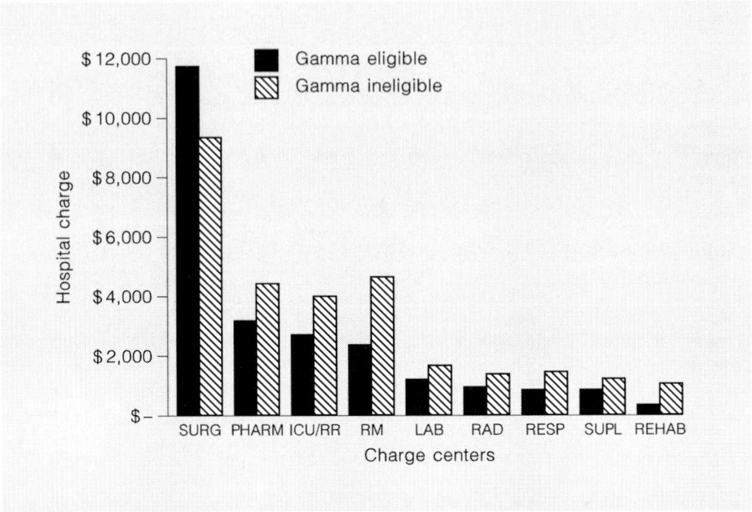

Fig. 1. Hospital cost center charges for Gamma-Knife-eligible and -ineligible patients. Shown are charges for surgery (SURG), pharmacy (PHARM), intensive care/recovery room (ICU/RR), hospital room (RM), laboratory (LAB), radiology (RAD), respiratory care (RESP), supplies (SUPL) and hospital rehabilitation (REHAB).

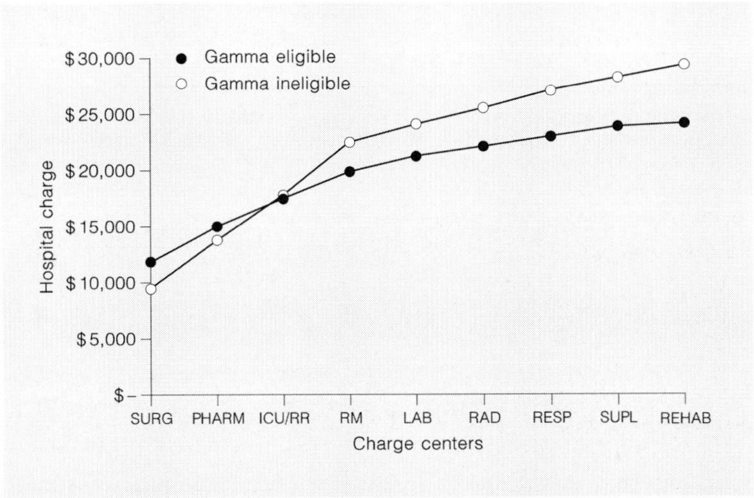

Fig. 2. Accumulated cost center charges for Gamma-Knife-eligible and -ineligible patients. Abbreviations as in figure 1.

Discussion

Managed health care places strong demands for economy, efficiency and, finally, quality in health care. San Diego County contains 2.85 million people. Most individuals are covered by some form of health insurance: 82% are insured, 3% are in active duty military, while 15% are uninsured. During the past 5 years, managed care with its various acronyms (e.g. PPO, HMO, POS, PGP) has come to dominate health care in San Diego. Currently, 65% of the population's health needs are managed by health maintenance organizations or preferred provider organizations. The prepaid capitated health maintenance organizations dominate the market. During the past 5 years, their penetration has risen from 28% to 37%, nearly twice the penetration in the United States as a whole.

In this study, a surprisingly large proportion (44%) of individuals who underwent a nontrauma craniotomy or a transsphenoidal procedure during a 4-year period was felt to have been eligible for Gamma Knife radiosurgery. Their eligibility was determined from commonly accepted criteria in the literature adopted by protocols of the San Diego Gamma Knife Center. There were only eight metastatic tumors operated during the 4 years. Five were felt to have been eligible for Gamma Knife surgery. Altogether, 56% of cases were judged to have been ineligible for various reasons. These included lesion size, pathological diagnosis, acute hemorrhage and a poor Karnofsky performance score, amongst others. These ineligible patients had more acute hospital care and required more hospital resources, as reflected in a longer length of stay, greater complication rate and higher hospital charges. For these reasons, they were eliminated from the charge and cost comparison with elective Gamma Knife surgery.

The institutional charge for Gamma-Knife-surgery eligible patients is 14% greater than the nominal charge for Gamma Knife surgery at the San Diego Gamma Knife Center ($ 25,149 versus $ 22,000). Nominal hospital charges have not changed appreciably in the last 5 years, but institutional charges have no comparative value in a managed care setting, since the majority of care is contracted at a discounted fee which provides the basis for competition in the community. Managed health care has put downward pressure on these discounted fees, but not on hospital charges.

The average receipts for Gamma-Knife-eligible cases were $ 13,894 or 55% of charges. Although the ineligible patients generated $ 5,892 in greater charges than Gamma-Knife-eligible patients, this resulted in only $ 497 greater income for the hospital, a reflection of the influence of per diem and capitated contracting. This community hospital has no cost accounting system, but in view of the narrow (and decreasing) margin of net income compared to net revenue each year, it is likely that the average receipts for this group of patients closely approaches the actual hospital costs. For the year 1995, the rate of return for this hospital was only 2.7%. Rutigliano et al. [3] estimated the cost of a hospital stay for an uncomplicated surgical resection to be $ 16,710 using the 1992 Medicare Provider Analysis and Review database and average cost to charge ratios. In view of the short hospital stay of Gamma-Knife-eligible patients (average 5.5 days) and the fact that the majority of hospital charges occur in charge centers over which surgeons have little control (surgery, pharmacy, intensive care unit/recovery room), it is unlikely that the hospital can profit from improved efficiency of physician practice patterns.

The average annual operating costs for a Gamma Knife center are approximately $ 1,468,050 [3]. This amounts to a cost per procedure of $ 10,486 in a unit treating 140 patients per year, which compares quite favorably with estimated hospital costs of $ 13,000–16,000 per procedure. Since Gamma Knife units operate under relatively fixed costs, the cost per patient is largely determined by the number of patients treated each year. The success of Gamma Knife surgical centers in a managed care setting will depend on a convincing demonstration of the safety, effectiveness and cost-effectiveness of radiosurgery to the providers of managed health care. The reduction in complication rate, rapid return to normal lifestyle, patient acceptance and satisfaction add undeniable value to its use. Success may also depend on the Gamma Knife center becoming a community resource shared by all qualified oncologists and neurosurgeons.

References

1 Lunsford LD, Flickinger JC, Lindner G, Maitz A: Stereotactic radiosurgery of the brain using the first United States 201 cobalt-60 source Gamma Knife. Neurosurgery 1989;24:151–159.

2 Pollock BE, Lunsford LD, Kondziolka D, Maitz A, Flickinger J: Gamma Knife stereotactic radiosurgery for acoustic tumors: What we have learned. Neurosurgery 1995;36:215–229.

3 Rutigliano MJ, Lunsford LD, Kondziolka D, Strauss MJ, Khanna V, Green M: The cost-effectiveness of stereotactic radiosurgery versus surgical resection in the treatment of solitary metastatic brain tumors. Neurosurgery 1995;37:445–455.

4 Mehta M, Noyes W, Levin AB, Kinsella T: Cost comparison of radiosurgery and surgery for treatment of brain metastasis. Int J Radiat Oncol Biol Phys 1994;30(suppl 1):265.

Proc 7th Int Meeting Leksell Gamma Knife® Society,
Island of Lana'i, Hawaii, November 1995
Stereotact Funct Neurosurg 1996;66(suppl 1):365–369

Stereotactic and Functional Neurosurgery

Evolution and Organization of a Regional Gamma Knife Center

Gene H. Barnett

Northeast Ohio Gamma Knife Center, The Cleveland Clinic Foundation,
Cleveland, Ohio, USA

Key Words

Gamma Knife · Radiosurgery · Public health · Medical economics

Abstract

The Gamma Knife is considered by many to be the 'gold standard' radiosurgery unit throughout the world. However, its benefits must be weighed against its cost and availability. A comparison was made between two tertiary-care, not-for-profit, medical-school-affiliated medical centers located in northeastern Ohio. Both applied for a certificate of need for a Leksell Gamma Knife. A requirement for on-site imaging and anesthesia support at one site resulted in considerable extra costs. One center then altered its application for a Gamma Knife to be used by its own four neurosurgeons. The other center modified its proposal to create a Gamma Knife center at the perimeter of its medical center, yet attached to existing imaging facilities. It would also allow regional hospitals, patients, health plans and qualified physicians and researchers to have access to the unit. This plan resulted in a marked reduction in costs. Moreover, it was estimated that this plan would greatly increase the volume of treated patients. This was the proposal endorsed by the regional Health Systems Agency by a vote of 19 to 1. The proposal from the other center for a closed system was rejected.

Introduction

Stereotactic radiosurgery using the Gamma Knife is considered by many to be the 'gold standard' to which other radiosurgical devices are compared. However, the cost of this equipment is high – of the order of US$ 3–4 million. The

KARGER

E-Mail karger@karger.ch
Fax + 41 61 306 12 34
http://www.karger.ch

1011–6125/96/0665–0365$10.00/0

Gene H. Barnett, MD
Department of Neurological Surgery S80
The Cleveland Clinic Foundation
9500 Euclid Avenue
Cleveland, OH 44195 (USA)

current milieu is characterized by contracting reimbursement and a heightened awareness of the need to optimize access to expensive medical resources. Thus, it would seem desirable to design and operate a Gamma Knife unit as a regional resource. A description of the evolution and organization of a regional Gamma Knife center follows.

Background

Northeast Ohio State has a population of 4.5 million people (11.1 million including secondary service areas). It is served by three linear accelerator radiosurgery units located in Cleveland, its principal city. Approximately 100 radiosurgery cases are treated annually by these institutions. No Gamma Knife unit is in operation in the state, the nearest being in Pittsburgh.

In the middle of 1994, two tertiary-care, non-profit-making, medical-school-affiliated medical centers (centers 1 and 2) applied to the state for a certificate of need (CON) for a Leksell Gamma Knife unit. The projected cost of each unit and its building was US$ 4.2 million. The projected patient throughput was 150 per year, to be achieved during the third year of operation. The state instructed the centers to modify their applications to provide a better, more rational service by allowing patients and physicians access to a single regional unit. Joint committees were formed to set equipment and construction standards for a jointly run stand-alone center. Two neutral sites (NS) were considered. NS-1 would be an addition to an existing stand-alone lithotripsy unit. This unit was operated jointly by the two institutions applying for the CON. NS-2 required renovations to an existing rehabiliation center to be owned and operated by the two institutions. Neither site had imaging facilities and only NS-1 had anesthesia.

Results

The joint committees agreed that there was a need for on-site imaging and anesthesia support. On-site anesthesia support was needed because both institutions considered that 10–15% of their patients would be children. On-site neuroimaging facilities were considered mandatory due to the risk of transporting patients (especially under anesthesia). Although the presence of computerized tomography (CT), magnetic resonance imaging (MRI) and angiography were desirable, the parties agreed to have only CT and MRI at the facility. Nonetheless, the projected costs for these joint ventures soared to US$ 8.8 and 9.1 million dollars, respectively (tables 1, 2). Patient volumes were projected to nearly double. Moreover, there were Nuclear Regulatory Commission safety issues which

Table 1. Cost analyses of NS-1 and NS-2

	NS-1, US$	NS-2, US$
Projected facility construction costs		
Structural and finish work	856,000	1,457,550
Mechanical systems	615,000	850,000
Site work	68,000	150,000
Special equipment	414,000	110,000
Contingency	219,000	260,000
Contractor and A&E	484,000	418,000
Subtotal	2,656,000	3,245,550
Projected equipment costs		
Gamma Knife	3,560,000	3,560,000
MRI	1,400,000	1,100,000
CT scan	716,000	850,000
Other	500,000	348,850
Subtotal	6,176,000	5,858,850

Table 2. Comparative costs (US$)

	NS-1	NS-2	NEOGKC
Facility	2,656,000	3,245,550	720,000
Equipment	6,176,000	5,858,850	3,605,000
Total capital	8,832,000	9,104,400	4,325,000

remained unresolved. Specifically, it remained unclear which of the two institutions would be accountable for safety.

After a while, center 2 reverted to its original application for a Gamma Knife unit to be used by its own four neurosurgeons. On the other hand, center 1 sought alternative options for a joint venture and modified its proposal. It suggested creating a Northeastern Ohio Gamma Knife Center (NEOGKC) located at the perimeter of its medical center which already had existing imaging facilities on site. This location allowed a variety of advantages. There would be on-site imaging. The signs would be neutral because the unit would not be identified as belonging to a single center. Radiation safety staff would be available on site, and accountability would not be a problem. Moreover, there would be institutional backup for medical emergencies. In addition to the above, the NEOGKC would

Table 3. Comparison between single hospital Gamma Knife versus NEOGKC

Item	Single hospital	NEOGKC
Projected volume		
Year 1	70	100
Year 2	100	200
Year 3	150	317
Percent year 3 utilization[a]	29	61
Financial projections – year 3, US$		
Gross technical charge	13,781	10,500
Net revenue	10,294	7,093
Cost per case	7,055	4,231
Contribution margin	3,329	2,862

[a] Using 260 days (52 weeks × 5 days × 2 patients) = 520 patients.

allow regional (i.e., all 88 counties of Ohio) hospitals, patients, health plans, qualified physicians and researchers access to and use of the unit. A credentialing committee composed of regional neurosurgeons and an educational program to train physicians inexperienced in radiosurgery was devised. The projected costs of this plan reverted to US$ 4.3 million, while the projected patient volume increased 250% (table 3). This would reduce charges to patients.

The two CON proposals were evaluated by the regional Health Systems Agency (HSA), charged with ensuring that such projects are in the public interest of patients in the region. The HSA endorsed the center 1 proposal and rejected that of center 2 by a vote of 19 to 1. Editorial comment by the largest regional newspaper, although expressing the desire for institutional cooperation, also favored center 1. Response by regional neurosurgeons and neurologists has been favorable. Center 2 continues to press for its proposal. A final decision by the state remains pending.

Comment

The organization of a Gamma Knife unit as a regional resource has several inherent advantages over a unit limited to the patient and medical population of a single hospital. By increasing patient access, the health needs of the region are better addressed. In addition, the increased patient volume results in a reduction in cost per case. These savings can be passed on to patients or providers or taken into account when negotiating managed care contracts.

Although the benefits of increased volume would also apply to a free-standing joint Gamma Knife unit venture, no such unit exists in North America, probably due to the perceived and real issues of patient and nuclear safety. Adequate anesthesia and imaging support raises the costs of a free-standing unit to more than equal the cost of two hospital-sited systems. Clearly the best use of regional resources and health care dollars while maximizing safety is to situate the unit at a major medical center, but provide access to all patients and allow treatment by all qualified physicians. To improve physician access further, an apprenticeship along with didactic training programs will allow credentialing of regional neurosurgeons interested in providing gamma Knife services to their patients. Research opportunities to regional investigators are also intended.

A final decision by the state of Ohio with regard to these proposals is anticipated in early 1996.

Author Index Vol. 66, Suppl. 1, 1996

Stereotactic and Functional Neurosurgery

KARGER

E-Mail karger@karger.ch
Fax + 41 61 306 12 34
http://www.karger.ch

Subject Index Vol. 66, Suppl. 1, 1996

Stereotactic and Functional Neurosurgery

E-Mail karger@karger.ch
Fax + 41 61 306 12 34
http://www.karger.ch